PHILOSOPHICAL AND THEORETICAL PERSPECTIVES FOR ADVANCED NURSING PRACTICE

Second Edition

The Jones and Bartlett Series in Nursing

PHILOSOPHICAL AND THEORETICAL PERSPECTIVES FOR ADVANCED NURSING PRACTICE

Second Edition

Edited by

Janet W. Kenney, RN, PhD

Professor
Arizona State University
College of Nursing
Tempe, Arizona

JONES AND BARTLETT PUBLISHERS
Sudbury, Massachusetts
BOSTON   TORONTO   LONDON   SINGAPORE

World Headquarters

Jones and Bartlett Publishers
40 Tall Pine Drive
Sudbury, MA 01776
(978) 443-5000
info@jbpub.com
www.jbpub.com

Jones and Bartlett Publishers Canada
P.O. Box 19020
Toronto, ON M5S 1X1
Canada

Jones and Bartlett Publishers International
Barb House, Barb Mews
London W6 7PA
UK

Library of Congress Cataloging-in-Publication Data

Philosophical and theoretical perspectives for advanced nursing
   practice / edited by Janet W. Kenney.—2nd ed.
      p.   cm.
      Includes bibliographical references and index.
      ISBN 0–7637–0917–4
      1. Nursing—Philosophy. 2. Nursing models.   I. Kenney, Janet W.
      [DNLM: 1. Nursing Theory. 2. Philosophy, Nursing. 3. Nursing—
   trends. 4. Nursing Research.   WY 86 P569 1999]
   RT84.5.P53   1999
   610.73'01——dc21
   DNLM/DLC
   for Library of Congress   98–43152
                                                      CIP

Acquisition Editor: Greg Vis
Production Director: Linda S. DeBruyn
Manufacturing Director: Therese Bräuer
Editorial Production Service: Modern Graphics, Inc.
Typesetting: Modern Graphics, Inc.
Cover Design: Dick Hannus
Printing and Binding: Malloy Lithographing, Inc.
Cover Printing: Malloy Lithographing, Inc.

Printed in the United States of America

03 02 01 00 99   10 9 8 7 6 5 4 3 2 1

Contents

Preface

The foundation of a discipline is its unique body of specialized knowledge. Practice disciplines, such as nursing, must continually expand their knowledge base, effectively disseminate new knowledge, and determine effective ways to use and apply this knowledge. Over the decades, scholars in most disciplines develop new and different philosophical and methodological perspectives, which may change or modify formerly accepted theories of practice. In the nursing discipline, theorists, researchers, and scholars continuously present new perspectives and viewpoints in the literature for consideration, discussion, and dialogue. As some new worldviews and theories are supported and tested, they become accepted over time. Thus, nursing's theoretical knowledge base and practice change and nursing science continuously evolves.

Since the early 1980s, models and theories developed by nurse theorists have gained greater acceptance and understanding as more research studies have supported their usefulness and application in practice. Also, nursing theory courses have been required in graduate nursing programs, and as a result, advanced nurse practitioners have a better knowledge of nursing theories and how to effectively apply them. Recognition that traditional scientific methods alone were inadequate to provide holistic nursing care, and the necessity of using all four "ways of knowing"—empirics, ethics, esthetics, and personal knowledge—has radically challenged and changed nursing theories, education, research, and practice. A major paradigm shift occurred as several nurse scholars presented their philosophies based on humans as rational, free-willed persons continually interacting with and dynamically changing with their environment through their own personal lived experiences. Traditional cause–effect scientific methods were ineffective in addressing research questions related to nonlinear interactive processes. Thus, new research methodologies were created to increase our understanding of humans' experiences from lived perspectives.

As these new philosophical, theoretical, and methodological perspectives were described and debated in the nursing literature, the nursing discipline began evolving in a new direction. Eventually, graduate nursing education, research and advanced practice nursing began to shift their perspectives accordingly. Nursing education and practice focused on developing nurses' critical thinking skills, theory-based practice, and research utilization as humanistic nursing science gained acceptance. However, the multi-complex, interrelated factors described in nursing journals that influenced nursing's paradigm shift to a humanistic science were not readily available in graduate nurses' textbooks.

While teaching nursing theory development at several universities over the last two decades, it was apparent that graduate students had difficulty understanding the changes in nursing philosophies and methodologies, leading to the evolution of nursing science. Instead of only learning how theory develops and analyzing various nurse theorists' models and theories, today graduate nurses also need to comprehend the historical evolution of nursing science, the current philosophical and methodological issues, and how to select and apply appropriate theories from the health and behavioral sciences in advanced nursing practice.

The second edition of this book is a collection of 33 classic articles by nurse leaders: 19 chapters were from the first edition, and 14 new articles by nurse scholars were added, including an original chapter by the editor. These articles will assist graduate nurses to understand the historical, philosophical, and theoretical foundation and evolution of nursing science. Nursing theory, research, practice, and education are dynamically interrelated. As changes occur in one arena, all other areas are influenced simultaneously. Our future nurse leaders need a foundation in how these arenas are interrelated and have evolved over time to understand the dynamic nature of the nursing paradigm and how it influences nursing practice and research.

The book is organized into eight parts, each with an overview describing the essence of the ensuing chapters. Part I, "The Nursing Discipline and Development of Knowledge," explains the criteria for a professional discipline, including the structure of nursing knowledge and relevant "ways of knowing" applicable to nursing's knowledge base. The six chapters in Part II, "History and Evolution of Nursing Science," describe factors that influenced development of the nursing discipline and discuss methodological research issues and the nature and scope of nursing science.

Parts III through VI focus on the four major concepts in nursing's metaparadigm. Contemporary nurse scholars are redefining and sometimes broadening the meanings of nursings' major concepts—person/client, environment, health, and nursing. These authors' views may be controversial, yet they challenge nurses to rethink how they define these concepts and how their definitions affect nursing practice and research. Part III, "Nursing's Metaparadigm: Conceptualizations of Client and Environment," includes a chapter on aggregate clients, such as families and communities, to encourage nurses to look beyond individual clients. Two chapters describe how social, political, and economic factors influence the environment, and may ultimately contribute to clients' health problems. Part IV, "Nursing's Metaparadigm: Conceptualizations of Health," presents several nurse scholars' and theorists' unique definitions of health. These four chapters challenge nurses to rethink how our definitions of health may be different from the client's view of health, yet they guide our nursing actions, and may thus be ineffective in altering the client's health problems or lifestyle. Part V, "Nursing's Metaparadigm: Conceptualizations of Nursing," examines several scholars' and theorists' views of 'what is nursing' while Part VI, "Contemporary Perspectives of Nursing," explores the nursing paradigm shift toward a 'Humanistic Nursing Science.' As a Humanistic Science, nursing is defined as caring and nurturing clients through understanding their changing life patterns reflected in their dynamic human-environment lived experiences. Nurses may be confused, frustrated, or delighted with these nontraditional views of nursing and wonder whether any are congruent with reality in the health care system.

The "Interrelationships among Nursing Theory, Research, and Practice," are explored in Part VII. These chapters discuss whether nursing theories, along with theories or models from other disciplines, can be used in nursing practice or tested in research. Criteria for determining whether research studies actually test theories are also analyzed and applied to some research studies. Part VIII, "Application of Theory in Advanced Nursing Practice," explains why critical thinking and use of theories from various disciplines are essential and relevant in nursing practice. How to select appropriate theories or models to guide nursing practice and ways to apply these theories are discussed to enhance nurses' credibility and advance nursing science.

Authors

Gayle J. Acton, RN, MSN

Evelyn Adam, RN, MN

Ellen C. Birx, RN, PhD

Anne Boykin, RN, PHD

Patricia G. Butterfield, RN, MS

Barbara A. Carper, RN, EdD

Peggy L. Chinn, RN, PhD, FAAN

William K. Cody, RN, MSN

Dorothy M. Crowley, RN, PhD

Sue K. Donaldson, RN, PhD

Joan Engebretson, RN, DrPH

Jacqueline Fawcett, RN, PhD, FAAN

Susan R. Gortner, RN, PhD, FAAN

Barbara A. Hopkins, RN, MSN

Mary H. Huch, RN, PhD

Barbara L. Irvin, RN, MN

Joy L. Johnson, RN, PhD

Janet W. Kenney, RN, PhD

Shaké Ketefian, RN, EdD, FAAN

Dorothy Kleffel, RN, DNSc

Violet M. Malinski, RN, PhD

Afaf Ibrahim Meleis, RN, PhD, FAAN

Gail J. Mitchell, RN, MScN

Margaret A. Newman, RN, PhD, FAAN

Marilyn E. Parker, RN, PhD

Nola J. Pender, RN, PhD, FAAN

John R. Phillips, RN, PhD

Steven Pryjmachuk, RMN, MSc

Dianne Pelletier Raymond, RN, MSN

Richard W. Redman, RN, PhD

Pamela G. Reed, RN, PhD, FAAN

Rozella M. Schlotfeldt, RN, PhD, FAAN

Savina O. Schoenhofer, RN, PhD

Phyllis R. Schultz, RN, PhD

Karen L. Schumacher, RN, MS

Kristen M. Swanson, RN, PhD

Toni Tripp-Reimer, RN, PhD

Madelon A. Visintainer, RN, PhD

Judith Wuest, RN, MN

John Wolfer, RN, PhD

Part I

THE NURSING DISCIPLINE AND DEVELOPMENT OF KNOWLEDGE

To be considered a discipline, nursing must meet several requirements. Each discipline determines the structure, nature, and scope of its knowledge base, the rules and procedures for acceptable methods of research, the purposes for conducting research and desired outcomes, and how to educate professionals in the discipline. To be accepted as a professional discipline, nursing is expected to have a unique body of knowledge based on credible methods for discovering knowledge, appropriate methods for applying that knowledge, and an established process for educating and socializing students into the profession. Society must also value nursing's knowledge and believe in nurses' integrity.

Over the last 40 years, in their quest to become a recognized professional discipline, nurse scholars have sought to define the nature and structure of nursing and to define acceptable research methods to advance nursing's knowledge base. For several decades, nurse scientists relied on empirical methods to create a base of nursing knowledge and achieve credibility as a legitimate discipline. In the 1970s, there was general agreement that the scope of the nursing discipline was clients or persons, health, environment, and nursing. However, nurse scholars have not reached consensus on how to structure and define these concepts, or on acceptable methods for conducting research to expand nursing knowledge.

Part I of this book includes five chapters that describe renowned nurse scholars' viewpoints on the need to structure nursing knowledge for development of a professional nursing discipline. In her chapter, "Structuring Nursing Knowledge: A Priority for Creating Nursing's Future," Rozella Schlotfeldt identified and prioritized five areas for systematic inquiry. She begins with a discussion of the criteria for a profession and advocates for nurses to reach agreement on the knowledge base essential to nurse practitioners. Schlotfeldt believes that professional knowledge includes nursing science, history, philosophy, and strategies, along with factors influencing human health. She describes the focus of inquiry and the necessity for developing knowledge in these areas to advance the science and discipline of nursing.

In their classic article, "The Discipline of Nursing," Sue Donaldson and Dorothy Crowley identified three major themes to guide nursing research in developing a unique knowledge base. These themes are relevant today and include: "principles and laws governing optimal function of human beings; patterns of human and environment interaction; and, processes to effect positive changes in health status." They also explained how the structure of knowledge leads to differences in how academic and professional disciplines define and develop practice, education, and research. Lastly, these authors describe the structure of the nursing discipline and major concepts that are needed in nursing theories and research studies.

During the evolution of nursing science and theory development, nurse authors often used terms such as theory, frameworks, and conceptual models interchangeably, and some of these terms have multiple meanings. In her effort to reduce confusion and enhance understanding, Evelyn Adam wrote, "Toward more clarity in terminology: Frameworks, theories, and models." She cites definitions of philosophy, theory, and models reflected in the nursing literature, and provides a diagram depicting differences in these terms. Adams illustrates how nursing science is based on the development of nursing theories that are derived from broader conceptual nursing models.

From her research in the 1970s, Barbara Carper identified four areas of knowledge nurses use in practice, three of which had previously been criticized and undervalued. Her chapter, "Fundamental Patterns of Knowing in Nursing," describes these four patterns as (1) empirics, the science of nursing; (2) esthetics, the art of nursing; (3) ethics, the moral knowledge in nursing; and (4) personal knowledge, the inner experience of nursing. Most disciplines integrate these four patterns of knowing to provide a complete picture of reality, yet nursing emphasized empirics to gain credibility as a profession, and devalued the other forms. Each pattern requires a different method for discovering knowledge and for validating that knowledge. Carper discusses the importance of developing and applying all four patterns of knowing in nursing and acknowledged the value of nurse's personal knowledge, which usually increases with experience in nursing practice. Her work stimulated nurse scientists to explore knowledge beyond empirics.

Nurse scholars continue to debate the values of different philosophies, paradigms and research methods in nursing. Some scholars describe the contradictions of combining different philosophical and methodological perspectives. Other nurses express concern that nurse scholars are out of touch with the reality of practice in health care delivery systems. In his chapter, "Aspects of 'Reality' and Ways of Knowing in Nursing: In Search of an Integrating Paradigm," John Wolfer explains the need for complementary types of knowledge, theory, and research, based on multiple modes of inquiry. He believes a paradigm that includes the body-mind-spirit reality would be most useful in nursing practice and lead to improved integration and application of nursing knowledge. These chapters will assist the reader to understand the development of nursing knowledge within the nursing discipline.

1

Structuring Nursing Knowledge: A Priority for Creating Nursing's Future

ROZELLA M. SCHLOTFELDT, RN, PhD, FAAN

Nursing's future will be created only as the discipline underlying nursing practices is identified, structured, and continuously updated by systematic inquiry. The kinds of knowledge contained within the discipline are identified and an approach to its structure is proposed.

There can be little doubt that one of the highest priorities for creating an appropriate future for nursing is that of identifying, structuring, and continuously advancing the knowledge that underlies the practices of professionals in the field. That statement can be made because a consensus has not yet been attained concerning the subject matter that must be mastered by those who seek to practice general and specialized nursing. Surely by the beginning of the twenty-first century, nursing's body of knowledge will be identified, selected, verified, and agreed upon by qualified professionals in the field, effectively structured, and continuously updated to reflect newly discovered knowledge. Also, knowledge judged to be erroneous, inadequate, and outdated should be deleted. This knowledge will be derived from basic and clinical scientific nursing research, both quantitative and qualitative, from philosophic and historical inquiries, and from evaluation research designed to establish valid criterion measures, devices, and approaches to establishing the efficacy and value of nursing's caring functions as they are relevant to the health, function, comfort, well-being, productivity, self-fulfillment, and happiness of human beings.

The thesis of this chapter is that only qualified professionals in the field, including general and specialist practitioners, educators, administrators, investigators, historians, philosophers, and theorists, should be given responsibility by the profession (however that is defined) to identify, verify, structure, and continuously update the extant content or subject matter that, at the minimum, should be included in the intellectual armamentaria of all professional nurses. This responsibility of the profession is essential to four functions: (a) the creation of comparable programs of study at the first professional degree level, (b) control of the profession's goals, mission, and accomplishments, (c) a valid procedure for licensing (not registering) all who quality as professionals in the field, and (d) certification of bona fide nursing specialists.

NURSING AS A PROFESSION

Two major criteria must be fulfilled by any occupational group whose members earn and

Source: Schlotfeldt, R. (1989). Structuring nursing knowledge: A priority for creating nursing's future. *Nursing Science Quarterly, 1* (1):35-38. Reprinted with permission from Chestnut House Publications.

achieve the status of a profession, or more appropriately for nursing, a learned helping profession. First, a profession must have an institutionalized goal or social mission. Learned professions are valued by the societies whose members give them positive sanction for two major reasons: (a) the services learned professionals render are judged to be essential and beneficial for all members of society during particular times in their lives and (b) members of each learned profession have identified and come to a consensus about the knowledge that practitioners must master and use selectively, creatively, humanely, effectively, and ethically in providing those essential services. As a second criterion, each profession must support a cadre of investigators whose role is to continuously advance its knowledge with a view toward improving its practices.

The traditional learned professions have included the clergy, lawyers, and physicians. The clergy have been valued and supported because they are expected to be knowledgeable and skillful in providing spiritual comfort and well-being for all those who consult them. Lawyers are expected to master coded law and to apply their discipline fairly and skillfully in fulfilling the goal of preserving social harmony and justice. Physicians have been valued because knowledge of human ills and disabilities and their causes and knowledge of the means to eliminate, attenuate, or manage them and alleviate their noxious consequences are considered essential to the well-being of society. Are the caring functions and mission of nurses, namely, appraising and optimizing the health, function, comfort, independence, and potential of human beings, any less valued than spiritual comfort and well-being? Are they any less desirable than social harmony and justice? Are they any less important than finding causes for, diagnosing, and treating human ills?

Unfortunately, the caring functions typically provided by nurses were for too long considered to be mere extensions of the duties and obligations of wives and mothers, for which large amounts of professional knowledge were not considered essential (Reverby, 1987). Lay members of societies have typically not recognized, and nurses themselves have been remarkably tardy in identifying and organizing the several kinds of professional knowledge that are fundamental to executing the caring functions that nurses typically provide.

The essential and often crucial nature of nurses' caring functions in promoting the health and well-being of all human beings is finally being recognized by thinking people, including scholarly nurses. There is now general agreement (at least verbal agreement) that nursing's social mission is to appraise and assist human beings in their quest to optimize their health status, health assets, and health potential (Fawcett, 1983). Furthermore, general agreement exists that there is or should be a body of structured knowledge that professionals in the field agree represents the discipline that is fundamental to general and specialty nursing practices.

Nursing scholars have discussed, described, and characterized the discipline (Donaldson & Crowley, 1978), and in the recent past the American Association of Colleges of Nursing (1986) has reported findings from a "national effort to define the essential knowledge, practice, and values that the baccalaureate nurse should possess" (p. 1). Panel members expressed the belief that the essentials so delineated can be achieved within the traditional baccalaureate degree program in nursing and that the baccalaureate represents first-level professional preparation in nursing.

The efforts that have been made toward establishing the discipline represent significant steps toward achieving the goal of identifying, organizing, and achieving a consensus concerning the specific body of extant knowledge that underlies nursing practices. It must be noted, however, that there has not yet been a concerted effort to identify and obtain agreement about the currently available knowledge that is fundamental to nursing's growing number of declared specialties or even to obtain a consensus about the requisite knowledge and skills that define what nursing's specialties are. It must be recognized also that the subject matter that constitutes the discipline has not yet been identified and structured, and agreement has not been reached concerning appropriate and needed inclusions from qualified professionals in the field. This paper presents an approach to organizing the several kinds of knowledge contained within the discipline, a possible next step toward having qualified professionals select and structure the specific extant subject matter of the discipline about which agreement is needed.

KNOWLEDGE OF THE DISCIPLINE

Figure 1.1 shows the kinds of professional knowledge contained within the discipline, which is depicted as a large sphere having a permeable and expandable membrane (represented by the second sphere) to permit the continuous addition of newly discovered knowledge and the deletion of that found through systematic inquiry to be erroneous, inadequate, or irrelevant.

The largest segment of the sphere (*a*) represents nursing's scientific subject matter. Therein belongs all of nursing science, (ie, the verified facts, principles, and laws that have been discovered through scientific inquiry to be valid, relevant, and useful for nursing practice); included also are extant scientific theories that guide scientific investigations in nursing and those that have been proposed by scholarly nurses as promising explanations of phenomena that are of particular concern to nurses.

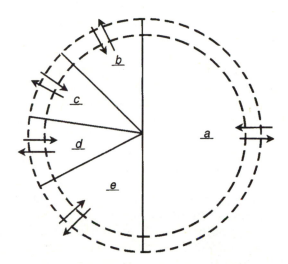

FIGURE 1.1.   The nursing discipline.
a, Nursing science; *b,* nursing history; *c,* nursing philosophy; *d,* nursing strategies; *e,* factors influencing human health. Arrows denote addition and deletion of knowledge. Personal knowledge is excluded.

To date, much of nursing science has been discovered by basic scientists and subsequently found through empirical evidence and systematic study to be relevant. Nurse investigators have also been adding to nursing's scientific knowledge by testing the relevance and utility of theories generated by basic scientists in clinical nursing situations (Chinn, 1984). Few investigations have yet been reported that test scientific theories regarding human phenomena that are of particular concern to nurses but not to basic scientists (Silva, 1986). A plausible reason is that there is little agreement among nurses concerning the human phenomena that are of concern to nurses and how they should be characterized and classified and how knowledge of them should be advanced.

In general, nurses accept the notion that human beings are biopsychosocial beings (Engel, 1977). It is proposed here that the subjects nurses serve also exemplify assets of the human spirit of which relevant knowledge is inadequate. Those assets surely include human spirituality and other qualities of the human spirit, such as determination, verve, courage, beliefs, hope, and aspiration. Nurses surely hold responsibility for advancing knowledge of those health-seeking assets. In sum, human beings' health-seeking mechanisms and behaviors, beliefs, and propensities can be classified as biological, psychological (both emotional and cognitive), and sociocultural and as assets of the human spirit; all of them are directly relevant to the natural efforts by humans to seek and attain optimal health. Because so much scientific nursing knowledge remains to be discovered, it is safe to predict that nursing science will likely always represent the largest and most rapidly changing aspect of the discipline. Furthermore, nurses are increasingly recognizing the relevance of scientific knowledge from disciplines not traditionally judged to be relevant for nursing. Included, for example, are concepts, principles, and theories from economics, political science, administration and management, and computer science. The science fundamental to education has long been incorporated as an integral part of the discipline of nursing.

A second important segment of the sphere representing the nursing discipline is historical knowledge (Figure 1.1b). Included is knowledge of the heritage of the occupation and the developing profession of nursing, including knowledge of people, circumstances, and events that have shaped that development. Included also is the history of nursing knowledge as it has been transmitted to generations of practitioners.

The third section of the sphere (Figure 1.1c) represents philosophic nursing knowledge. Included are the profession's accepted values and codes of professional behavior. Included also should be the several philosophic theories that have been tested, found useful and relevant to nurses' work, and accepted as philosophic guides to practice. Illustrative are selected theories of value, justice and morality,

and ethical theories. Because nurses are encountering increasing numbers of moral and ethical dilemmas and because nurses are increasingly manifesting interest in becoming scholars in the discipline of philosophy, it is predicted that nursing knowledge henceforth will include increasing amounts of tested and relevant philosophic knowledge that will be incorporated into the discipline.

The fourth section of the sphere (Figure 1.1d) represents knowledge of nursing strategies, approaches, and technologies along with the scientific and artistic principles essential to their execution. Included also is knowledge of the prevailing health-care system. Relationships between the goals and caring functions of nurses and the goals and practice functions of other health professionals in the existing health-care systems represent another important segment of the discipline.

Another significant segment of nursing's body of knowledge has always been knowledge of factors that influence the health status, health assets, and health potential of human beings, both favorably and unfavorably (Figure 1.1e). Included is knowledge of biological, physical, and cognitive abilities with which people are naturally endowed and knowledge of environmental factors, economic and social circumstances, and changes associated with normal development, including the aging process. In the nursing perspective presented here, pathologies and medical diagnoses and treatments are factors that affect the health of human beings. Nurses must have adequate knowledge of these factors: such knowledge is an integral part of the discipline that must be mastered by nurse practitioners.

There is yet another kind of knowledge that is directly relevant to and essential for nursing practice. It is the knowledge that professionals must gain from relevant data concerning each person being served and that obtained through astute and perceptive observations. Personal knowledge of individuals and groups of persons is needed for nurses to respect the uniqueness of those for whom they provide exemplary services. For that reason, there can be no prescriptive nursing practice theories nor professional approaches to nursing care that are universally generalizable.

In summary, conceptualizing the discipline of nursing as an expandable and permeable sphere made up of segments of varying size provides an approach to classifying and organizing the several kinds of knowledge that constitute the nursing discipline. Such an approach demonstrates the vast and growing amounts of knowledge that professionals in the field must master and be able to use selectively, creatively, artistically, humanely, and skillfully to provide exemplary care.

Nursing should be recognized as a learned helping profession and a respected academic discipline. Surely nursing scholars will ensure the attainment of those goals by the beginning of the twenty-first century. Crucial to their attainment is identifying and attaining agreement about the human phenomena that are of particular concern to nurses, enhancing scholarly clinicians' involvement in generating promising relevant theories, and testing those theories as the means to discover knowledge through which to continuously improve nursing practices. Such an approach will ensure the availability of valid nursing knowledge in the twenty-first century and its currency during all centuries to come.

REFERENCES

American Association of Colleges of Nursing. (1986). *Essentials of college and university education for professional nursing*. Washington, DC: Author.

Chinn, P. (1984). From the editor. *Advances in Nursing Science, 6* (2), ix.

Donaldson, S., & Crowley, D. (1978). The discipline of nursing. *Nursing Outlook, 26*, 113-120.

Engel, G. (1977). The need for a new medical model: A challenge for biomedicine. *Science, 196*, 129-136.

Fawcett, J. (1983). Hallmarks of success in nursing theory development. In P. Chinn (Ed.), *Advances in nursing theory development* (pp. 3-17). Rockville, MD: Aspen.

Reverby, S. (1987). A caring dilemma: Womanhood and nursing in historical perspective. *Nursing Research, 36*, 5-11.

Silva, M. (1986). Research testing nursing theory: State of the art. *Advances in Nursing Science, 9* (1), 1-11.

2

The Discipline of Nursing

SUE K. DONALDSON, RN, PhD

DOROTHY M. CROWLEY, RN, PhD

All enquiry undertaken by nurses is not research that contributes to the discipline of nursing; to be nursing research, studies must be undertaken from a nursing perspective.

When one considers the gamut of research that nurses are undertaking, all of it is clearly important to the nursing profession, but the knowledge represented by the research problems and methodologies appears to be global. By definition, however, a discipline is not global; it is characterized by a unique perspective, a distinct way of viewing all phenomena, which ultimately defines the limits and nature of its inquiry.

This is the problem that plagues all of us: identification of the essence of nursing research and of the common elements and threads that give coherence to an identifiable body of knowledge. As nurse researchers, we seem to function primarily with tacit rather than explicit knowledge of the broad conceptualizations unique to nursing. We take for granted the nursing perspective as generally accepted and understood, until explanation of the particulars is required. Moreover, nursing authors tend to emphasize speculative formulations and theoretical reflections aimed at deriving the nature of nursing rather than explicating the structure of the body of

knowledge that constitutes the discipline of nursing.

Rather than expending a disproportionate amount of effort in the quest for *the* definition of the nature of nursing, it might behoove us—at least at this time—to seek relationships and commonalities in the ideas of writers whose work has influenced (and continues to influence) tacit knowledge of the scope of the field. At least since the time of Nightingale, there has been a remarkable consistency in the recurrent themes that nurse scholars use to explain what they conceive to be the essence or the core of nursing. Three general themes for enquiry emerge:

1. *Concern with principles and laws that govern the life processes, well-being, and optimum functioning of human beings—sick or well.* For example, a concern with the discovery of laws that govern health, knowledge of reparative processes, and prevention was manifest in the late nineteenth or early twentieth century in Nightingale's writings and certainly in Rogers' concern with laws and principles governing life processes in the past two decades.

2. *Concern with the patterning of human behavior in interaction with the environment in crit-*

Source: Donaldson, S. K., & Crowley, D. M. (1978). The discipline of nursing. *Nursing Outlook, 26* (2): 113-120. Used with permission from Mosby-Year Book, Inc.

ical life situations. As evidence of this theme, Rogers' writings reflect a concern with life rhythms and their relationship to environmental rhythms. Similarly, Johnson's writings in the 1960s focused attention on systems of behavior, pattern-maintenance, and pattern-disruption. The conceptual frames for most nursing curricula today include coping processes, adaptation, and supportive and non-supportive environments.

3. *Concern with the processes by which positive changes in health status are affected*. Peplau addressed herself to nursing as an interpersonal process, an educative and maturing force; whereas, Kreuter as well as Leininger and others addressed the particular type of process of support system seen as nursing's unique contribution.

These themes suggest boundaries of an area for systematic enquiry and theory development with potential for making the nature of the discipline of nursing more explicit than it is at present.

Integration of nursing research from the level of a conceptual framework for a particular study to the level of more general theories and ultimately to that of a unified body of nursing knowledge has not been pursued to any large extent. Nor have there been widespread efforts on the part of those doing research in nursing to relate individual studies to one another and, thereby, build a larger context for reference. This has contributed to fragmentation of knowledge and confusion about a perspective for nursing research.

As was the case in considering different ideas about the nature and themes of nursing, however, the goal is not to identify a single theory of nursing—rather, we would advocate pluralism. Nevertheless, it would seem desirable to be able to place such theories within the context of a discipline of nursing. More explicit identification of what we are

doing in nursing research is imperative if we are to truly function as nurse researchers, rather than as nurses conducting research in other disciplines, and if we are to have nursing theories for the professional practice of nursing. There is also a crucial need for identification of the structure of the discipline of nursing in our educational program. How can we justify doctoral programs in nursing if the discipline of nursing is not defined? Perhaps of even greater importance is the content of these doctoral programs. In fact, the very survival of the profession may be at risk unless the discipline is defined. As Armiger noted: "There exists today an unprecedented need for identification of the uniqueness of nursing science and practice, lest overriding forces in contemporary society lead to disintegration of nursing as a distinct profession."[1]

What is needed is the thinking of nurse philosophers and also some philosophizing on the part of the nurse researchers. The problem is not to devise the structure of the discipline of nursing, but to make this structure explicit. Our purpose is to make a beginning along these lines. Throughout this paper, the term *nursing* will refer to the discipline, unless otherwise clarified, and *structure* will refer to the broad conceptualizations and syntax of the discipline, rather than the theories generated within this structure.

CLASSIFICATION OF HUMAN KNOWLEDGE: DISCIPLINE

Traditionally, human knowledge and enquiry have been considered in the context of disciplines. Disciplines reflect true distinctions between bodies of knowledge per se and, as such, become the realm of learning. The *Oxford English Dictionary* defines discipline as "a branch of instruction or education, a department of learning or knowledge." Institutions of higher education are organized around these branches of knowledge into colleges, schools, and departments. Typically, disciplines have evolved as a consequence of a distinct perspective and syntax, which determine what phenomena or abstractions are of interest, in what context such phenomena are to be viewed, what questions are to be raised, what methods of study are to be used, and what canons of evidence and proof are to be required.

As a result of the complex way in which disciplines evolve, disciplines can be and have been identified and organized around a variety of characteristics and combinations of characteristics. Mathematics, for example, has been viewed as distinct from all other disciplines in that its subject matter appears to have no material existence; logic has been set apart because it is concerned with the development of canons of reasoning and evidence, which are utilized in the other disciplines. Thus, it is the unique relationship of logic to the other disciplines that sets it apart, rather than a peculiarity of its subject matter, as was the case for mathematics.

In identifying disciplines and classifying them, we are dealing with the nature and structure of the whole of human knowledge. It should be kept in mind that the number and membership of the disciplines are not agreed upon and that there is no single accepted organization of even the well-accepted disciplines. This is reflected in the diversity of organization of branches of learning in universities and colleges. The broadest classifications of disciplines depend upon a view of the inherent nature of all phenomena. A distinction on the part of the philosophers between the generality of natural phenomena and the particularity of human events leads to a distinction between such sciences as physics and sociology, which seek general laws for repeating behavior, and such disciplines as history, which

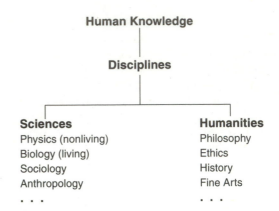

FIGURE 2.1. **Structuring of human knowledge.**

focuses on unique events, or ethics, which deals with human choices and value orientations (as shown in Figure 2.1). Among the sciences themselves, the biological sciences become distinct from physics and chemistry because they deal with the recognition of the phenomena of life and with living as opposed to nonliving things.

Nursing has both scientific aspects and aspects akin to the arts. For example, human health is considered within nursing in terms of political issues and history as well as in terms of inexorable laws of health. Therefore, nursing as a discipline is broader than nursing science and its uniqueness stems from its perspective rather than its object of enquiry or methodology.

You might well ask, Why bother with pursuing this discussion, especially since there is no agreement as to a single structure of human knowledge? There are at least two reasons: First, the discipline of nursing was not created *per se solum*, but emerged within the context of the other disciplines. Therefore, we must know its relationship to other disciplines in addition to its structure. Second, it must be remembered that the family of disciplines, be-

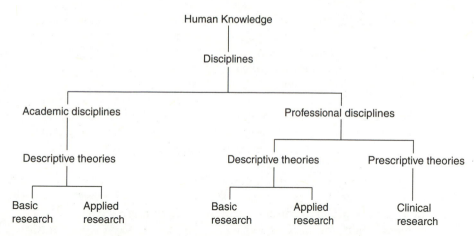

FIGURE 2.2. **Theories and research characteristics of academic and professional disciplines.**

cause each of its members represents knowledge derived within a particular conceptual structure, is subject to revision in the form of fusion, extinction, and multiplication of its members as new conceptualizations emerge. Nursing as a discipline is also subject to change based upon changes in its structural conceptual base; in fact, nurse researchers and scholars have the responsibility of questioning and revising nursing's structure.

According to Shermis, the accepted academic disciplines are all characterized by an impressive body of enduring works, suitable techniques, concerns which are significant and relevant to humans, unifying and inspiring traditions, and considerable scholarly achievements. Although these are not criteria for distinguishing disciplines from nondisciplines, they do provide a basis for acceptance of a branch of learning as a discipline.

But what of emerging disciplines? In the professional field, there typically is an evolutionary process that occurs as the field moves from a vocational level, in which the art and technology are preeminent, to the rationalization of practice and the establishment of a cognitive base for professional practice. It is im-

portant to recognize that a discipline emerges as a result of creative thinking related to significant issues. Because of the vital significance of nursing's perspective, its concern with human hea-lth and well-being, and its growth through research and scholarly work, nursing will gain full acceptance in time.

For purposes of this discussion, a distinction between academic disciplines and professional disciplines will be utilized (as illustrated in Figure 2.2). The academic disciplines include sciences such as physics, physiology, and sociology, as well as liberal arts disciplines such as mathematics, history, and philosophy. The aim of academic disciplines is to know, and their theories are descriptive in nature. In contrast, professional disciplines such as law, medicine, and nursing are directed toward practical aims and thus generate prescriptive as well as descriptive theories.

For academic disciplines, the goal is to know, regardless of whether the research is basic or applied. In fact, the distinction between applied and basic research seems appropriate only in relation to descriptive theories, since applied research answers questions related to the applicability of basic theories in practical situations, rather than questions related to *how* basic theories are to be applied. Thus, applied physicists test the practical limits of theories of physics but would not derive information as to the best design for a bridge, for example.

Fields that emphasize applied research would be more correctly termed applied disciplines, or applied branches of academic disciplines, rather than professional disciplines, which have prescriptive theories in addition to descriptive ones. The prescriptive theories characteristic of professional disciplines deal with the actual implementation of knowledge in a practical sense. As Johnson has stated, ". . . professional knowledge does not consist of basic science theory which has been validated in practice."[2] In this regard, it is not correct to view professional disciplines simply as applied sciences.

Within the professional discipline there is a need "to know" and to work from descriptive theories in addition to prescriptive ones. As Gortner has pointed out, "some of the work is basic, in that it is applicable to a general understanding of human behavior or responses to illness," and other studies of nursing are applied.[3] Basic and applied research are both needed in a professional discipline because each discipline has a different practical aim which influences the perspective of that field, the way it conceptualizes the relevant world, and the questions it poses for investigation. Therefore, because of the uniqueness of each discipline's perspective and the context in which knowledge from each discipline fits, it is not possible to simply "borrow" theory or knowledge from other disciplines.

Schwab has noted that in general the statements of a given discipline are like single words of a sentence; their meanings derive more from their context than from their dictionary sense. In other words, statements of disciplines, their conclusions, are properly understood only in the context of the enquiry that produced them. They are true only in that they fit the criteria for truth in the given discipline. From this standpoint, nurse scientists may help in utilization of information from other disciplines, but this will not eliminate the need for undertaking basic research in nursing from nursing's perspective. Viewing phenomena from the perspective of healthy functioning of individuals in interaction with their environments will generate distinctive research at all levels and a defined, structured body of knowledge.

Even when useful information might be derived from the research of another discipline, the studies are not pursued, either because of lack of interest or because the conditions used invalidate the results for nursing's purpose. For example, a physiologist studying mechanisms underlying a given cellular process may work with intact cells but at a very low temperature, say 0°C, to slow the process down to allow measurement of its kinetic properties. The low temperature does not invalidate the physiologist's conclusions, but may make the data inappropriate in terms of knowing exact rates characteristic of the process at in vivo temperatures. Furthermore, animal and suborganismal, even subcellular, research is valid in its own right in physiology, whereas in nursing the information is ultimately being sought in relation to intact human beings.

Nursing cannot rely upon the academic disciplines to supply its total requirement for knowledge of laws and processes. Rather, appropriately prepared nurse researchers must generate and test descriptive theories as necessary and develop their own technology, as has been recommended for other professionals.

Another very important issue is the extent to which each discipline is dependent upon the development of the others. The Comtian view of the sciences, which is a hierarchical one, is noteworthy in this regard, since it has

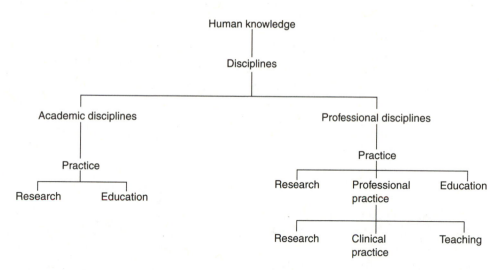

FIGURE 2.3.   Practice realms of disciplines.

influenced curricula; in turn, these curricula can lead to unwarranted views of the dependence of some disciplines on the others.

Comte held that not only human knowledge in general but also each branch of knowledge passes through states or stages of progress on its way to becoming scientific. He also conceived of the branches of knowledge as evolving in an increasingly complex organizational hierarchy ranging from the physical to the social. As a result of an arbitrary interpretation of Comte's hierarchy in curricula, physics and chemistry have been required, for example, for the mastery of biology, and so on. Although there may be increased efficiency of instruction following this plan, it should be remembered that learners influenced by such curricula may come to view all knowledge as hierarchical. Yet, the hierarchical nature of knowledge has not been demonstrated; in fact, acceptance of hierarchical structuring of knowledge can be very limiting and should be questioned.

In the first place, there is the danger that one conceive all knowledge of scientific quality as being encompassed by the academic dis-

ciplines, with the professions resting on these disciplines for their cognitive base. Second, if even the potential for professional disciplines is conceded, it is difficult for proponents of the hierarchical view to envision how professional disciplines could expand their respective bodies of knowledge independently. In contrast, professional disciplines can be viewed as emerging *along with* rather than *from* academic disciplines.

This is not to imply that disciplines are totally independent of each other. Certainly, logical formulations in one discipline cannot ignore the "truths" of the others. The quality of theories and research designs and the validity of conclusions drawn within one discipline are dependent upon their congruence with all of knowledge. Therefore, knowledge in one discipline may set constraints on or enhance the process of enquiry in another. Perhaps the most obvious interrelationship of disciplines is in their associated practice realm.

Every discipline exists in part to provide knowledge which is to be utilized and thus has an associated practice realm (Figure 2.3). Accordingly, every discipline has educators and researchers who function in this realm to impart the knowledge base to others and expand the knowledge base through research. In addition, professional disciplines have practitioners who deliver a service by engaging in professional practice in the form of clinical service, education, and research.

Sharing of knowledge from many disciplines occurs in the realm of practice associated with each discipline. For example, researchers affiliated with academic disciplines may borrow relevance or reality orientation from observations of professional practitioners and use prescriptive or practice theories from professional disciplines and practice. Similarly, professional disciplines derive knowledge from academic disciplines.

RELATIONSHIP OF THE DISCIPLINE TO PRACTICE

Although the discipline and the profession are inextricably linked and greatly influence each other's substance, they must be distinguished from each other. Failure to recognize the existence of the discipline as a body of knowledge that is separate from the activities of practitioners has contributed to the fact that nursing has been viewed as a vocation rather than a profession. In turn, this has led to confusion as to whether the discipline of nursing exists.

Part of the problem in viewing a professional discipline as distinct from professional practice stems from the fact that both the discipline and practice evolved interdependently in response to societal needs; as a result, both possess a common practical aim related to these needs (Figure 2.4). Professions evolved because the service they provided was valued. Given the emphasis placed upon science and rationality in the postindustrial age, it is not surprising that there was a strong impetus for establishing a scientific and theoretical base for professional practice. The process of upgrading professional prac-

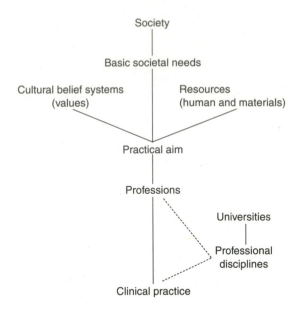

FIGURE 2.4. Interdependent evolution of discipline and practice of a profession.

tice also entailed the establishment of closer relations between knowledge serving as the basis of professional practice and knowledge in the academic disciplines. Since the university traditionally has been the locus of development of theoretical knowledge, the professional disciplines were eventually housed there along with the academic disciplines.

The location of professional disciplines such as nursing in institutions such as universities, which are primarily concerned with human knowledge as a product rather than service, does not change the accountability of these disciplines for societal needs and the practical aim of their associated professions. As Johnson has noted, the decisions of what to study and what questions to ask necessarily have stemmed from social decisions about the profession's realm of responsibility in giving services or in clinical practice.

Florence Nightingale defined the discipline in terms of the responsibility of nursing's practitioners to promote human health based on systematic enquiry into nature's "laws of health."[4] Part of the reason for nursing's struggle in evolving stems from the slow emergence of the recognition of its social relevance. Nurses give service related to the quality of human life; this service is only recently being valued. After all, why should quality of life be considered before biological survival can be assured?

Ethical and moral values inherent in clinical practice have profoundly influenced the perspective and value orientation of the discipline. Thus, nursing has traditionally valued humanitarian service. But in addition, the self-respect and self-determination of clients are to be preserved. The goal of nursing service is to foster self-caring behavior that leads to individual health and well-being. These values and goals, which are intrinsic to professional practice, have shaped the value orientation of the discipline. As a result of this value orientation, knowledge of the basis of human choices and of methods for fostering individual independence are sought, rather than knowledge of interventions that control and directly manipulate the person per se into a societally determined state of health.

The clinical practice of nursing requires the development of prescriptive theories on the part of the discipline. Much of the early research related to the nursing profession consisted of investigations about nurses, their characteristics and behavior, but these investigations could not actually be considered nursing research. In recent years, the amount of research concerned with theories fundamental to clinical practice has increased.

A key point, however, is that the discipline of nursing should be *governing* clinical practice rather than being defined by it. Of necessity, clinical practice focuses on the individual in the here and now who has a problem requiring relevant and appropriate action. The discipline, in contrast, embodies a knowledge base relevant to all realms of professional practice and which links the past, present, and future. Its scope goes far beyond that required for current clinical practice. If the discipline were so narrowly defined, professional nursing could be limited to functioning in the realm of disaster relief rather than serving as a force in the promotion of world health. This is not meant to diminish the importance of problems encountered by nurses in current clinical practice. These problems deserve attention, but they are not the only concern of the discipline.

Part of the problem is that "clinical practice" is too often used synonymously with "professional practice," and clinical practice is narrowly defined. Professional competency goes beyond that required for delivery of health care to individuals, preparation of future practitioners, and conduct of systematic enquiry. For example, McGlothlin believes that competency includes the need on the part of professionals for social understanding of sufficient breadth to place the practice in the context of society and the need for leadership skills.

Some of the knowledge required for achieving these competencies can only come from the discipline of nursing. Prescriptive theories essential to clinical practice and the appropriate design of nursing research can only be derived from the discipline of nursing. Similarly, although knowledge from political science, history, philosophy, and other disciplines is very important for social understanding, the professional nurse cannot put nursing into a societal context without knowledge derived from the discipline of nursing. This knowledge is obtained in part from nurse philosophers and nurse historians who view nursing as it relates to other disciplines and can articulate how nursing's heritage relates to its perspective. The discipline of nursing must also provide essential components of the knowledge base for preparation of world leaders in the field of health.

The need for philosophical, historical, and similar types of enquiry within the discipline of nursing is crucial not only in terms of providing the knowledge base for professional preparation but also for the development of the discipline. It must be remembered that the discipline is defined by social relevance and value orientations rather than by empirical truths. Thus, the discipline and profession must be continually reevaluated in terms of societal needs and scientific discoveries. Similarly, the entire structure of the discipline may need to be revamped in time, and this should be done by nurse researchers.

For this reason we have been very careful not to equate the discipline of nursing with the science of nursing. As mentioned earlier, only part of nursing employs scientific method. We need doctoral preparation for nurse historians as well as nurse scientists. As Schlotfeldt has pointed out: "Nursing faculties rarely have among their members scholars who are concerned with establishing the history of nursing science and with identifying the philosophies of conceptualizations of nursing that have influenced the structure of that knowledge at various times in nursing's history."[5] Once again, the purpose in having nurse philosophers and historians is not to duplicate the efforts of other disciplines, but rather to provide these approaches from the perspective of nursing.

It should be remembered that although nursing requires researchers and scholars who utilize a variety of approaches, all research that is important to the profession of nursing is not derived from the discipline of nursing. Only information and theories stemming from nursing's perspective come from nursing per se. Nursing educators utilize information and theories from education. Even clinical practice should not be viewed as being grounded solely in the discipline of nursing.

In delivering health care, practitioners must in fact draw from many disciplines, such as business administration, medicine, education, and basic sciences. Rarely, if ever, does the skilled clinician rely only on knowledge from one discipline or even rely solely on scientific knowledge. Clinical practice is always to some extent empirical, pragmatic, intuitive, and artistic.

Once we agree that the discipline of nursing does not have to embody all, the entire whole, or knowledge utilized by the profession of nursing, then we can begin to define the discipline. Nursing is not global in its subject matter and therefore does not subsume part of any other disciplines—for example, education—just because practitioners are educated. Similarly, studies of higher education in nursing that deal with the educational process are not nursing research but educational research. In contrast, a study of the effects of educational techniques on clients' achievement of self-care is within nursing per se. Even though nursing care delivery is greatly affected by attitudes of nurses administration policies, such problems may be studied appropriately in other disciplines.

The purpose in excluding some research from nursing is not to create a ranking of importance or prestige, but rather to make the essence of nursing explicit. Nurses who conduct administrative or educational research may contribute as much to the professional practice of nursing as nurses who conduct nursing research.

In summary, the discipline and clinical practice of nursing share a common social relevance and practical aim. However, the discipline, which is a body of knowledge, must not be confused with its associated practice realm, which embodies the processes of conducting research, giving service, and educating. Furthermore, some members of the profession must engage in enquiry that is not immediately applicable to current clinical practice. As

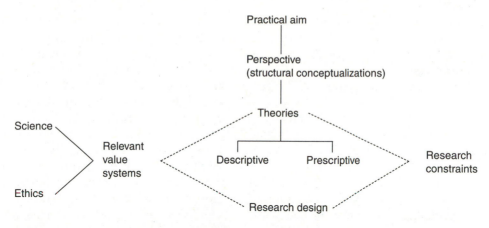

FIGURE 2.5. **Structure of a professional discipline.**

a branch of knowledge, the discipline embodies more than the science of nursing and requires researchers who employ a variety of approaches from nursing's perspective. Although the discipline provides crucial and unique content for nurse researchers, clinicians, and educators, these practitioners draw on many disciplines. Appropriately prepared nurses may elect to conduct research within other disciplines because of the critical importance of this non-nursing research to professional practice or the growth of the discipline.

STRUCTURE OF THE DISCIPLINE OF NURSING

We are now at the point of examining the structure of the discipline. According to Schwab, disciplines have both substantive and syntactical structures. The substantive structure is composed of conceptualizations which are borrowed or invented, but their inclusion is always based on their fit with the perspective of the discipline. The syntax of a discipline refers to the research methodologies and criteria used to justify the acceptance of

statements as true within the discipline (see Figure 2.5).

We have incorporated the syntax of nursing as value systems (both of science and of professional ethics) and research constraints. Such constraints include consideration of accessibility of controls, congruity with existing knowledge, manifest and latent consequences, and technological feasibility. Both values and constraints influence theory generation and actual research design. In effect, they function to ensure that enquiry will result in conclusions and statements that are appropriate, reliable, and valid for the purpose of the discipline.

Thus, the substantive structure determines primarily the scope and subject of enquiry—what is of interest; and the syntactical structure determines primarily the procedure for conducting research and criteria for acceptability of findings as truth. The findings generated by enquiry are then incorporated into the structure as concepts, theories, and facts—the statements of the discipline. In this paper, we have focused upon the structural conceptualizations, but it should be remembered that the syntax of the discipline is also important, since the syntax determines the extent to which the truth of statements of the discipline is war-ranted. In contrast, the substantive structure relates to the subject matter of the enquiry. The structural conceptualizations are selected for inclusion in a given discipline with its per-spective as a screen.

From its perspective, nursing studies the wholeness or health of humans, recognizing that humans are in continuous interaction with their environments. Nursing's perspective evolves from the practical aim of optimizing of human environments for health. Examples of major conceptualizations in nursing deal with:

1. Distinctions between human and nonhu-man beings
2. Distinctions between living and nonliving
3. Nature of environments and human-envi-ronmental interactions from cellular to so-cietal levels
4. Illness versus health and well-being
5. Functioning of the whole human organ-ism versus functioning of the parts
6. Levels of functioning of whole organisms
7. Human characteristics and natural pro-cesses, such as consciousness, abstraction; adaptation and healing; growth; change; self-determination; development; aging; dying; reproducing; drive satisfaction; and relating.

The structural conceptions are being uti-lized, but they are usually not identified or clarified, and rarely questioned. It is impor-tant, for example, to know whether health is viewed, in the context of a given theory or de-sign, as a specific state, or as it is defined by each individual.

Depending upon the particular structural conceptualizations utilized, or combinations of them, widely different theories are proposed for testing. Such variation in theories does not lead to different bodies of knowledge, but to different aspects of a single body.

Pluralism of theories promotes productiv-ity; in fact, without testing of a wide variety of theories, progress towards "truth" cannot be made. In physiology, for example, where knowledge of the functions and nature of vital processes of living organisms is sought, a pluralism of theories exists. Many physiolo-gists conceive the functioning of the organism as explainable in terms of the functioning of its parts, whereas others propose an explana-tion utilizing a conception that the whole is more than the sum of its parts. This dual ap-proach is very useful, regardless of the cor-rectness of the theories, since testable theories are generated that yield empirical evidence related to knowledge of the nature of and mechanisms underlying behavior of living systems. The goal in generating theories is not just to propose an all-encompassing theory but to provide testable theories.

Research designed to test hypotheses stem-ming from theories is very important to the discipline and practitioners when the relation-ship of nursing theories to the structure of the discipline is explicit. This is the type of research that is easily identified as nursing research. Schwab calls this stable enquiry, in that there is no hesitation about what questions to ask or what structural conceptualizations to employ. For example, if the current principles of physi-ology are organ and function, the researcher engaged in stable enquiry discovers the func-tion of one organ after another.

This type of stable research tends to be the most rewarded, but there is another very im-portant realm of enquiry which must be ex-panded. We refer to questions relating to the structural conceptualizations and value orien-tations of the discipline. For example, What is the nature of health? Is health on a contin-uum with illness? Is health for every person a reasonable goal for society?

At least two major benefits are derived from this second type of research. First, the structural conceptualizations are clarified or altered to make them consistent with reality. They should not be accepted as givens. Second, the discipline will be continually shaped according to significant themes, those which are of vital significance to man [*sic*]. If nurse researchers are to provide the knowledge base for societal directions in relation to health, they must engage in this type of research.

For the continued growth, significance, and utility of the discipline of nursing, researchers must place their research within the context of the discipline. Theories must also be viewed in terms of the basic structural conceptualizations of the discipline. The responsibility for revising and clarifying the structural conceptions, the very framework, of the discipline of nursing rests with nurse researchers. This means lessening our preoccupation with the process of nursing and pedagogy and placing emphasis on content as substance.

REFERENCES

1. Armiger, Sister Bernadette. Scholarship in nursing. *Nurs. Outlook* 22:160-164, Mar. 1974.
2. Johnson, D. E. Development of theory: A requisite for nursing as a primary health profession. *Nurs.Res.* 23:373, Sept.-Oct. 1974.
3. Gortner, S. R. Scientific accountability in nursing. *Nurs.Outlook* 22:765, Dec. 1974.
4. Nightingale, Florence. *Notes on Nursing: What it is and What it is not.* London, Harrison, 1860.
5. Schlotfeldt, R. M. Nursing research: Reflection of values. *Nurs.Res.* 26:8, Jan.-Feb. 1977.

BIBLIOGRAPHY

Argyris, Chris, & Schon, D. A. *Theory in Practice: Increasing Professional Effectiveness.* San Francisco, Jossey-Bass, 1974.

Davies, J. T. *The Scientific Approach.* New York, Academic Press, 1965.

Gortner, S. R., & Nahm, Helen. An overview of nursing research in the United States. *Nurs.Res.* 26:10-33, Jan.-Feb. 1977.

Greenwood, E. The practice of science and the science of practice. In *The Planning of Change*, 2d edition, edited by W. G. Bennis and others. New York, Holt, Rhinehart and Winston, 1969.

Haldane, J. S. *The Sciences and Philosophy.* Garden City, N.Y., Doubleday, Doran and Co., 1929.

Henderson, Virginia. The nature of nursing. *Am. J.Nurs.* 64:62-68, Aug. 1964.

Hyde, A. The phenomenon of caring. *Nurs.Res.Rep.* 10:2-3ff, Oct. 1975.

Johnson, D. E. The significance of nursing care. *Am. J.Nurs.* 61:63-66, Nov. 1961.

Kreuter, F. R. What is good nursing care? *Nurs.Outlook* 5:302-304, May 1957.

Leininger, M. The phenomenon of caring; Part 5. Caring: the essence and central focus of nursing. *Nurs.Res.Rep.* 12:2, 14, Feb. 1977.

McGlothlin, W. J. *Patterns of Professional Education.* New York, G. P. Putnam's Sons, 1960.

Merton, R., & Lerner, D. Social scientists and research policy. In *The Planning of Change*, 2d edition, edited by W. G. Bennis and others. New York, Holt, Rhinehart and Winston, 1969.

Parsons, Talcott, & Platt, G. M. *The American University.* Cambridge, Mass., Harvard University Press, 1973.

Peplau, H. E. *Interpersonal Relations in Nursing, A Conceptual Frame of Reference for Psychodynamic Nursing.* New York, G. P. Putnam's Sons, 1952.

Rogers, M. E. *Introduction to the Theoretical Basis of Nursing.* Philadelphia, F. A. Davis Co., 1970.

Schwab, J. Structure of the disciplines: Meanings and significances. In *The Structure of Knowledge and the Curriculum*, ed. by G. W. Ford and Lawrence Pugno. Chicago, Rand McNally, 1964.

———. The structure of the natural sciences. In *The Structure of Knowledge and the Curriculum*, ed. by G. W. Ford and Lawrence Pugno. Chicago, Rand McNally, 1964.

Shermis, S. On becoming an intellectual discipline. *Phi Delta Kappan* 44:84-86, 1962.

3

Toward More Clarity in Terminology: Frameworks, Theories, and Models

EVELYN ADAM, RN, MN

Lack of precision in a person's choice of words, which perhaps indicates a lack of clarity and accuracy in ideas, may become a subtle form of negative teaching. It is suggested that such terms as conceptual frame of reference *and* theoretical framework *should be used as broad terms for conceptions of reality, reserving* philosophy, theory *and* conceptual model *as more restricted terms for conceptions of reality.*

Nurse authors do not agree that nursing theory exists, that nursing has its own body of knowledge, that nursing is a science or even a discipline. Yet nursing is fully equipped to justify its claim to such terms. Starting from a nursing perspective rather than from a borrowed one, nursing theory can be developed, nursing knowledge can be accumulated, and nursing science can be advanced, all in the interests of a worthwhile contribution to society's health.

Reviewing the multitude of ways that certain terms are used in the nursing literature, one cannot but notice the lack of agreement among authors and even a number of contradictions in the writings of the same person. Nurses sometimes define words in a restricted sense and then proceed, within the same context, to attribute to those words a much broader meaning.

The effect of this confusion on learning has not been demonstrated. It may well convince the student to always define his or her terms; it may also be a form of negative teaching in that it implicitly condones and perpetuates imprecision. On the assumption that multiple contradictions in terminology are not necessarily conducive to learning, the purpose of this article is to review some of the meanings attributed to oft-used words in nursing, and to offer a modest suggestion for greater clarity in terminology as well as for some new light on nursing's future.

The confusion surrounding terminology in nursing has not diminished since Lewis (1974) cautioned us that failure to attend to the exact meaning of a word may indicate not only a lack of precision in a writer's choice and use of words but inaccuracy and imprecision in her ideas as well. Vincent (1975), on the other hand, questions nursing's concern about lack of agreement on the meaning of terms such as *data collection* and *assessment*.

Words are of course always evolving and changing in meaning and any attempt to establish a "one word, one meaning" rule would be undesirable indeed. It is also true that the exact

Source: Adam, E. (1985). Toward more clarity in terminology: Framework, theories, and models. *Journal of Nursing Education, 24* (4): 151-155. Reprinted with permission from SLACK, Inc.

meaning of a word varies according to the context. "The ignoring of contexts in any act of interpretation is at best a stupid practice. At its worst, it can be a vicious practice" (Hayakawa, 1963, p. 62). Many terms have a variety of meanings, each one legitimate. Conceptual and theoretical frameworks are the same, or very different, depending on the writer, and even more concrete terms such as *nursing care plan* and *nursing problem* mean many things to many people. It is generally accepted that the *nursing process* (the four-, five-, or six-step method) is not the *process of nursing*—defined by Orlando (1961) as the interaction between patient behavior, the nurse's reaction and the nurse's action. There is also some agreement that *nursing practice* (as opposed to education and research) is not *the practice of nursing* (the pursuing of that particular field); the distinction between *nursing need* and *need of nursing* is however less clear and that between *nursing theory* and *theory of nursing* even less so.

Some "tidying up" of terminology may be worthwhile if nurses are to communicate effectively with each other.

FRAMEWORKS AND MODELS: CONCEPTUAL AND THEORETICAL

Reilly (1975) and Peterson (1977) state that a conceptual framework is not a theoretical framework, and Fawcett (1978a, b) makes a distinction between conceptual and theoretical models. In explaining the difference between the two types of frameworks, Reilly (1975) declares that a conceptual model provides a perspective or a way of looking at nursing and does not constitute reality; she adds that a theoretical model "does constitute reality since it has a scientifically accepted base" (p. 567). Peterson (1977) defines a theoretical framework as a conceptual model which contains both structure and detail. Peterson (1977) and Faw-

cett (1978a, b) agree that a conceptual model is the precursor of a theory.

Other writers however seem to use conceptual and theoretical frameworks as synonyms. In an editorial comment, Notter (1968) states that research must be based on a conceptual or theoretical framework. Johnson (1978) deplores the misunderstanding of the difference between, on the one hand, theories of nursing and, on the other hand, "what are variously called conceptual frameworks, conceptual models, and theoretical frameworks" (p. 5). Johnson refers to the need for a conceptualization that would provide a useful framework for practice, education, and research—a conceptual model or theoretical framework. Newman (1979) uses conceptual framework and conceptual model interchangeably but sees theory, in contrast, as "testable and therefore refutable and alterable" (p. 6); she notes that "a conceptual model (framework) specifies the focus of inquiry for the discipline" (p. 13).

Seeking a common denominator, it can be argued that frameworks and frames of reference (as well as philosophies, theories, and conceptual models) can all be defined as abstractions, conceptions (the products of conceptualization), mental images, and ways of looking at, or conceptualizing, reality. This writer believes that a case can be made for considering theoretical frames of reference and conceptual and theoretical frameworks as broad terms for conceptions of reality, while reserving *philosophy*, *theory*, and *conceptual model* as more specific and more restricted terms for conceptions of reality. In other words, philosophies are always frames of reference or conceptions of reality but frames of reference are not always philosophies. All theories are abstract frameworks or conceptual entities but not all frameworks are theories. Conceptual models are always mental images but again the converse is not necessarily true (Figure 3.1).

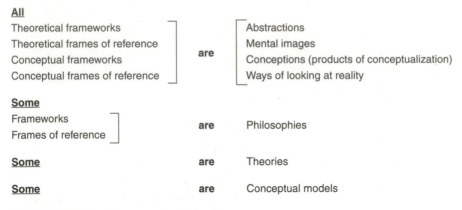

FIGURE 3.1.   Concepts of reality.

PHILOSOPHY, THEORY, AND CONCEPTUAL MODEL

Philosophy

Dickoff and James (1970), while chiding nurses that their so-called philosophy of nursing is rather a dogmatic religion of nursing, define *philosophy* as a habitual approach or a set of mind. Such highly abstract notions are fascinating to ponder; some nurses may be idealistic and others realistic in their approach to life and nursing; some may have an existential, some a pragmatic set of mind. It could be argued that statements such as "nursing is caring" or "nursing provides comfort and concern" are more religious than "philosophical"; in any case, no nurse is likely to quarrel with such statements and they are so abstract that they are difficult to operationalize. Examining the intrinsic aspects of nursing, Watson (1979) proposes that the basic core of nursing comprises the "philosophy and science of caring" (p. xv).

Theory

When discussing theory, Fawcett (1978a, b) and Bush (1979) quote Kerlinger's definition,

while Riehl and Roy (1980) and Johnson (1978) use the one offered by Dickoff and James. Hardy (1978a) refers to Kaplan's definition. As already stated, Johnson (1978) disagrees with the widespread labeling of conceptual models as "theories of nursing." For Johnson (1978), a theory of nursing is as impossible or unnecessary as would be a theory of medicine or of law, since a theory of nursing would have to describe and explain nursing as a scientific discipline; theory in nursing, that is, theory that describes and explains that which is of concern to nursing, is what is needed (p. 7).

More recently, Lancaster and Lancaster (1981) state that *model* is not a synonym for theory; they add that all theories are models but that the converse is not true. This position seems contrary to the one that holds that models are the precursors of theory (Bush, 1979; Fawcett, 1978a, b; Newman, 1979; Peterson, 1977).

Dickoff and James (1968) point out that nursing theory must be theory at the fourth or highest level (situation-producing level), which presupposes the existence of three prior levels. Dickoff, James, and Wiedenbach (1968) note that the first level—that of isolating and naming factors—is one so basic as to be often overlooked. Johnson (1978) also suggests that nurses may be neglecting the first levels of theory development.

Roy and Roberts (1981) define *theory* as "a system of interrelated propositions used to predict, explain, understand, and control a part of the empirical world" (p. 5). Nurses disagree however about the existence of nursing theory. Fawcett (1978a) believes that nursing theory "is practically nonexistent" (p. 58). Johnson (1974), discussing the difficulties facing nurse scientists, states that "there is no circumscribed body of knowledge" (p. 372). Flaskerud and Halloran (1980), observing that progress in developing nursing theory has slowed, remark that practitioners often have not heard of nursing theory, educators circumvent or argue about it, and researchers use frameworks from other disciplines. Hardy (1978b) suggests that nursing is in a preparadigm stage where confusion prevails as to what entities are of particular concern to nursing; research is therefore often poorly focused and unsystematic. In the preface to her book about nursing theory, Stevens (1979) concedes that "even to talk about "nursing theory" requires a suspension of precision" (p. x).

Meanwhile, theories from other fields are useful to several disciplines. General systems theory is used, for example, in nursing, sociology, and engineering, and different theories of stress and of adaptation are as valuable to nurses as they are to psychologists and physicians. The day may come when nursing theory will be as useful to related disciplines as existing theories, developed in other fields, are today useful to nurses.

Conceptual Model

The word *model* without the adjective *conceptual* has many and varied meanings (Adam, 1980). For Riehl and Roy (1980), a conceptual model for nursing is "a mental image of the realm of nursing" (p. 6). Fawcett (1978b) defines a conceptual model as a perspective that tells the scientist what to look at. Newman (1979) states that a conceptual model also provides direction, to the practitioner, for the observations necessary for assessment and intervention. In that regard, Chin (1976) holds that no practitioner can carry on thought processes without concepts; "indeed, no observations or diagnoses are ever made on 'raw facts,' because facts are really observations made within a set of concepts" (p. 90). Bush (1979) points out that in education, practice, and research, a model for nursing serves to unify, to give direction, and to simplify. Stevens (1979) refers to the "discipline model," which must be made evident to the student, as "the image of nursing conveyed to the student by the faculty" (p. 130), and to the "curriculum model" as the vehicle whereby the student is introduced to the discipline model.

A conceptual model for nursing is therefore a conception of nursing. Again, all conceptions of nursing are not conceptual models: indeed many private and personal conceptions of nursing are not sufficiently clear as to be made explicit, and for a mental image to be called a conceptual model it must be explicit and clear. Johnson (Riehl & Roy, 1980) presents the essential components of a conceptual model: assumptions, values, and major units.

Conceptual models for nursing are conceptual frames of reference which are specific to nursing. Conceptual frameworks are conceptual models of nursing only if they are specific to nursing and if they are made up of the assumptions, values, and major units essential to a conceptual model. A conceptual model for nursing, in providing a particular perspective, offers direction for practice, research, and education in nursing, but not, for example, in medicine nor in psychology; the converse is equally true. All three disciplines may, of course, use some of the same philosophies and theories, but each discipline has a conception of its distinct goal and of the phenomena that concern it particularly. In other words, each discipline is guided by a broad perspective of its own social mission even as it uses various philosophies and theories in the pursuit of that social mission.

The confusion between the terms *theory* and *conceptual model* may explain the reluctance of some nurses to make explicit their conceptual base. This writer has encountered two areas of misunderstanding. It is often thought that a model indicates what nursing is, when indeed a model is rather a conception of what nursing should be or could be. The day may come when nurses can say what nursing is, that which today they can merely say it should or could be. The misconception that a conceptual model indicates what nursing is, engenders feelings that a model is limiting and restrictive and therefore threatening to a nurse's personal and academic liberty. Making clear to the students the mental image of nursing that underlies the curriculum seems to be, for some educators, tantamount to teaching a dangerous dogma.

The second area of misunderstanding is the expectation that conceptual models for nursing should be tested—in the same way that theories are tested—before they warrant adoption or even serious consideration. A conceptual model for a discipline provides a very broad perspective of that discipline's focus of inquiry, and that broad perspective does not lend itself to "testing" in the way that propositions do. Yet nurses seem to want assurance that one of the conceptual models is the "right" one, the best one, forgetting perhaps that their personal conception of nursing, the one that is currently guiding their practice or teaching or research, has not only not been proven "right" but is not even very clear. Criteria do exist for evaluating a conceptual model but they are not the same as those used for judging a theory. Johnson (1974) has de-

veloped criteria extrinsic to the substance of the model: social utility, social congruence, and social significance. Social decisions, of this nature, about a particular model, obviously cannot be made until that conceptual model becomes the basis of nursing practice, research, and education; until those social decisions are made, there is room for several conceptual models. It is therefore unrealistic to demand that a conceptual model be "tested" or "validated"; it is, however, entirely realistic to demand that the service which derives from it be congruent with society's expectations, significant to society's health, and useful in giving clear direction for research, practice, and education.

The two areas of misunderstanding lead educators to argue that a conceptual model may be appropriate for one level of nursing education but not for another. Yet wherever the subject matter is nursing, a mental image of the discipline is conveyed to the students. If that mental image is not clear enough to be made explicit, students may be learning that their chosen profession does not have an explicit conceptual base.

DISCIPLINE, PROFESSION, SCIENCE

Discussion of the terms *discipline* and *profession* often centers less on their meaning than on the criteria that must be met for a group to claim the status of discipline or of profession. In the discussion, the words *theory* and *science* are inevitably invoked.

Roy and Roberts (1981) define *discipline* as a field of inquiry "characterized by a unique perspective, a distinct way of viewing all phenomena" (p. 21); they add that when the discipline of nursing defines its body of knowledge, there will be a science of nursing. Donaldson and Crowley (1978) note that disciplines are departments of learning and knowledge;

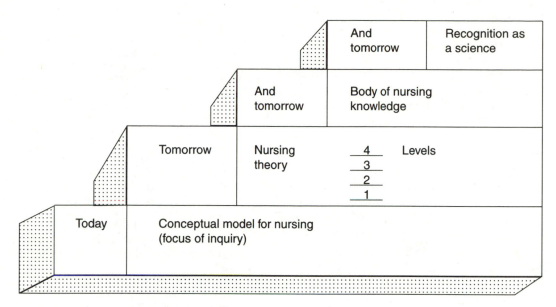

FIGURE 3.2.   The Path Ahead

they reflect true distinctions between bodies of knowledge and have evolved as a result of a distinct perspective and syntax. The same authors distinguish between academic disciplines, whose goal is to know, and professional disciplines, which are directed toward practical aims.

A discipline then has its own perspective. If it is true that a discipline will be known as a science when it has developed its body of knowledge, it must be recalled that a body of knowledge is also considered an essential attribute of a profession. The word *profession*, of course, may be used in the sense of an organized association of persons; it is used here in the sense of a field of human endeavor involving advanced learning. *Profession* has long been defined as a learned vocation (Cogan, 1953, p. 34).

There is some agreement among nurse authors that science is a body of organized systematic knowledge (Greene, 1979; Johnson, 1974; Roy & Roberts, 1981). Johnson (1974) adds that sciences differ from one another inasmuch as they study different phenomena that

have been selected from a distinctive perspective. Greenwood (1961) states that the scientific activity within a given discipline produces "a system of internally consistent propositions which describe and explain the phenomena that constitute the subject matter of that discipline" (p. 75).

CONCLUSION

One might be tempted to draw a dreary conclusion. Because at least some authors claim that nursing has, as yet, no theoretical body of knowledge, then perhaps nursing is not really a profession. Since there is no agreement that nursing theory exists, then nursing is perhaps not a science and because nursing often uses a borrowed perspective, it follows that nursing is not a discipline. Nurse educators should therefore avoid using those terms.

This writer prefers a positive conclusion. If indeed for nursing to be recognized as a science (and as a profession) it must have a body of knowledge; if to have a body of knowledge there must be theory development; if to develop theory one must begin at the first level of factor isolating; if factor isolating cannot be done except from a broad perspective; nursing is in the enviable position of having several broad perspectives (conceptual models for nursing), any one of which provides a conceptual departure point for practice, research, and education. Nursing is prepared to justify the claims of those who already refer to nursing theory and nursing science (Figure 3.2). At the same time as it offers a distinct and explicit service to society, nursing is equipped to move forward to leadership in the health arena. Rather than explaining and excusing the confusion in terminology, educators face the challenge of helping students learn the intellectual excitement of a strong commitment to nursing.

REFERENCES

Adam, E. (1980). *To be a nurse*. Toronto: W.B. Saunders.

Bush, H.A. (1979). Models for nursing. *Advances in Nursing Science, 1*(2), 13-21.

Chin, R. (1976). The utility of system models and developmental models for practitioners. In W.G. Bennis, K.D. Benne, & R. Chin (Eds.), *The Planning of Change* (3rd ed., pp. 90-102). New York: Holt, Rinehart & Winston.

Cogan, M.L. (1953). Toward a definition of profession. *Harvard Educational Review, 23*:33-50.

Dickoff, J. & James, P. (1968). A theory of theories: A position paper. *Nursing Research, 17*(3), 197-203.

Dickoff, J., James, P., & Wiedenbach, E. (1968). Theory in a practice discipline, Part I. Practice oriented theory. *Nursing Research, 17*(5), 415-435.

Dickoff, J. & James P. (1970). Beliefs and values: Bases for curriculum design. *Nursing Research, 19*(5), 415-427.

Donaldson, S.K. & Crowley, D.M. (1978). The discipline of nursing. *Nursing Outlook, 26*(2), 113-120.

Fawcett, J. (1978a). The relationship between theory and research: A double Helix. *Advances in Nursing Science, 1*(1), 49-62.

———. (1978b). The "what" of theory development. In *Theory development: What, why, how?* (pp. 17-33). New York: National League for Nursing, No. 15-1708.

Flaskerud, J.H. & Halloran, E.J. (1980). Areas of agreement in nursing theory development. *Advances in Nursing Science, 3*(1), 1-7.

Greene, J.A. (1979). Science, nursing and nursing science: A conceptual analysis. *Advances in Nursing Science, 2*(1), 57-64.

Greenwood, E. (1961). The practice of science and the science of practice. In W.J. Bennis, K.D. Benne, & R. Chin (Eds.), *The planning of change* (pp. 73-82). New York: Holt, Rinehart & Winston.

Hardy, M.E. (1978a). Evaluating nursing theory. In *Theory development: what, why, how?* (pp. 75-86). New York: National League for Nursing, No. 15-1708.

———. (1978b). Perspectives on nursing theory. *Advances in Nursing Science, 1*(1), 37-48.

Hayakawa, S.I. (1963). *Language in thought and action* (2nd ed.). New York: Harcourt, Brace & World.

Johnson, D.E. (1974). Development of theory: A requisite for nursing as a primary health profession. *Nursing Research, 23*(5), 372-377.

———. (1978). State of the art of theory development in nursing. In *Theory development: what, why, how?* (pp. 1-10). New York: National League for Nursing. No. 15-1708.

Lancaster, W. & Lancaster, J. (1981). Models and model building in nursing. *Advances in Nursing Science, 3*(3), 31-42.

Lewis, E.P. (1974). Pretentious prose (editorial). *Nursing Outlook, 22*(7), 431.

Newman, M.A. (1979). *Theory development in nursing*. Philadelphia: F.A. Davis Co.

Notter, L.E. (1968). The theoretical framework: An essential characteristic of research (editorial). *Nursing Research, 17*(4), 291.

Orlando, I.J. (1961). *The dynamic nurse-patient relationship*. New York: Putnam's Sons.

Peterson, C.J. (1977). Questions frequently asked about the development of a conceptual framework. *Journal of Nursing Education, 16*(4), 22-32.

Reilly, D.E. (1975). Why a conceptual framework? *Nursing Outlook, 23*(8), 566-569.

Riehl, J.P. & Roy, C. (1980). *Conceptual models for nursing practice* (2nd ed.). New York: Appleton-Century-Crofts.

Roy, C. & Roberts, S. (1981). *Theory construction in nursing. An adaptation model*. Englewood Cliffs, NJ: Prentice-Hall.

Stevens, B.J. (1979). *Nursing theory. Analysis, application, evaluation.* Boston: Little, Brown & Co.

Vincent, P. (1975). Some crucial terms in nursing—a second opinion. *Nursing Outlook, 23*(1), 46-48.

Watson, J. (1979). *Nursing. The philosophy and science of caring.* Boston: Little, Brown & Co.

4

Fundamental Patterns of Knowing
in Nursing

BARBARA A. CARPER, RN, EdD

It is the general conception of any field of inquiry that ultimately determines the kind of knowledge the field aims to develop as well as the manner in which that knowledge is to be organized, tested, and applied. The body of knowledge that serves as the rationale for nursing practice has patterns, forms, and structure that serve as horizons of expectations and exemplify characteristic ways of thinking about phenomena. Understanding these patterns is essential for the teaching and learning of nursing. Such an understanding does not extend the range of knowledge, but rather involves critical attention to the question of what it means to know and what kinds of knowledge are held to be of most value in the discipline of nursing.

IDENTIFYING PATTERNS OF KNOWING

Four fundamental patterns of knowing have been identified from an analysis of the conceptual and syntactical structure of nursing knowledge.[1] The four patterns are distinguished according to logical type of meaning and designated as (1) empirics, the science of nursing; (2) esthetics, the art of nursing; (3) the component of a personal knowledge in nursing; and (4) ethics, the component of moral knowledge in nursing.

Empirics: The Science of Nursing

The term *nursing science* was rarely used in the literature until the late 1950s. However, since that time there has been an increasing emphasis, one might even say a sense of urgency, regarding the development of a body of empirical knowledge specific to nursing. There seems to be general agreement that there is a critical need for knowledge about the empirical world, knowledge that is systematically organized into general laws and theories for the purpose of describing, explaining, and predicting phenomena of special concern to the discipline of nursing. Most theory development and research efforts are primarily engaged in seeking and generating explanations which are systematic and controllable by factual evidence and which can be used in the organization and classification of knowledge.

The pattern of knowing which is generally designated as "nursing science" does not presently exhibit the same degree of highly integrated abstract and systematic explanations characteristic of the more mature sciences, although nursing literature reflects this as an ideal form. Clearly there are a number of co-existing, and in a few instances competing, conceptual structures—none of which has achieved the status of what Kuhn calls a scien-

Source: Carper, B. A. (1978). Fundamental patterns of knowing in nursing. *ANS, 1* (1): 13-24. Reprinted with permission from and copyright © 1978 Aspen Publishers, Inc.

tific paradigm. That is, no single conceptual structure is as yet generally accepted as an example of actual scientific practice "which include[s] law, theory, application, and instrumentation together . . . [and] . . . provide[s] models from which spring particular coherent traditions of scientific research."[2(p10)] It could be argued that some of these conceptual structures seem to have greater potential than others for providing explanations that systematically account for observed phenomena and may ultimately permit more accurate prediction and control of them. However, this is a matter to be determined by research designed to test the validity of such explanatory concepts in the context of relevant empirical reality.

New Perspectives

What seems to be of paramount importance, at least at this stage in the development of nursing science, is that these preparadigm conceptual structures and theoretical models present new perspectives for considering the familiar phenomena of health and illness in relation to the human life process; as such they can and should be legitimately counted as discoveries in the discipline. The representation of health as more than the absence of disease is a crucial change; it permits health to be thought of as a dynamic state or process which changes over a given period of time and varies according to circumstances rather than a static either/or entity. The conceptual change in turn makes it possible to raise questions that previously would have been literally unintelligible.

The discovery that one can usefully conceptualize health as something that normally ranges along a continuum has led to attempts to observe, describe, and classify variations in health, or levels of wellness, as expressions of a human being's relationship to the internal and external environments. Related research has sought to identify behavioral responses, both physiological and psychological, that may serve as cues by which one can infer the range of normal variations of health. It has also attempted to identify and categorize significant etiological factors which serve to promote or inhibit changes in health status.

Current Stages

The science of nursing at present exhibits aspects of both the "natural history stage of inquiry" and the "stage of deductively formulated theory." The task of the natural history stage is primarily the description and classification of phenomena which are, generally speaking, ascertainable by direct observation and inspection.[3] But current nursing literature clearly reflects a shift from this descriptive and classification form to increasingly theoretical analysis which is directed toward seeking, or inventing, explanations to account for observed and classified empirical facts. This shift is reflected in the change from a largely observational vocabulary to a new, more theoretical vocabulary whose terms have a distinct meaning and definition only in the context of the corresponding explanatory theory.

Explanations in the several open-system conceptual models tend to take the form commonly labeled *functional* or *teleological*.[4] For example, the system models explain a person's level of wellness at any particular point in time as a function of current and accumulated effects of interactions with his or her internal and external environments. The concept of adaptation is central to this type of explanation. Adaptation is seen as crucial in the process of responding to environmental demands (usually classified as stressors), and enables an individual to maintain or reestablish the steady state which is designated as the goal of the system. The developmental models often exhibit a more genetic type of explanation in that certain events, the developmental tasks, are believed to be causally relevant or necessary conditions for the normal development of an individual.

Thus the first fundamental pattern of knowing in nursing is empirical, factual, descriptive, and ultimately aimed at developing abstract and theoretical explanations. It is exemplary, discursively formulated, and publicly verifiable.

Esthetics: The Art of Nursing

Few, if indeed any, familiar with the professional literature would deny that primary emphasis is placed on the development of the science of nursing. One is almost led to believe that the only valid and reliable knowledge is that which is empirical, factual, objectively descriptive, and generalizable. There seems to be a self-conscious reluctance to extend the term *knowledge* to include those aspects of knowing in nursing that are not the result of empirical investigation. There is, nonetheless, what might be described as a tacit admission that nursing is, at least in part, an art. Not much effort is made to elaborate or to make explicit this esthetic pattern of knowing in nursing—other than to vaguely associate the "art" with the general category of manual and/or technical skills involved in nursing practice.

Perhaps this reluctance to acknowledge the esthetic component as a fundamental pattern of knowing in nursing originates in the vigorous efforts made in the not-so-distant past to exorcise the image of the apprentice-type educational system. Within the apprentice system, the art of nursing was closely associated with an imitative learning style and the acquisition of knowledge by accumulation of unrationalized experiences. Another likely source of reluctance is that the definition of the term *art* has been excessively and inappropriately restricted.

Weitz suggests that art is too complex and variable to be reduced to a single definition.[5] To conceive the task of esthetic theory as definition, he says, is logically doomed to failure in that what is called art has no common properties—only recognizable similarities. This fluid and open approach to the understanding and application of the concept of art and esthetic meaning makes possible a wider consideration of conditions, situations, and experiences in nursing that may properly be called esthetic, including the creative process of discovery in the empirical pattern of knowing.

Esthetics versus Scientific Meaning

Despite this open texture of the concept of art, esthetic meanings can be distinguished from those in science in several important aspects. The recognition "that art is expressive rather than merely formal or descriptive," according to Rader, "is about as well established as any fact in the whole field of esthetics."[6(pxvi)] An esthetic experience involves the creation and/or appreciation of a singular, particular, subjective expression of imagined possibilities or equivalent realities which "resists projection into the discursive form of language."[7] Knowledge gained by empirical description is discursively formulated and publicly verifiable. The knowledge gained by subjective acquaintance, the direct feeling of experience, defines discursive formulation. Although an esthetic expression required abstraction, it remains specific and unique rather than exemplary and leads us to acknowledge that "knowledge—genuine knowledge, understanding—is considerably wider than our discourse."[7(p23)]

For Wiedenbach, the art of nursing is made visible through the action taken to provide whatever the patient requires to restore or extend his [sic] ability to cope with the demands of his [sic] situation.[8] But the action taken, to have an esthetic quality, requires the active transformation of the immediate object—the patient's behavior—into a direct, nonmediated perception of what is significant in it—that is, what need is actually being expressed by the behavior. This perception of the need expressed is not only responsible for the action taken by the nurse but reflected in it.

The esthetic process described by Wiedenbach resembles what Dewey refers to as the difference between recognition and perception.[9] According to Dewey, recognition serves the purpose of identification and is satisfied when a name tag or label is attached according to some stereotype or previously formed scheme of classification. Perception, however, goes beyond recognition in that it includes an active gathering together of details and scattered particulars into an experienced whole for the purpose of seeing what is there. It is perception rather than mere recognition that results in a unity of ends and means which gives the action taken an esthetic quality.

Orem speaks of the art of nursing as being "expressed by the individual nurse through her creativity and style in designing and providing nursing that is effective and satisfying."[10(p155)] The art of nursing is creative in that it requires development of the ability to "envision valid modes of helping in relation to 'results' which are appropriate."[10(p69)] This again invokes Dewey's sense of a perceived unity between an action taken and its result—a perception of the means of the end as an organic whole.[9] The experience of helping must be perceived and designed as an integral component of its desired result rather than conceived separately as an independent action imposed on an independent subject. Perhaps this is what is meant by the concept of nursing the whole patient or total patient care. If so, what are the qualities that enable the creation of a design for nursing care that eliminate or would minimize the fragmentation of means and ends?

Esthetic Pattern of Knowing

Empathy—that is, the capacity for participating in or vicariously experiencing another's feelings—is an important mode in the esthetic pattern of knowing. One gains knowledge of another person's singular, particular, felt experience through empathic acquaintance.[11,12] Empathy is controlled or moderated by psychic distance or detachment in order to apprehend and abstract what we are attending to, and in this sense is objective. The more skilled the nurse becomes in perceiving and empathizing with the lives of others, the more knowledge or understanding will be gained of alternate modes of perceiving reality. The nurse will thereby have available a larger repertoire of choices in designing and providing nursing care that is effective and satisfying. At the same time, increased awareness of the variety of subjective experiences will heighten the complexity and difficulty of the decision making involved.

The design of nursing care must be accompanied by what Langer refers to as sense of form, the sense of "structure, articulation, a whole resulting from the relation of mutually dependent factors, or more precisely, the way the whole is put together."[7(p16)] The design, if it is to be esthetic, must be controlled by the perception of the balance, rhythm, proportion, and unity of what is done in relation to the dynamic integration and articulation of the whole. "The doing may be energetic, and the undergoing may be acute and intense," Dewey says, but "unless they are related to each other to form a whole," what is done becomes merely a matter of mechanical routine or of caprice.[9]

The esthetic pattern of knowing in nursing involves the perception of abstracted particulars as distinguished from the recognition of abstracted universals. It is the knowing of a unique particular rather than an exemplary class.

The Component of Personal Knowledge

Personal knowledge as a fundamental pattern of knowing in nursing is the most problematic, the most difficult to master and to teach. At the same time, it is perhaps the pattern most essential to understanding the meaning of health in terms of individual well-being. Nursing considered as an interpersonal process involves interactions, relationships, and transactions between the nurse and the patient-client. Mitchell points out that "there is growing evidence that the quality of interpersonal contacts has an influence on a person's becoming ill, coping with illness and becoming well."[13(p4950)] Certainly the phrase "therapeutic use of self" which has become increasingly prominent in the literature implies that the way in which nurses view their own selves and the client is of primary concern in any therapeutic relationship.

Personal knowledge is concerned with the knowing, encountering, and actualizing of the concrete, individual self. One does not know *about* the self; one strives simply to *know* the self. This knowing is a standing in relation to another human being and confronting that human being as a person. This "I-Thou" encounter is unmediated by conceptual categories or particulars abstracted from complex organic wholes.[14] The relation is one of reciprocity, a state of being that cannot be described or even experienced—it can only be actualized. Such personal knowing extends not only to other selves but also to relations with one's own self.

It requires what Buber refers to as the sacrifice of form, i.e., categories or classifications, for a knowing of infinite possibilities, as well as the risk of total commitment.

> Even as a melody is not composed of tones, nor a verse of words, nor a statue of lines—one must pull and tear to turn a unity into a multiplicity—so it is with the human being to whom I say You. . . . I have to do this again and again; but immediately he is no longer You.[14(p59)]

Maslow refers to this sacrifice of form as embodying a more efficient perception of

reality in that reality is not generalized nor predetermined by a complex of concepts, expectations, beliefs, and stereotypes.[15] This results in a greater willingness to accept ambiguity, vagueness, and discrepancy of oneself and others. The risk of commitment involved in personal knowledge is what Polanyi calls the "passionate participation in the act of knowing."[16(p17)]

The nurse in the therapeutic use of self rejects approaching the patient-client as an object and strives instead to actualize an authentic personal relationship between two persons. The individual is considered as an integrated, open system incorporating movement toward growth and fulfillment of human potential. An authentic personal relation requires the acceptance of others in their freedom to create themselves and the recognition that each person is not a fixed entity, but constantly engaged in the process of becoming. How then should the nurse reconcile this with the social and/or professional responsibility to control and manipulate the environmental variables and even the behavior of the person who is a patient in order to maintain or restore a steady state? If a human being is assumed to be free to choose and chooses behavior outside of accepted norms, how will this affect the action taken in the therapeutic use of self by the nurse? What choices must the nurse make in order to know another self in an authentic relation apart from the category of patient, even when categorizing for the purpose of treatment is essential to the process of nursing?

Assumptions regarding human nature, McKay observes, "range from the existentialist to the cybernetic, from the idea of an information processing machine to one of a many splendored being."[17(p399)] Many of these assumptions incorporate in one form or another the notion that there is, for all individuals, a characteristic state which they, by virtue of membership in the species, must strive to assume or achieve. Empirical descriptions and classifications reflect the assumption that being human allows for prediction of basic biological, psychological, and social behaviors that will be encountered in any given individual.

Certainly empirical knowledge is essential to the purposes of nursing. But nursing also requires that we be alert to the fact that models of human nature and their abstract and generalized categories refer to and describe behaviors and traits that groups have in common. However, none of these categories can ever encompass or express the uniqueness of the individual encountered as a person, as a "self." These and many other similar considerations are involved in the realm of personal knowledge, which can be broadly characterized as subjective, concrete, and existential. It is concerned with the kind of knowing that promotes wholeness and integrity in the personal encounter, the achievement of engagement rather than detachment; and it denies the manipulative, impersonal orientation.

Ethics: The Moral Component

Teachers and individual practitioners are becoming increasingly sensitive to the difficult personal choices that must be made within the complex context of modern health care. These choices raise fundamental questions about morally right and wrong action in connection with the care and treatment of illness and the promotion of health. Moral dilemmas arise in situations of ambiguity and uncertainty, when the consequences of one's actions are difficult to predict and traditional principles and ethical codes offer no help or seem to result in contradiction. The moral code which guides the ethical conduct of nurses is based on the primary principle of obligation embodied in the concepts of service to people and respect for human life. The discipline of nursing is held to be a valuable and essential social service responsible for conserving life, alleviating suffering, and promoting health. But appeal to the

ethical "rule book" fails to provide answers in terms of difficult individual moral choices, which must be made in the teaching and practice of nursing.

The fundamental pattern of knowing identified here as the ethical component of nursing is focused on matters of obligation or what ought to be done. Knowledge of morality goes beyond simply knowing the norms or ethical codes of the discipline. It includes all voluntary actions that are deliberate and subject to the judgment of right and wrong—including judgments of moral value in relation to motives, intentions, and traits of character. Nursing is deliberate action, or a series of actions, planned and implemented to accomplish defined goals. Both goals and actions involve choices made, in part, on the basis of normative judgments, both particular and general. On occasion, the principles and norms by which such choices are made may be in conflict.

According to Berthold, "goals are, of course, value judgments not amenable to scientific inquiry and validation."[18(p196)] Dickoff, James, and Wiedenbach also call attention to the need to be aware that the specification of goals serves as "a norm or standard by which to evaluate activity . . . [and] . . . entails taking them as values—that is, signifies conceiving these goal contents as situations worthy to be brought about."[19(p422)]

For example, a common goal of nursing care in relation to the maintenance or restoration of health is to assist patients to achieve a state in which they are independent. Much of the current practice reflects an attitude of value attached to the goal of independence, and indicates nursing actions to assist patients in assuming full responsibility for themselves at the earliest possible moment or to enable them to retain responsibility to the last possible moment. However, valuing independence and attempting to maintain it may be at the expense of the patient's learning how to live with physical or social dependence when necessary—for example, in instances when prognosis indicates that independence cannot be regained.

Differences in normative judgments may have more to do with disagreements as to what constitutes a "healthy" state of being than lack of empirical evidence or ambiguity in the application of the term. Slote suggests that the persistence of disputes, or lack of uniformity in the application of cluster terms, such as *health*, is due to "the difficulty of decisively resolving certain sorts of value questions about what is and is not important." This leads him to conclude "that value judgment is far more involved in the making of what are commonly thought to be factual statements than has been imagined."[20(p220)]

The ethical pattern of knowing in nursing requires an understanding of different philosophical positions regarding what is good, what ought to be desired, what is right; of different ethical frameworks devised for dealing with the complexities of moral judgments; and of various orientations to the notion of obligation. Moral choices to be made must then be considered in terms of specific actions to be taken in specific, concrete situations. The examination of the standards, codes, and values by which we decide what is morally right should result in a greater awareness of what is involved in making moral choices and being responsible for the choices made. The knowledge of ethical codes will not provide answers to the moral questions involved in nursing, nor will it eliminate the necessity for having to make moral choices. But it can be hoped that:

> The more sensitive teachers and practitioners are to the demands of the process of justification, the more explicit they are about the norms that govern their actions, the more personally engaged they are in assessing surrounding circumstances and potential consequences, the

more "ethical" they will be; and we cannot ask much more.[21(p221)]

USING PATTERNS OF KNOWING

A philosophical discussion of patterns of knowing may appear to some as a somewhat idle, if not arbitrary and artificial, undertaking having little or no connection with the practical concerns and difficulties encountered in the day-to-day doing and teaching of nursing. But it represents a personal conviction that there is a need to examine the kinds of knowing that provide the discipline with its particular perspectives and significance. Understanding four fundamental patterns of knowing makes possible an increased awareness of the complexity and diversity of nursing knowledge.

Each pattern may be conceived as necessary for achieving mastery in the discipline, but none of them alone should be considered sufficient. Neither are they mutually exclusive. The teaching and learning of one pattern do not require the rejection or neglect of any of the others. Caring for another requires the achievements of nursing science, that is, the knowledge of empirical facts systematically organized into theoretical explanations regarding the phenomena of health and illness. But creative imagination also plays its part in the syntax of discovery in science, as well as in developing the ability to imagine the consequences of alternative moral choices.

Personal knowledge is essential for ethical choices in that moral action presupposes personal maturity and freedom. If the goals of nursing are to be more than conformance to unexamined norms, if the "ought" is not to be determined simply on the basis of what is possible, then the obligation to care for another human being involves becoming a certain kind of person—and not merely doing certain kinds of things. If the design of nursing care is to be more than habitual or mechanical, the capacity to perceive and interpret the subjective experiences of others and to imaginatively project the effects of nursing actions on their lives becomes a necessary skill.

Nursing thus depends on the scientific knowledge of human behavior in health and in illness, the esthetic perception of significant human experiences, a personal understanding of the unique individuality of the self, and the capacity to make choices within concrete situations involving particular moral judgments. Each of these separate but interrelated and interdependent fundamental patterns of knowing should be taught and understood according to its distinctive logic, the restricted circumstances in which it is valid, the kinds of data it subsumes, and the methods by which each particular kind of truth is distinguished and warranted.

The major significances to the discipline of nursing in distinguishing patterns of knowing are summarized as (1) the conclusions of the discipline conceived as subject matter cannot be taught or learned without reference to the structure of the discipline—the representative concepts and methods of inquiry that determine the kind of knowledge gained and limit its meaning, scope, and validity; (2) each of the fundamental patterns of knowing represents a necessary but not complete approach to the problems and questions in the discipline; and (3) all knowledge is subject to change and revision. Every solution of an existing problem raises new and unsolved questions. These new and as yet unsolved problems require, at times, new methods of inquiry and different conceptual structures; they change the shape and patterns of knowing. With each change in the shape of knowledge, teaching and learning require looking for different points of contact and connection among ideas and things. This clarifies the effect of each new thing known

on other things known and the discovery of new patterns by which each connection modifies the whole.

REFERENCES

1. Carper, B. A. "Fundamental Patterns of Knowing in Nursing." PhD dissertation, Teachers College, Columbia University, 1975.
2. Kuhn, T. *The Structure of Scientific Revolutions* (Chicago: University of Chicago Press 1962).
3. Northrop, F. S. C. *The Logic of the Sciences and the Humanities* (New York: The World Publishing Co. 1959).
4. Nagel, E. *The Structure of Science* (New York: Harcourt, Brace and World, Inc. 1961).
5. Weitz, M. "The Role of Theory in Aesthetics" in Rader, M., ed. *A Modern Book of Esthetics* 3rd ed. (New York: Holt, Rinehart and Winston 1960).
6. Rader, M. "Introduction: The Meaning of Art" in Rader, M., ed. *A Modern Book of Esthetics* 3rd ed. (New York: Holt, Rinehart and Winston 1960).
7. Langer, S. K. *Problems of Art* (New York: Charles Scribner and Sons 1957).
8. Wiedenbach, E. *Clinical Nursing: A Helping Art* (New York: Springer Publishing Co., Inc. 1964).
9. Dewey, J. *Art as Experience* (New York: Capricorn Books 1958).
10. Orem, D. E. *Nursing: Concepts of Practice* (New York: McGraw-Hill Book Co. 1971).
11. Lee, V. "Empathy" in Rader, M., ed. *A Modern Book of Esthetics*, 3rd ed. (New York: Holt, Rinehart and Winston 1960).
12. Lippo. T. "Empathy, Inner Imitation and Sense-Feeling" in Rader, M., ed. *A Modern Book of Esthetics* 3rd ed. (New York: Holt, Rinehart and Winston 1960.)
13. Mitchell, P. H. *Concepts Basic to Nursing* (New York: McGraw-Hill Book Co. 1973).
14. Buber, M. *I and Thou*. Translated by Walter Kaufman (New York: Charles Scribner and Sons 1970).
15. Maslow, A. H. "Self-Actualizing People: A Study of Psychological Health" in Moustakas, C. E., ed. *The Self* (New York: Harper and Row 1956).
16. Polanyi, M. *Personal Knowledge* (New York: Harper and Row 1964).

17. McKay, R. "Theories, Models and Systems for Nursing." *Nurs Res* 18:5 (September-October 1969).
18. Berthold, J. S. "Symposium on Theory Development in Nursing: Prologue." *Nurs Res* 17:3 (May-June 1968).
19. Dickoff, J., James P., and Wiedenbach, E. "Theory in a Practice Discipline: Part I." *Nurs Res* 17 (September-October 1968).
20. Slote, M. A. "The Theory of Important Criteria." *J Philosophy* 63 (April 14 1966).
21. Greene, M. *Teacher as Stronger* (Belmont, Calif.: Wadsworth Publishing Co., Inc. 1973).

5

Aspects of "Reality" and Ways of Knowing in Nursing: In Search of an Integrating Paradigm

JOHN WOLFER, RN, PhD

Types of knowledge, theory and research needed in a practice-oriented discipline are considered in relation to different "aspects of reality." Major changes in nursing epistemology are reviewed to show an expanding model of inquiry. It is argued that a paradigm which recognizes a spectrum of reality from "body" through "mind" to "spirit" provides a philosophical basis for understanding the necessity of multiple modes of inquiry and multiple types of knowledge and theory. From this perspective, fundamentally different modes of inquiry are seen as complementary rather than competitive or inherently superior or inferior. [Keywords: epistemology, theory construction]

One way to approach the question of what types of knowledge, theory and research a practice-oriented discipline such as nursing needs is to ask with what "aspects" of "reality" is the discipline concerned? "Reality" here refers to what people experience and more or less share as "real," that is, consensual reality. A familiar way of conceptualizing reality or existence in Western culture has been to identify three fundamental aspects: body, mind and spirit. Body refers to the material world. Mind refers to the "mental" world and spirit refers to the "transcendental" world. The material refers to all we know about the physical world as experienced through the senses and organized by rational thought. The mental refers to all we know about the "human world" primarily through conceptual/symbolic processes. The transcendental refers to all we directly experience of the world through contemplative modes. Metaphorically speaking, the way we know and experience these aspects of reality is through the "eye of flesh" (sensory based), the "eye of mind" (cognitively based) and the "eye of contemplation" (non-cognitively mediated direct experience) (Wilber, 1990).

A central point of this paper is that the distinction between aspects of reality which require fundamentally different ways of knowing to access and understand phenomena within the domains has not been recognized or made explicit in the nursing literature. The arguments for the need for, or the superiority of, some methodologies over others (usually cast as quantitative vs. qualitative approaches) have essentially boiled down to a recognition that basically different types of "problems" require different methods (the "problem-method fit" issue). Recog-

Source: Wolfer, J. (1993) Aspects of "Reality" and Ways of Knowing in Nursing: In Search of an Integrating Paradigm. IMAGE: *Journal of Nursing Scholarship* 25 (2):141–146. Reprinted with permission from Sigma Theta Tau International.

nition that fundamentally different types of problems require very different types of methods has been necessary and extremely helpful in our evolving understanding of the nature and process of knowledge development especially in liberating us from the early constraint of trying to force all problems into a positivistic straight-jacket. The claim here is that the recognition of the necessity of a proper problem-method fit can be strengthened by also recognizing the ontological differences underlying basically different types of problems (e.g., "body" problems vs. "mind" problems) which lead to different epistemologies and hence general methodologies and specific methods.

The intent of this paper is to review the ontological and epistemological arguments for an "aspects of reality" approach in the nursing literature for critical discussion, not as a competing or merely semantic alternative to the problem-method-fit approach, but as an additional way of understanding why we need multiple ways of knowing and multiple types of knowledge. This additional way of understanding has emerged as an explicit and formally developed philosophical perspective in the relatively new field of transpersonal psychology as represented in the work of one of its leading theorists, Ken Wilber (1977, 1984). Wilber has synthesized a vast amount of knowledge from both Eastern and Western traditions along with the work of many recent scholars in philosophy and the social and behavioral sciences. The present paper is based primarily on the paradigm developed in *Eye to Eye*, (Wilber, 1990).

If we can tentatively accept an "aspects of reality" paradigm as a "map" for representing part of the broad spectrum of human experience that nurses work with at one time or another, then we can examine the relationship between this paradigm and the major forms of knowledge, theory and research ("ways of knowing") identified in nursing literature.

Table 5-1 presents the paradigm. The main focus of this paper will be on the first two aspects, body and mind. That is not to imply the spiritual aspect is not relevant and important, even central from some perspectives (e.g., Watson, 1975).

SCIENCE OF BODY AND MIND

The primary academic model for knowledge generation in nursing has been the familiar analytic/empirical model of the traditional "hard" or "basic" sciences that provides knowledge of physical reality. Empirical data are obtained through the senses (the "eye of the flesh") and organized through rational thinking into theories about structures, processes, mechanisms and relationships that lead to causal explanations about "natural" phenomena. The investigator's primary purpose is to produce accurate descriptions, explanations and predictions in the interest of understanding for its own sake (satisfaction of curiosity, so-called "pure" science) and/or for a "technical" interest (Allen, 1985) in controlling the physical world. The theories can be characterized as relatively objective, deterministic, reductionistic, mechanistic, universal, quantitative and relatively "value-free." They are free in this context because scientific theories survive in the long run primarily on the basis of how well they work in solving scientific problems and not primarily on the basis of the investigator's personal moral/ethical values. (The choice of problem, the allocation of scarce resources for certain research, the social problems created by science and the applications of knowledge are not, of course, value-free. The "value problem" in science is also beyond the scope of this paper.) The "truth value" of any theory is determined through the "canons of science" which incorporate the methodological

TABLE 5.1. A Spectrum of Reality and Modes of Inquiry

	Aspects of Reality		
	Body--------------------	**Mind**--------------------	**Spirit**
Type of Phenomena	material/physical	mental/symbolic	transcendental transcognitive
Type of Data	sensory-based	language-based	trans-data
Type of Knowledge	theories about structures functions relationships cause/effect	theories of processes relationships experience meaning	direct, non-cognitive experience
Knowledge Characteristics	objective deterministic reductionistic mechanistic universal quantitative less value oriented	interpretive indeterminate holistic dynamic/organic historical/contextual qualitative value-oriented	non-cognitive, immediate experience
Interest/Purpose	technical description explanation prediction control/ application	understanding description explanation empowerment emancipation justice	salvation/ enlighten-ment peace
Validation/Credibility	precision prediction replication serve purpose	relevance persuasive expert consensus serve purpose	experiential confirmation
Types of Discource	linear-discursive rational-analytic mathematical	linear-discursive rational-analytic narrative	paradoxical negation mythical
Methods/Ways of Knowing	observation classification measurement experiment quantitative-analysis	observation phenomenology ethnography grounded theory critical/feminist inquiry philosophical inquiry hermeneutical analysis	contemplate prayer/ mediation
Examples	physiological-nursing physics biology behavioral-psychology astronomy etc.	transcultural-nursing transpersonal-psychology sociology history philosophy etc.	spiritually supportive care

principles and specific methods and objective observation/description, accurate measurement, quantification of variables whenever possible, mathematical and statistical analysis, experimental methods and verification through replication. Validation/verification of theoretical propositions comes through precision of observation and measurement, successful prediction, replication, and in the final analysis, the theory works to solve the problems scientists are interested in (Lauden, 1977). That is, the theory serves its intended purpose. The main types of discourse in this area are linear-discursive, rational-analytic and mathematical.

For the material world, this model or paradigm has worked well. In accordance with the nature of physical reality, the world view and methods of the traditional physical sciences have served their intended purposes in extraordinary ways. In spite of the inhumane uses of scientific methods and knowledge at times, the physical sciences have been fantastically successful in describing, explaining, predicting and controlling many facets of biophysical reality. This obvious point is often overlooked in most of the recent criticisms of traditional scientific methodology. Characteristics of scientific theory about the physical world, such as reductionism, universality and quantification are positive attributes that are crucial for the intended purposes of the physical sciences (causal explanation, prediction and control). Reducing certain physical wholes to their parts (e.g., in molecular biology) in order to describe and understand how the parts determine, at least to a large extent, what is going on with the whole, has resulted in accurate prediction and control in the biophysical world. Reductionism works for much of physical reality even though complex wholes such as human bodies cannot be totally explained and controlled by knowing and manipulating the physical parts only. Nursing investigations related primarily to as-

pects of physical care fall into this part of the spectrum. Other obvious examples of "basic" sciences are listed in Table 5-1.

Jumping across the continuum to a clearly different aspect level of reality is the domain or realm of "mind." Everything individual and collective minds do and produce as part of human experience falls within this area of the continuum. Roughly speaking, we are moving from the physical sciences to the "interpretative sciences" (Allen, 1985) and "human sciences" (Watson, 1985). The phenomena are "mental" and symbolic, not merely material or physical. Something new has been added that is distinctly human, namely the creation of intersubjective "meaning." To describe, understand and participate in this realm of meaning, one must engage the phenomena with some form of language. Hence the "data" are language-based where language is used in a very broad way to include not only rational, linear, discursive language, but also nondiscursive, metaphoric language as well as non-verbal forms of communicating meaning. In other words, this is primarily the domain of the "qualitative." The primary modes of knowing here are experiential in addition to "empirical" in the more limited physical sense, participatory, intersubjective, rational, analytic and for certain phenomena, intuitive-empathic. These modes of knowing result in understanding the meaning and intent of individual and collective human experience. Systematic knowledge here takes the form of descriptive theories regarding structures, processes, relationships, and traditions that underlie psychological, social, and cultural aspects of reality. In order to make sense, that is, derive meaning and understanding of individual and collective human experience, the raw data must be *interpreted* within the appropriate context (Allen, 1985; Allen, Benner, & Diekelmann, 1986; Lincoln & Guba, 1985). Interpretation leads to generalization in the form of theories that describe and elucidate structures, processes, and relationships within a limited historical and social-cultural context. Hence the theories can be characterized as interpretive, indeterminate, holistic, dynamic/organic, historical/contextual, qualitative, and for some types of inquiry toward the right side of this part of the spectrum such as feminist and critical theory, strongly value-oriented. The theories are value-oriented in the sense that humanistic values are often central at this level of investigation. Typically but not exclusively, the primary purpose of the investigator is producing descriptions and interpretations that, in addition to satisfying curiosity, result in understanding the nature of human experience in the interest of freeing people from unnecessary suffering, ignorance, constraint and oppression. Procedures for strengthening the "trustworthiness" and "credibility" of the more empirical types of research in this domain have been worked out and articulated (Lincoln & Guba, 1985). For the less strictly "empirical" forms of inquiry such as critical theory, consensual agreement among qualified investigators over time plays a very important role for establishing "truth" where truth is taken as "useful" for understanding certain human phenomena in such a way as to lead to the possibility of liberation, empowerment and justice. In other words, in addition to whether the theory serves its knowledge development purpose, there may be an additional criterion regarding the degree to which the theoretical understanding is embodied in practice and leads to relief from suffering, ignorance, constraint and oppression.

Nursing literature regarding the evolving self-understanding of theory and knowledge development in the discipline shows a shift from thinking about theory primarily in terms of traditional "hard" scientific theory with a positivistic bias (Jacox, 1974; Fawcett, 1978) to the recognition of the legitimacy and neces-

sity of "soft" or "interpretative," or "phenomenological" or "human" sciences (Allen 1985; Allen et al. 1986; Silva & Rothbart, 1984). This distinction has often been oversimplified as "quantitative vs. qualitative" research. Much necessary effort has been expended to justify theory based on a post-positivistic model of theory and research which a practice profession especially needs. As a result, the methods and principles of "qualitative research" have been clarified and well articulated (Lincoln & Guba, 1986; Sandelowski, 1986). In effect, the definition or model of what is considered legitimate science has been expanded from a narrow, essentially positivistic one, more appropriate for the physical and behavioristic sciences, to a much broader and more appropriate one for many aspects of the reality in nursing.

VALUE THEORY

While the model of science has been expanding, there also has been an increasing recognition of the need for some other forms of theory and knowledge which are not "scientific" in either the strict, traditional sense or the liberal, expanded sense of the human sciences. One of the first milestones of this trend was the work of Dickoff, James, and Wiedenbach (1968) which developed the understanding that a practice profession such as nursing needs something more than, and different from, "mere" scientific theory, namely, "practice" or "prescriptive" theory. The significant addition here was the explicit recognition that scientific theory from any level of investigation must be organized at a "higher" level of theory which is grounded in practice and incorporates *goals* based on *values*. Most of nursing practice is directed towards the achievement of outcomes that are held to be desirable and valuable. The choice of, and prioritization of goals in a clinical setting is not itself a "scientific" activity or product of scientific research in the usual sense and is based (often implicitly) on beliefs and feelings about what is valuable and right for people needing nursing care.

Although Dickoff et al. (1968) did not emphasize or expand the need for, and nature of, normative/ethical theory, this type of theory would seem to be an inherent and necessary part of theory at the prescriptive level. By implication then, the systematic explication and clarification of the values and ethics underlying nursing care goals, and how they lead to what are primarily nursing goals, should be an integral part of nursing practice theory. Therefore, practice theory requires the development and articulation of relevant normative and ethical theory. Systematic theory which articulates the normative/ethical rationale for goals and priorities in practice is not based on empirical fact *per se* and does not involve the empirical methods of either quantitative or qualitative research. Depending on one's definition of "science," such theory, although the work of the trained and qualified "mind's eye," is not the direct product of scientific research in either the traditional or expanded sense. Methods of inquiry for the development of value theory as an intrinsic part of practice theory are referred to as philosophical, intellectual, or scholarly research (Donaldson & Crowley, 1978; Ellis, 1984). Risking social stigma for advocating what some might call "non-scientific" research and theory development in an age of scientism, the new paradigm in concert with the "realities" of nursing as a practice and professional discipline calls for and justifies it. Within this paradigm human values are seen as real and as important as empirical aspects of reality. Accordingly, a practice discipline needs "researchers" articulating normative and ethical theory in nursing through the appropriate "methods" of scholarly, philosophical and hermeneutical inquiry. The new paradigm

recognizes and makes legitimate these modes of inquiry as absolutely essential for developing knowledge regarding these aspects of human reality. It should not be necessary to call this type of systematic inquiry "science" (Watson, 1985) in order to justify it.

Another landmark in the nursing literature which added something significantly new to our understanding of the types of knowledge and theory needed in a practice oriented discipline was Carper's (1978) paper on "patterns of knowledge." Although other authors in nursing have recognized the need for theory and knowledge which is not strictly scientific according to either positivistic or postpositivistic definitions (Donaldson & Crowley, 1978; Ellis, 1984; Schultz & Meleis, 1988), Carper's epistemological study of nursing knowledge as an example of philosophical inquiry, identified three patterns of nursing knowledge in addition to empirical knowledge. Ethical, esthetic and "personal" knowledge were seen as part of, and required in, nursing's "body of knowledge" or theoretical base. By implication this requires "investigators" reporting the "results" of their "research" where the "methods" and principles of "intellectual inquiry" involve the "mind's eye" at the mental/symbolic level of human experience and understanding.

Failure to clearly distinguish the fundamental difference between phenomena at the physical level and phenomena at the mental/symbolic level runs to the core of the limited view of reality expressed in a positivistic model of analytic/empiric science. The early positivistic model held, in effect, that any proposition about reality which could not be expressed in strictly empirical terms was either meaningless or unimportant. When the goal is to explain physical reality, this position might not be so absurd. But as it happened, the positivistic view was overgeneralized in such a way as to claim, in effect, that there was no other reality, at least one that could be known "scientifically." What was in the beginning a narrow and inaccurate philosophy of science (Webster & Jacox, 1981) became a cultural bias now known as "scientism." The fallacy of scientism went from saying, "That which cannot be seen by the eye of flesh cannot be empirically verified" to "That which cannot be seen by the eye of flesh does not exist." It went from saying, "There is an excellent method for gaining knowledge in the realm of the five senses" to "Thus the knowledge gained by mind and contemplation is invalid" (Wilber, 1990, p. 23). Scientism is the world view that holds only the physical is real and the "true" business of science is to learn about this reality through the strict methods of traditional science. In other words, scientism became an ideology with a very limited view of reality and how it is known. But when we turn to the mental/symbolic realm of human discourse, the epistemology and methods of the physical sciences are inappropriate. No amount of scientific rigor and quantification can discover the meaning, intention and value of human interaction at the symbolic level. ". . . values, life meanings, purposes and qualities slip through physical science like sea slips through the nets of fishermen" (Smith, 1976, p. 16).

To assume that the symbolic world can be known through the methods of physical science is to commit a "category error." A category error is made when the modes of knowing in one domain (e.g., the physical with the eye of the flesh) are used in an attempt to "see" in a different domain (symbolic) which requires different modes of knowing (the eye of the mind) or vice versa (attempting to know the physical realm through rational thought without an empirical data base). To hold that nursing research should only use the eye of the flesh (so called quantitative research) or only the eye of the mind (so called qualitative research) is a form of category error in that either position categorically negates the reality and importance of the other. Much of the recent criticism of the epis-

temology and methodology of traditional hard science concerns their inappropriate application to mental/symbolic phenomena of the social sciences which it can not access. This criticism usually does not make the ontological distinction between physical and mental/symbolic aspects of reality. Consequently, it fails to acknowledge the necessity and effectiveness of the physical sciences for solving problems in their proper domain.

A NEW PARADIGM

In order to avoid category errors in any direction and at any level, the new paradigm holds that there are three fundamental components or strands of valid knowledge attainment for all three aspects of reality (Wilber, 1990).

(1) The "instrumental" strand is a set of instructions which tell the "investigator" what must be done in order to know something at any level. These are the specific methods and general principles of inquiry for physical science, interpretative/phenomenological science, all types of intellectual/philosophical inquiry, and contemplative/spiritual experience. One must know and follow the methods correctly (i.e., be properly "trained" and "disciplined") in a domain in order to arrive at the "truth" in that domain. No proper training and discipline, no valid knowing.

(2) The "illuminative" strand refers to what is experientially known when one has followed the methods and principles correctly. Examples would be confirmation of an hypothesis from a replicated experiment on pain reduction in patients with AIDS, a shared understanding of what it "means" and "feels like" subjectively phenomenologically for people who are dying of AIDS, the clarification of patient care goals for patients with AIDS reached by logically, dialogically and empathetically working through relevant normative and ethical understandings, or the direct, non-cogni-

tively mediated experience of a spiritual "truth" after following the "methods" of a given spiritual tradition.

(3) The "communal" strand is the confirmation of (or lack of) what is known by checking it out with others who have adequately completed the injunctive and illuminative strands in a given domain. This is the "public" confirmation of a "truth" through the community of "experts" who arrive at consensual agreement through systematic and shared experience within a domain. The specific methods of confirmation/validation differ across the domains, but the principle of systematic consensual confirmation holds. The major category error of our time has been for the strict empiricists to claim that only their methods of consensual validation were valid. The consensual agreements reached by experts over time after systematic study about truths at the mental/symbolic level in the interpretative sciences and scholarly disciplines, or at the transcendental level in the spiritual/contemplative traditions, were meaningless and invalid from that restricted world view. The scholastics and churchmen of the early 1600s refused to look through Galileo's telescope on the grounds that pure rational thought had already arrived at the "truth" about the earth and celestial bodies (Wilber, 1990).

Recognition that there are different but systematic and legitimate ways of knowing (methods and principles) for different aspects of reality which lead to publicly validated theories or knowledge or direct experience of the phenomena in a given realm is consistent with the full spectrum of human experience. This full spectrum, including the transcendental or spiritual is what nursing practice engages (or desires to engage) in the course of providing "holistic" care. Presently, this "new" paradigm, as an epistemological map of the types of possible knowledge and the multiple ways of producing or engaging that knowledge, is rough and incomplete. Many types of research and

theory do not fall neatly into any one of the three aspects and there are many intriguing questions in the intersections and across areas of the spectrum. For example mind-body interaction research obviously spans the physical and mental and critical social and feminist inquiry or "critical scholarship" in nursing (Thompson, 1987) will at times span large areas of the spectrum from the physical to the spiritual. The real territories are multidimensional continua which can be mapped many different ways for many different purposes. The different maps are tools for achieving different ends. No single map depicts the one and absolute "truth" about the territory. For our purposes we seek maps that will enable us to develop and use theory and knowledge that is appropriate and useful for understanding the full multidimensional continuum of nursing practice, education and research.

This map enables us to see that different research methodologies must be different to address the fundamental differences in the nature of the phenomena being investigated. To say different investigators use different methods simply because they address different problems and questions is only partially correct. They *must* use different methods because fundamentally different phenomena (aspects of reality) *require it.* Methods strictly from the eye of flesh will not permit "seeing" the *meaning* of dying from AIDS or what the ethical and empathetical rationale is for changing care priorities. These aims require methods from the eye of the mind (and heart). Methods from the eye of the mind will not "see" whether one physical care procedure is more effective than another which requires methods from the eye of the flesh. Minds eye methods will not give the bedside nurse the transcendental "knowledge" to "be there" for the patient in a "spiritual" way. All of these modes of knowing will be needed to improve the quality of caring for the whole patient (and the whole nurse). In other words, this map offers a way of looking at the reality of nursing which "sees" different types of knowledge, theory and research as complementary rather than competitive or exclusionary. To nurse the whole patient (or educate the whole student) we must have knowledge about the whole spectrum of the patient's (and student's) reality in the nursing care (education) situation. From this perspective so called qualitative compared to quantitative approaches do not have to be seen in opposition (Munhall, 1982) or seen as one inherently better than the other (Moccia, 1988; Tinkle & Beaton, 1983) without taking into account the fundamental differences in the nature of the phenomena or part of the spectrum under investigation. To advocate the exclusive or primary justification for one set of approaches over another is a form of category error which negates one aspect or the other of the full spectrum of the nurse's and patient's body-mind-spirit reality. This is not to say that in a given clinical area at a given time there may be normative and ethical arguments for doing one kind of research rather than another because of scarce resources and compelling human needs. That is a value decision, not strictly an ontological or epistemological one. When the motivating interest of nursing inquiry is to help make things "better" for patients and clients (or staff or students), this interest can lead to any type of research at any level of investigation for any aspect of reality. Although the interpretative sciences in general, and critical and feminist theory in particular, begin with an explicit interest in making things better for people (e.g., freedom from ignorance and oppression), this does not mean that a nurse researcher cannot use the methods of biological science to find more effective nursing techniques for reducing pain in the interest of "making things better," humanly speaking.

REFERENCES

Allen, D. (1985). Nursing research and social control: Alternative models of science that emphasize understanding and emancipation. *Image, 17,* 58–64.

Allen, D., Benner P. & Dielkelmann, N.L. (1986). Three paradigms for nursing research: Methodological implications. In P.L. Chinn (Ed.), *Nursing research methodology: Issue and implementation,* (23–37). Rockford, MD: Aspen.

Carper, B. (1978). Fundamental patterns of knowing in nursing. *Advances in Nursing Science, 1,* 13–23.

Dickoff, J., James, P. & Wiedenbach, E. (1968). Theory in a practice discipline: Part 1. *Nursing Research, 17,* 415–435.

Donaldson, S.K. & Crowley, D.M. (1978). The discipline of nursing. *Nursing Outlook, 26,* 113–120.

Ellis, R. (June, 1984). Nursing knowledge development. Paper presented at the National Forum on Doctoral Education in Nursing. Denver, CO.

Fawcett, J. (1978). The relationship between theory and research: A double helix. *Advances in Nursing Science, 1,* 49–62.

Jacox, A. (1974). Theory construction in nursing. *Nursing Research, 23,* 4–13.

Laudan, L. (1977). *Progress and its problems: Towards a theory of scientific growth.* Berkeley: University of California Press.

Lincoln, Y.S. & Guba, E.G. (1985). *Naturalistic inquiry.* Beverly Hills: Sage Publications.

Moccia, P. (1988). A critique of compromise: Beyond the methods debate. *Advances in Nursing Science, 10,* 1–9.

Munhall, P.L. (1982). Nursing philosophy and nursing research: In apposition or opposition? *Nursing Research, 31,* 176–181.

Sandelowski, M. (1986). The problem of rigor in qualitative research. *Advances in Nursing Science, 8,* 27–37.

Schultz, P.R. & Meleis, A.I. (1988). Nursing epistemology: Traditions, insights, questions. *Image, 20,* 217–221.

Silva, M.C. & Rothbart, D. (1983). An analysis of changing trends in philosophies of science on nursing theory development and testing. *Advances in Nursing Science, 1,* 1–13.

Smith, H. (1976). *Forgotten truth.* New York: Harper & Row.

Thompson, J. (1987). Critical scholarship: The critique of domination in nursing. *Advances in Nursing Science, 10,* 17–37.

Tinkle, M.B. & Beaton, J.L. (1983). Toward a new view of science: Implications for nursing research. *Advances in Nursing Science, 5,* 27–36.

Watson, J. (1985). *Nursing: Human science and*

human care. Norwalk, CT: Appleton-Century-Crofts.

Webster, G. & Jacox, A. (1981). Nursing theory and the ghost of the received view. In J.C. McCloskey & H.K. Grace (Eds.) *Current issues in nursing* (26–35). Boston: Blackwell Scientific Publications.

Wilber, K. (1977). *The spectrum of consciousness*. Wheaton, IL: Theosophical Publishing House.

Wilber, K. (1984). *Quantum questions*. Boston: Shambhala.

Wilber, K. (1990). *Eye to eye: The quest for the new paradigm*. Boston: Shambhala.

Part II

HISTORY AND EVOLUTION OF NURSING SCIENCE

Historically, nursing practice was learned during a hospital apprenticeship by performing technical skills. Gradually nursing education moved from hospital programs to academic institutions, and students were taught the medical model, which separates the mind and body, and focuses on treatment of physical problems. In their search for professional recognition, nurses adopted the nursing process to identify client problems, and began conducting empirical research to establish a scientific base for practice. Some nurses sought graduate degrees in other disciplines, and several scholars developed conceptual models to represent their views of nursing. The evolution of nursing science has been influenced by many factors, including graduate nurses' education in other disciplines, belief in the supremacy of empiricism to illuminate the 'truth,' dogmatic beliefs that nursing theories and models must be rigorously 'tested' before they are applied in practice, the gap between application of research findings to nursing practice, and the lack of support for new research methodologies, among other things.

The six chapters in this part explore different authors' views of factors that have and continue to influence the development of nursing science. Judith Wuest compares the historical development of the nursing discipline with changes in the women's movement and feminist perspectives. She believes, as do many others, that nurse scholars were overly influenced by masculine beliefs as they strived for professional recognition. This chapter provides an excellent history lesson, along with recognition of how society's values have shaped nursing's evolution.

In an effort to reduce nurses' reliance on empirical research, Peggy Chinn's chapter, "Debunking Myths in Nursing Theory and Research," explores seven myths about the superiority of empirically based knowledge, and logically explains the fallacies of these myths. She describes how myths that empirical science represents the ultimate "truth" are unfounded since the findings are based on assumptions that the research is unbiased, objective, and value-free. In her analysis of these myths, Chinn identifies the limitations of male-dominated traditional science, levels the playing field for recognizing that all four patterns of knowing are relevant in nursing, and opens the door for nurses to design new research methods to explore other "patterns of knowing" relevant to nursing.

As several nurse theorists developed more esoteric philosophical views and theories of humanistic nursing science, they shifted from emphasizing empirical research to qualitative methodologies. Some scholars expressed concern about the value of these "less credible" methods for developing nursing's knowledge base. In their chapter, "(Mis)Conceptions and Reconceptions about Traditional Science," Karen Schumaker and Susan Gortner discuss different world views of science, and compare the philosophical bases of nursing in traditional science with a contemporary, postpositivistic philosophy of science. They analyze three relevant misconceptions in the nursing literature, which have discredited traditional science and caution nurse researchers not to abandon empirical methods in studies that explore humanistic nursing science.

Another philosophical debate among nurse scholars is whether nursing is a science, an art, or an applied science. How nursing is defined determines and influences research priorities and methodologies. Several nurse authors have discussed the need for basic and/or applied research to expand nursing knowledge. In her chapter, "Nursing Science: Basic, Applied, or Practical? Implication for the Art of Nursing," Joy Johnson discusses the differences of these scientific methods. She presents a strong argument that nursing science must ultimately pursue a practical science to achieve the goal of nursing.

In the nursing literature, various scholars have provided different perspectives on the scope and nature of nursing science. In his article, "What Constitutes Nursing Science?," John Phillips describes the shifting perspectives of recognized nurse scholars over the last three decades. He advocates that nurses design new methods through creative synthesis of science to enhance our understanding of human processes and nursing, and thus expand the science of nursing.

In looking toward the future, Shake Ketefian and Richard Redman challenge nurse leaders to expand nursing knowledge beyond our parochial and ethnocentric boundaries. In their chapter, "Nursing Science in the Global Community," these authors describe the historical influence of three perspectives—contextual, quantitative, and qualitative—on shaping nursing theory development, and nursing science. They explain how Western values and our social environment have led to assumptions that theories developed by American nurse scholars are universal and acultural. In closing, they offer suggestions on how to address internationally relevant nursing concerns and test nursing models and theories in other countries. Collectively, these chapters reflect many factors that continue to influence the evolution of nursing science.

6

Professionalism and the Evolution of Nursing as a Discipline: A Feminist Perspective

JUDITH WUEST, RN, MN

The evolution of nursing knowledge and nursing as a practice discipline has been stunted by the quest for professionalism. Liberal and socialist feminist theory clarifies the hazards inherent in the masculine institution of professionalism for a predominately female discipline. Socialist feminist theoretical perspectives facilitate a vision of nursing that includes altering social structure such that caring is valued. (Index words: Feminism; Knowledge development; Nursing discipline; Theory) J Prof Nursing 10:357–367, 1994. W.B. Saunders Copyright © 1994

The development of nursing as a discipline has been dominated by the hegemony of the patriarchal institutions of professionalism. Feminism can broadly be defined as seeking to end the domination of women (Jaggar, 1983). Nursing, historically a women's occupation, has been a vehicle of both liberation and oppression. The lens of liberal and socialist feminist theory provides a perspective for examining the evolution of nursing as a discipline. Professionalism has played a key role in marginalizing nursing and in constraining knowledge development. Feminism with its emphasis on praxis illuminates possible future directions in knowledge development for nursing as a practice discipline.

FEMINIST THEORETICAL PERSPECTIVES

Feminist theories have defined the causes of women's oppression and offer a means for eliminating it (MacPherson, 1991). Alison Jaggar (1983) clearly distinguished between liberal and socialist feminism.

Liberal Feminist Theory

"Liberal feminism rests on a conception of human nature that is radically individualistic" (Jaggar, 1983, p 355). Impartiality is a key tenet of liberal feminism. Thus, all individuals should be treated equally, and women should receive no special privileges. The focus of liberal feminism is on eliminating oppression by seeking equal opportunity for women, not on determining the factors that lead to women's oppression (MacPherson, 1991). The major approach to knowledge development is logical positivism, a legacy of Cartesian dualism. Adequacy of scientific theory is based on objectivity, scientific method, and value-free criterion. Within the liberal tradition, judgments must be impartial to the perspective of a particular group or individual.

Source: Wuest, J. (1994) Professionalism and the Evolution of Nursing as a Discipline: A Feminist Perspective. *Journal of Professional Nursing*, 10(6):357–367. Reprinted with permission from W.B. Sanders. Copyright© 1994.

Socialist Feminist Theory

Socialist feminism adopts the Marxist view that individual existence requires interaction with other humans and the non-human world. Knowledge development occurs in the process of human activity that is influenced by society. Knowledge is not value free and is always shaped by the perspective of the class from which the knowledge emerges. In contrast to the Marxist view that the perspective of the working class is most adequate, socialist feminism asserts that the standpoint of women is most valid because women's social position gives them access to a reality not accessible to men, and because women have no vested interest in maintaining the status quo of a patriarchal society. Although this is a similar position to that of radical feminists, the difference lies in how the knowledge is acquired. Socialist feminists do not accept that the standpoint of women is expressed in "women's naive and unreflective worldview" (Jaggar, 1983, p 371) because this is distorted by male-dominated structure and ideology. Instead, women's standpoint is continually evolving through scientific and political struggle. Jaggar acknowledged that individual women's standpoints may differ especially by race and class but suggested that this diversity contributes to a representation of reality that is continuously unfolding. Women's standpoint evolves in a matrix operation in which women's distinctive social experience guides the pattern of research in a particular discipline and the outcomes of the research are then tested within the social reality of women. Knowledge is deemed useful if it helps to reconstruct a world in which women's interests are not subordinate to those of men.

FEMINISM, PROFESSIONALISM, AND NURSING

Until recently, nursing links with feminism have been tenuous. A brief historical look at both the women's movement and the growth of professionalism in North America will shed light on the development of the discipline of nursing. From a socialist feminist perspective, examining historical context is essential; however, this examination reveals that any links between nursing and feminism have largely been in the liberal feminist tradition of seeking equality.

Early Women's Movement

Cott (1987) identified three foci in the women's movement of the nineteenth century: service and social action performed by charitable, altruistic women who felt their gender gave them a special mandate and who found new strength in their collectivity and self-assertion; women's rights action performed by individually motivated women who wanted "rights equivalent to those men enjoyed on legal, political, economic, and civic grounds" (p 16); and action for self-determination through "emancipation from structures, conventions and attitudes enforced by law and custom" (p 16). Regardless of specific beliefs, "the spectrum of ideology in the women's movement had a see-saw quality" (Cott, 1987, p 19). At one end was elimination of limitations and the attainment of equal rights, a liberalist perspective. At the other was the desire to value the unique qualities and abilities that women had to offer society. This valuing resulted either in acceptance of the unique but subservient status of women's existing social order or in adoption of a socialist feminist approach to change the existing social order to one that valued women in different ways. "No collective resolution of these tensions occurred and seldom even did individuals resolve them in their own minds" (Cott, 1987, p 20).

Nursing's Early Development in North America

The three positions of maintaining the status quo, seeking equality, and seeking to change the social order can be seen in nursing's development. "Nursing's identity has been inextricably bound to the very word and notion of nurturance as well as to the *myth* that women exist to be mothers" (Church, 1990, p 7). Initially, nursing was simply one of the many domestic roles that women were expected to fulfill on the basis of love and obligation (Reverby, 1987). "To practice it [nursing] at home was to fulfil the true calling of womanhood" (O'Brien, 1986, p 14). By the mid-1800s in North America, despite the desire of middle class women to be ladies, many found themselves economically in need of work. The affluent could afford to hire others to take on many of their domestic responsibilities. Hence, the emergence of the professed nurse.

> They brought to the bedside only the authority their personalities and community stature could command. Neither credentials nor a professional identity gave weight to their efforts. Their womanhood and the experience it gave them, defined their authority and taught them to nurse. (Reverby, 1987, p. 6).

In contrast to factory work, "the nature of nursing with its roots deep in the domestic world of the family, muted the dramatic shift in self-perception that women in factory work experienced" (O'Brien, 1986, p 13). Reverby (1987) noted that within the hospital setting, working class women attempted to exert control on working conditions and relationships with physicians, despite their lack of formal training and subservient class position.

> The sense of rights of working class womanhood gave them authority to press their demands. The necessity to care, and their perception of its importance to patient outcome also structured their belief that demanding the right to be relatively autonomous was possible. (Reverby, 1987, pp 6–7).

Nevertheless, these women were unsuccessful largely because of class differences between nurses and hospital administrators, paternalism, and very demanding work.

Few nurses at this time were engaged in trying to change the social order. Lavinia Dock was a pioneer in nursing history who was labeled a suffragist, a pacifist, and a Marxist. Her overriding concern was self-determination for women, nurses, and nursing (Church, 1990). Throughout her life, she challenged nurses to fight against male dominance but was considered by the majority of nurses as deviant. Dock urged nursing leaders to involve public and political activism (Ashley, 1976). A more widely known nurse feminist was Margaret Sanger, birth control agitator, who championed women's rights to control their sexuality regardless of church or state (Cott, 1987). These nurses made a significant contribution to the development of nursing but were representative of a minority view within nursing.

During this time period, Nightingale's philosophy of nursing education, legitimated by her successes in the Crimea, was developing a following in North America. Her intentions were to establish autonomous schools of nursing, under the control of nurses who would ultimately share power with physicians in the health care setting. Although this approach was admirable from the liberalist feminist perspective, her intended hierarchy within the nursing school eliminated the possibility of equality among nurses (Reverby, 1987). Nightingale's vision was distorted in its implementation by the physicians and hospital superintendents in North America who viewed schools of nursing as vehicles for obtaining cheap labor. They supported the establishment of apprenticeship schools and in doing so gained control over nurse's labor (Melosh, 1982). Nightingale indicated that nurses were prepared by developing womanly virtue. Thus, she legitimized paid work by embodying in it nineteenth century social values and needs (O'Brien, 1986). From a socialist feminist perspective, nursing is an example of household work shifted to the outside world of production. Because this work was not valued when it took place within the home, it similarly received little economic or status reward when practiced publicly (Miller, 1991). Coburn (1987) noted that despite the desire of upper-class Nightingale nurses to attract refined women to nursing, the difficult working conditions and unpleasant work deterred many. The majority of recruits were working-class women whose only other option was factory work.

> The school's emphasis on high moral character constituted an imposition of upper-class values on working-class women. The socialization process during training rested largely in the hands of middle- and upper-class nursing educators—women whose financial and social position allowed them to receive the necessary qualifications to teach. (Coburn, 1987, p 447)

This was the beginning of a class system within nursing: the elite educators and administrators versus the bedside practicing nurses. From a socialist feminist perspective, many of the decisions made from this point forward ensured the continuation of this division.

Ashley (1976) suggested that the apprenticeship system of nursing educations entrenched the dominations of nurses by physicians and hospital administrators.

> Convinced of their inferiority and of the need for their subordination to the medical profession, many nurses identified with the system that oppressed them and worked to support its continuing existence. Nurses learned to believe in the virtues of hospital training. Early conditioning within these institutions intensified the capacity of women to aid the cause of their oppressors. (Ashley, 1976, p 32)

Nursing training was rigid, orderly, and disciplined and students were overworked. Nevertheless, standards of care were established, nurses developed pride in their skills, had their idealism nurtured, and felt empowered to care (Reverby, 1987).

> . . . nurses have emphasized perceived womanly qualities and differences from men by stressing a role complementary to that performed by men. This position, often labelled anti-feminist, has led present-day feminists to disregard nursing because it tends to epitomize a set of characteristics and problems from which women are attempting to distance themselves. (Kirkwood, 1991, p 53)

In this sense, nursing embodies the dilemma of early (and present day) feminists who, by seeking equality, deny the very uniqueness of their contribution to society. But nursing was being controlled by forces beyond simply their desire to care.

> . . . caring was shaped not simply by women's psychological identity but by the social and political context in which nursing developed. It was a duty to care directed by a male medical hierarchy, not an ethic of care in which nurses would be able to make more autonomous judgments about the kind of care patients should receive. (Baines, 1991, p 63)

Nurses and Physicians

At the turn of the century, the medical profession was not well established in North America and was open to competition from nurses, pharmacists, and other allied occupations

(Torrance, 1987). Medical students had no internship and nursing students in training schools had greater opportunity to observe and to care for the sick. Although the training system had established physicians as dominant, their position was not secure. In 1904 through 1905, Abraham Flexner, a sociologist, visited and assessed Canadian and American medical schools. His report, published in 1910, was highly critical of schools that lacked the facilities to teach laboratory-based scientific medicine and resulted in the closure or reorganization of 92 medical schools. "The Flexner Report . . . helped to consolidate the dominance of the allophatic practitioners and to establish laboratory-based scientific medical education and practice. This mechanistic-individualistic conception is currently pervasive in medical practice and research" (Bolaria, 1988, p 3). The alliance of medicine with science and the subsequent entrenchment of medical education in the university resulted in the definition and domination of the health care field by the physicians. Flexner's study led also to a definition of "profession" and that had significant implications for the future of nursing.

Professionalism

In 1915, Flexner presented a paper that identified the criteria for characterizing professions from an analysis of the universally acknowledged professions of law, medicine, and clergy (Parsons, 1986).

Professions involve essentially intellectual operations; they derive their raw materials from science and learning; this material they work up into a practical and definite end; they possess an educationally communicable technique; they tend to self-organization; they are becoming in-

creasingly altruistic in motivation. (Flexner, 1915, p 904)

This definition stressed rationalism, scientific standards, and objectivity, all characteristics that embodied the masculine ethos. His masculine, sociological view was never questioned and the criteria became the sociological standard for distinguishing professions (Parsons, 1986). Professions were dominated by men and "a culture developed that affirmed male-centered values of order, efficiency, and hierarchical division of labour" (Baines, 1991). Flexner's paper also suggested that occupations could alter their status and become professions by developing the traits that were lacking.

Professions, reinforced by their scientific credibility became sources of power and prestige. Professionalization offered white, middle-class men a means of carving out new roles and obtaining monopoly on their services (Baines, 1991). Women who entered women-dominated professions were more motivated by an ethic of service or care than by a desire for power (Baines, 1991). "The bases for women's special expertise and place within the professions continued to rest on an ideology of service that lionized caring as a virtue particular to women" (Baines, p 55). The norm of professionalism is historically and socially unacceptable to women because of their exclusion from its conception (Parsons, 1986). Cott (1987) noted that although women professionals were seen as leaders before obtaining the vote, once the vote was attained, the bond that held them together was gone. A barrier developed between women professionals and nonprofessionals. To progress within the professions, and hold the tenets of non-bias, objectivity, and impersonality, women were required to abandon allegiance to feminism and create a community of interest with professional men rather than nonprofessional women (Cott, 1987). Glazer and Slater (1987) noted that professionals scorned nurturant, expressive, and familial interaction, valuing expertise and monopoly over an ethic of service.

Nursing and Professionalism

"Prior to Flexner, American nurses . . . were secure in their identity as professionals" (Parsons, 1986, p 273). However, nursing did not measure up to Flexner's criteria. By 1936 there were articles in nursing journals that indicated nursing was a developing profession (Parsons, 1986). Nursing had a limited body of scientific knowledge defined as nursing and exclusive of other disciplines. Because the phenomena unique to nursing had not been articulated and studied, nursing lacked control over practice and was subordinate to the medical profession (Lyon, 1990). Varying levels of educational preparation resulted in the absence of pervasive ideology and monopoly over work. Roberts (1984) asserted that nurses, once autonomous, became oppressed through societal forces and now exhibit the characteristics of an oppressed group. "Nurses have also accepted the fact that if they could only attain the characteristics of the powerful, or professional status, they too would be powerful" (Roberts, 1984, p 26).

In the early twentieth century, women who wanted recognition for nurses as significant health care providers readily accepted Flexner's assertion that an occupation could become a profession. Acceptance of professional ideology can be viewed as a strength from a liberal feminist perspective. It pushed nurses to sever the link with domestic labor and establish standards of paid work, to refuse the limitations of gender in their own lives and in goals for nursing profession, and to challenge the traditional constraints on women in the workforce (Melosh, 1982). Because nursing was a women's profession, women had the potential monopoly and

power to effect change. What nurses and other women striving for more traditional professions failed to recognize was that the criteria that they were trying to meet were established by men. The rightness of these criteria was not questioned. In fact, by accepting these criteria, and striving to meet them, nursing was supporting the existing patriarchal order. This decision resulted in securing privileges for few nurses at the expense of many (Melosh, 1982).

KNOWLEDGE DEVELOPMENT

Professionalism and Knowledge Development

When nursing leaders decided to respond to the Flexner report by seeking to meet his criteria of profession, they recognized that nursing had to establish a scientific knowledge base. Because professionals had to be scientific, and the only academic preparation for nurses at that time was at the Columbia Teacher's College, most study and research related to education and administration and not to clinical practice (Baer, 1987). Thus, academically prepared nurses were further divided from those practicing at the bedside, and there was much debate about whose work was the most meaningful. This divisiveness is characteristic of the horizontal violence of oppressed groups. Roberts (1984) noted that whether nurses were in the hospital or the academic setting they were (and are) rewarded for being marginal and taking on the characteristics of the dominant groups. As nursing programs opened up in universities in Canada and the United States, nurses struggled to have their knowledge and experience validated as scholarship. "A knowledge base for nursing stemming from women's private, domestic sphere was suspect within the male-dominated culture of the university, which took pride in intellectual scientific achievements" (Kirkwood, 1991, p 54).

World War II opened opportunities for nurses to expand their practice roles and to have advanced university study in post-war years; however, Baer (1987) noted that all nurses were not enthusiastic about these openings. Nurses seeking professionalization were anxious to upgrade their educational preparation, but this was very threatening to nurses who had trained under the hospital system. Hospital educators, anxious to support apprenticeship, failed to grasp post-war opportunities for upgrading. This further developed the class system in nursing.

Research became an issue for nurses as they attempted to establish a scientific knowledge base. Nurses ignored gender issues and moved away from its domestic heritage. "Nurses believed that, if they met university demands to demonstrate nursing was a scholarly discipline with a unique scientific base, nurses would be accorded the same professional respect as others in the university" (Kirkwood, 1991, p 61). Hughes (1990, p 31) noted that the development of nursing as a discipline is often equated with its evolution as a profession but history "suggests that professional status is not likely to evolve passively from nursing's recognition as a scholarly discipline." However, it is significant that "by successfully developing and maintaining university nursing education, nurses have to some extent undermined the patriarchal structure of the university by locating work, traditionally assigned to women in the public sphere of higher education dominated by men" (Kirkwood, 1991, p 62).

In November 1951, the *American Journal of Nursing* announced the publication of *Nursing Research*, noting that research was essential for knowledge development in nursing (Baer,

1987). It was 1976 before over half the articles published focused on clinical practice rather than education, because most of the researchers were nursing faculty whose higher education had been in education. Whereas their institutions required that they participate in scholarly activity to meet criteria for tenure and promotion, service agencies and hospitals did not encourage such activity from practicing nurses (Baer, 1987). Hence, the gap widened with practitioners viewing educators as more and more removed from the real world of nursing.

> Nursing's major goal in fostering research was to achieve recognition of its professional status. Some individual nurses certainly saw research as a means, a method through which they could answer questions and expand their ideas. But for most nurses, it was an end, a criterion of professionalism they yearned to attain. (Baer, 1987, p 24)

Research and Theory Development

Early approaches to research followed the reductionistic methods of the biomedical model as the surest way to be credible as scientists (Nagle & Mitchell, 1991). Nursing adopted the empirical ethic of science through a research tradition "that concentrates on objectivity, facts, measurement of smaller and smaller parts, and issues of instrumentality, reliability, validity, and operationalization to the point that nursing is in danger of exhausting the meaning, relevance, and understanding of the values, goals, and actions that it espouses in its heritage and ideals" (Watson, 1988, p. 17). Researchers have only recently begun to recognize that the scientific method is insufficient for addressing many of nursing's concerns and are beginning to embrace more diverse, qualitative approaches to research.

Concern for nursing's lack of theory base developed in the 1960s when nurses began to study at a doctoral level in other disciplines. The embryonic nursing science was attached to other sciences and fed on their theories, methods, and instruments (Stainton, 1982). Much debate developed surrounding such issues as whether nursing theory should be borrowed from other disciplines, single versus multiple theories, and whether theories should influence or be influenced by practice.

At early nursing theory conferences, the views of theory development expressed by such leaders as Dickoff and James and Abdellah supported the logical empiricist tradition for the development of nursing science (Silva & Rothbart, 1983). "Early nurse theorists such as Roy and Orem maintained the status quo of objective reductionism by focusing on problems and defining health according to medical and/or societal norms" (Nagle & Mitchell, 1991, p 18). Although nurses were strongly supporting this approach, the philosophers of science from where this tradition stemmed were seriously questioning the limitations of this approach (Silva & Rothbart, 1983; Webster & Jacox, 1985). Nurse researchers and theorists recognized the limitations of the received view in theorizing about people's experiences with health and illness; however, the drive for professionalism and scientific legitimacy resulted in nursing, as an emerging discipline, holding on to this respectable approach.

> In the 1960s the unity and political and academic power of the received view theorists was sufficiently great that lip service had to be paid to their basic beliefs. Now we are free to choose among the insights of the received view and select only those which we find useful and sound for our purposes in constructing nursing theory. (Webster & Jacox, 1985, p 27)

These authors suggest that nursing is free to develop its own philosophy of science. Evidence of changing views about the philosophy of science is in the works of such theorists as Watson (1988) and Parse (1981).

Theory and Nursing Practice

Theory is argued to be important in the establishment of the unique body of knowledge essential for nursing to be recognized as a profession and as a means of fostering communication and improving patient care. Theory development through creative conceptualization expanded nursing knowledge. However, the language of theory is frequently abstract and there is much discussion among theorists and those attempting to understand and apply nursing theories to practice. "There are serious credibility gaps between the ideal prescriptive theory that is taught and the practical knowledge used by practitioners" (Aydelotte, 1990, p 10).

> Resultant debates have tended to develop into a vicious circle, with theorists berating practitioners for their lack of concern with the conceptual basis for their actions, whilst practitioners bemoan theoretical approaches which are seen as having little or no relevance to their daily work. (Nolan & Grant, 1992)

Fawcett (1992) asserted the existence of a reciprocal relationship between conceptual models and nursing practice, but she was adamant that the models come first and are tested for their credibility and refined in the field of clinical practice. This position fails to consider the fact that many practitioners find the conceptual model too obscure to enter into that reciprocity.

Nagle & Mitchell (1991) noted that nursing is being driven by professional licensing bodies and accreditation bodies to adopt a single theory as a base for practice within their agency. They suggested that this is a paternalistic action that denies nurses the autonomy of choosing their own theoretic base for practice consistent with their unique worldview. This suggestion assumes that most practicing nurses have articulated a worldview and is further evidence of the rift between practitioners and those nurses with advanced education. This imposition may give practicing nurses a means for voicing what they do and do not like about practicing within a specific, theoretical framework. This may be the key to Fawcett's reciprocity.

FEMINISM: LOOKING TO THE FUTURE FOR NURSING

The acceptance of patriarchal professionalism has resulted in nursing adopting liberalist traditions for the development of research and practice. "Feminism, in its liberal form, appears to give nursing a political language that argues for equality and rights within the given order of things" (Reverby, 1987, p 10). Nurses have often been criticized for rejecting liberal feminism.

> From a feminist perspective, the individualism and autonomy promised by this rights framework often fails to acknowledge collective social need, to provide a way for adjudicating conflict over rights, or to address the reasons for the devaluing of female activity. (MacPherson, 1991, p 30).

Reverby (1987) suggested that nursing will have to create the social climate that values caring. This implies the need for a socialist feminist approach in which nursing takes a more active role in altering social structure.

Professionalization has objectified those for whom nurses care. "A feminist ethos of professionalism needs to be based on an ideology that integrates an ethic of care and forms a more equal partnership with the cared for" (Baines, 1991, p 67). Feminism offers some revolutionary ideas for nursing (Chinn, 1987). "Feminism values and endorses women, critiques male thinking, challenges patriarchal systems, and focuses on creating self-love and respect for all others and all forms of life" (Chinn, 1987, p 23).

Knowledge Development

Dorothy Smith (1990) addressed the impact that hegemony has on knowledge development by influencing the issues that are valued and by dictating an approach to those issues based on the conceptual view of those institutions rather than the lived experienced of the people involved. As people are educated to take up roles within institutions, they are exposed to a "conceptual imperialism" (Smith, 1990, p 15) that ensures a perpetuation of the worldview of the institution under the guise of objectivity. People have two ways of knowing, experiencing and doing: one on a local, immediate, bodily level, and one that is at an objective, conceptual level. The objective account, giving the appearance of neutrality and impartiality in fact conceals class, gender, and race and puts forward the ideology of the governing groups. The objectified text has power because of the way it organizes social relations. People read the objectified text as fact and repress their own lived experience. Thus, people begin to see things the same way. "Objectified knowledge, as we engage with it, subdues, discounts, and disqualifies our various interests, perspectives, angles, and experience, and what we might have to say speaking from them" (Smith, 1990, p 80).

Smith's account sheds some light on the current division that exists between nursing theory and practice. Nursing theory has been developed by the elite and educated, the nurses who have wielded power in the development of nursing as a profession. The separation of these nurses from those at the bedside has been well documented. These nurses identified a professional route for the development of nursing knowledge and endorsed the patriarchal structure. Hence, the approaches to nursing theory reflect the dominant culture rather than the lived experience of nurses at the bedside.

Smith (1990) argued that women must create a reflexive critique through investigation that is grounded in the lives of women and people. This requires an exploration of women's everyday experience with socially organized practices and an examination of how women's practices contribute to and are articulated with the relations that rule our lives. This emphasis on praxis is most consistent for the development of nursing knowledge that reflects the human experience of nursing. However, a major barrier exists. Many nurses who wield educational and administrative power within nursing have a vested interest in maintaining their current positions of power and this is readily accomplished through Smith's "conceptual imperialism." For a significant change to occur nurse leaders and educators must be conscious of this oppression.

There is evidence that nursing is beginning to consider some more revolutionary approaches to knowledge development. Critical scholarship, a pattern of thought and action that challenges institutionalized power relations in the social reality of nursing has been suggested by Thompson (1987) as one means of addressing the issues that nursing faces. She urged nurses to question the assumption that underlie our liberal undergraduate education such as the logical positivist approach to science, the functionalist framework of the social world, and professional ideology because these assumptions foster acceptance of the status quo. "Critical scholarship in nursing can speak about the process of reweaving, regaining confidence in new reality, regaining a commitment to new definitions of nursing practice, and feeling grounded in new value orientations" (Thompson, 1987, p 37). Anderson (1991, p 2) noted that feminism and poststructuralist perspectives

> challenge us to extend our analysis of phenomena relating to the lives of clients or patients beyond the micro level of analysis to an examination of the broader social processes that influence health and illness behaviour. This has the potential for the development of nursing science that will be inclusive of the complex socioeconomic, historical, and political nexus in which human experience is embedded.

Silva and Rothbart (1983), drawing on the work of Laudan, suggested that nursing theory development is currently in a state of transition, that it will never result in a static set of truths but will always be evolving.

> Data for nursing theory development and testing will include the common practices of nurse clinicians, the social and psychological factors affecting the profession of nursing, the widely held beliefs of the community of nurses, and the reasoning patterns of individual nurse theorists. A result of integrating these data will be a nursing theory that more explicitly addresses the human dimension of nursing (Silva & Rothbart, 1983, p 11)

The test for adequacy of theory will be more focused on solution of nursing care problems than on truth and error. This is very consistent with socialist feminist theory for which the criteria of adequacy is usefulness. These approaches hold promise for future development of nursing research and theory development.

Feminist Epistemology and Research Methodology

Jaggar and Bordo (1989, p 4) indicated that feminist epistemology shares the critique of many philosophers that "the Cartesian framework is fundamentally inadequate, an obsolete and self-deluded world view badly in need of reconstruction and revisioning" borrowing from other traditions such as Marxist historicism, psychoanalytic theory, literary theory, and sociology of knowledge to support its claim. Contemporary feminism's arguments differ from others in the assertion that the Cartesian framework is not gender neutral. Feminist epistemology is not about women being able to conduct science in its current form as well as men can. "Rather its position is that women who have come to recognize and accept feminist assumptions about the world will practice science differently in a world that legitimates these assumptions . . ." (Farganis, 1989, p 208). Belenky, Clinchy, Goldberger, and Tarule (1986) have identified that the epistemological perspectives that influence how women see and know the world are different from those of men.

Farganis (1989) suggested that feminism acknowledges that each person has a different position from which they view the world but does not accept that each view is equally good. Feminism has a moral dimension that opposes normative relativism. Because of their experiences as marginal persons and their experiences of care and concern, "women can offer an epistemically sounder and politically and morally better position" (p 217). Rose (1986) supported this view urging that knowledge gained through the practice of caring be a base for a science that values people. Harding (1986) went one step further and suggested that the hierarchy of positivism should be re-versed with studies directed by such moral emancipatory interests as the elimination of sexist, racist, and classist understandings of social life being most valued.

In the health care field, patriarchal standards have reigned and the personal experience of professional caregiving has been devalued. "Feminist ideology holds that marginal persons in society are those whose roles threaten those in power" (Miller, 1991, p 49). Nursing can be considered marginal and this results in "the development of care modalities that are unspoken, unrecognized, and unappreciated by the dominant groups and, therefore, by society at large" (Miller, 1991, p 49). Feminist approaches to science support the development of a nursing science based on the knowledge that nurses have gained through practice.

A further contribution that feminism makes to nursing knowledge development is direction for research. Fonow and Cook (1991) distilled four common, interdisciplinary themes of feminist epistemology and methodology that are helpful for nursing research.

Reflexivity

This is the practice of reflecting on, examining critically, and exploring analytically the research process and using it to understand the underlying assumptions about gender relations. Consciousness raising is one method of reflexivity that is reflected in the increased consciousness of the researcher of the effects of the research process on the researcher's identity, the impact of the research on the subjects, and finally as a feminist research method. Collaboration between women researchers is another focus of reflexivity: ". . . there is also the expectation among some scholars that feminist collaboration will bring about a deeper intellectual analysis, an original approach to framing questions, with a mind-set of innovation to deal with the gendered context of research" (Fonow & Cook, 1991, p 5).

Action Orientation

The orientation of feminist research is toward social change. This can be accomplished by participating with people in an examination of positions and options, by historically analyzing the past for the purpose of future social change, or by focusing on the policy implications of research findings. "A personal commitment to feminism and to caring as a standard for professional nursing practice can only lead to the demand for major changes in the structure and provision of health care service to all human beings" (Gaut, 1991, p 6). This change can be accomplished by attention to research with an action orientation.

Attention to the Affective Components of the Research Act

Feminist research recognizes the affective dimension and sees emotion as a source of insight. This can be connected to the notion of reciprocity between researcher and the researched manifested either in friendship or in negative interactions.

Use of the Situation at Hand

This use of everyday, existing situations is particularly important for nursing research because nursing's major interest is the experiences of people in health and illness situations.

CONCLUSION

Professionalism has failed to bring nursing the power and prestige that were anticipated by nursing's early leaders. Professionalism is a patriarchal invention and by its very nature is alienating to women. By accepting the liberal tradition of knowledge development embodied in professionalism, nurses have not appreciated their own knowledge acquired through their caring experience. Rather than joining with other women to change the dominant social order to one that values women's unique differences, nurses have focused primarily on attaining professional status. Only recently have nurses begun to recognize that the received view of knowledge development is not sufficient for addressing the complex concerns of nursing as a human science. This realization has resulted in nursing seeking alternate approaches.

Feminism offers much to nursing through its focus on praxis. The liberalist feminist tradition of seeking equality is not sufficient to meet the challenges facing nursing. The socialist feminist perspective offers more direction. It suggests that nursing knowledge development should be directed toward creating a social order in which women are not subordinate to men. This means that our efforts should not be geared to maintaining the status quo within our field of practice but rather should be focusing on ways to alter public policy. Socialist feminism suggests that women as a social group have the more valid perspective because they have no vested interest in maintaining the status quo in society. Applying this view to nursing, nurses in practice have a more legitimate perspective of nursing than nurse leaders and educators. Thus, the distinctive experience of nursing practice should guide nursing research and the outcomes of research should be tested within the reality of practicing nurses because that reality may be quite different to that of the nurse researcher. The actual process of research should itself be dialectical, thus effecting some change in those participating. This approach may help to reduce the current chasm between nursing practice and research. Jean Watson urged nursing to "question its old dogmas, transcend its existing paradigms, and refocus its scientific attention to human phenomena that are consistent with the nature of nursing and preservation of humanity" (1988, p 22). Feminism, particularly socialist feminism, has the potential to help nurses to meet this challenge and to make a significant contribution to changing the existing social order of health care and gender relations.

REFERENCES

Anderson, J. (1991). Current directions in nursing research: Toward a poststructuralist and feminist epistemology. *The Canadian Journal of Nursing Research*, 23(3), 1–3.

Ashley, J. (1976). *Hospitals, paternalism, and the role of the nurse*. New York: Teachers College Press.

Aydelotte, M. (1990). The evolving profession: The role of the professional organization. In N. Chaska (Ed.) *The Nursing Profession: Turning Points*. (pp. 9–15) St. Louis, MO: Mosby.

Baer, E. (1987). 'A cooperative venture' in pursuit of professional nursing status: A research journal for nursing. *Nursing Research*, 36, 18–25.

Baines, C. (1991). The professions and the ethic of care. In C. Baines, P. Evans, and S. Neysmith (Eds.) *Women's caring: Feminist perspectives on social welfare*. (pp. 36–72) Toronto, Canada: McClelland & Stewart.

Belenky, M., Clinchy, B., Goldberger, N., & Tarule, J. (1986). *Women's ways of knowing*. New York: Basic Books.

Bolaria, B. S. (1988). Sociology, medicine, health, and illness: An overview. In B. S. Bolaria & H. Dickinson (Ed.). *Sociology of health care in Canada* (pp. 1–14). Toronto, Canada: Harcourt Brace Jovanovich.

Chinn, P. (1987). Response: Revision and passion. *Scholarly Inquiry for Nursing Practice*, 1(1): 21–24.

Church, O. (1990). Nursing's history: What it was and what it was not. In N. Chaska (Ed.). *The nursing profession: Turning points*. (pp. 3–8). St. Louis, MO: Mosby.

Coburn, J. (1987). I see and am silent. In D. Coburn, C. D'Arcy, G. Torrance, & P. New (Eds.). *Health care and Canadian Society: Sociological perspectives*. (pp. 441–462) Markham: Fitzhenry and Whiteside.

Cott, N. (1987). *The grounding of modern feminism*. New Haven, CT: Yale University Press.

Farganis, S. (1989). Feminism and the reconstruction of social science. In A. Jaggar & S. Bordo (Eds.). *Gender/Body/Knowledge: Feminist reconstructions of being and knowing*. (pp. 207–223). New Brunswick, NJ: Rutgers.

Fawcett, J. (1992). Conceptual models and nursing practice: The reciprocal relationship. *Journal of Advanced Nursing*, 17, 224–228.

Flexner, A. (1915). Is social work a profession? *School Soc*, 1, 901–911.

Fonow, M., & Cook, J. (1991). Back to the future: A look at the second wave of feminist epistemology and methodology. In M. Fonow & J. Cook (Eds.). *Beyond method: Feminist scholarship as lived research*. (pp. 1–15) Bloomington, IN: Indiana University Press.

Glazer, P., & Slater, M. (1987). *Unequal colleagues*. New Brunswick, NJ: Rutgers.

Gaut, D. (1991). Caring and nursing: Explorations in feminist perspectives-Introductory remarks. In R. Neil & R. Watts (Eds.). *Caring and nursing: Explorations in feminist perspectives*. (pp. 5–8). New York: National League of Nursing.

Harding, S. (1986). *The science question in feminism*. Ithaca, NY: Cornell University Press.

Hughes, L. (1990). Professionalizing domesticity: A selected synthesis of nursing historiography. *Advances in Nursing Science*, 12(4), 25–31.

Jaggar, A. (1983). *Feminist politics and human nature*. Totowa, NJ: Rowman & Allenhead.

Jaggar, A., & Bordo, S. (1989). *Gender/body/knowledge: Feminist reconstructions of being and knowing*. New Brunswick, NJ: Rutgers.

Kirkwood, R. (1991). Discipline discrimination and gender discrimination: The case of nursing in Canadian universities, 1920–1950. *Atlantis*. 16(2), 52–63.

Lyon, B. (1990). Getting back on track: Nursing's autonomous scope of practice. In N. Chaska (Ed.). *The nursing profession: Turning points*. (pp. 267–274). St. Louis, MO: Mosby.

MacPherson, K. (1991). Looking at caring and nursing through a feminist lens. In R. Neil & R. Watts (Eds.). *Caring and nursing: Explorations in feminist perspectives*. (pp. 25–43). New York: NLN.

Melosh, B. (1982). *The physician's hand: Work culture and conflict in American Nursing*. Philadelphia, PA: Temple University Press.

Miller, K. (1991). A study of nursing's feminist ideology. In R. Neil & R. Watts (Eds.). *Caring and nursing: Explorations in feminist perspectives*. (pp. 43–56). New York: NLN.

Nagle, L. & Mitchell, G. (1991). Paradigmatic issues in research and practice. *Advances in Nursing Science*, 14(1), 17–25.

Nolan, M., & Grant, G. (1992). Mid-range theory building and the nursing theory-practice gap: A respite care case study. *Journal of Advanced Nursing*, 17, 217–223.

O'Brien, P. (1986). 'All a woman's life can bring': The domestic roots of nursing in Philadelphia, 1830–1885. *Nursing Research*, 36, 12–17.

Parse, R. (1981). *Man-living-health: A theory of nursing*. New York: Wiley.

Parsons, M. (1986). The profession in a class by itself. *Nursing Outlook*, 34, 270–275.

Reverby, S. (1987). A caring dilemma: Womanhood and nursing in historical perspective. *Nursing Research*, 36, 5–11.

Roberts, S. J. (1984). Oppressed group behavior: Implications for nursing. *Advances in Nursing Science*, 5(4), 21–30.

Rose, H. (1988). Beyond masculine realities. In R. Bleier (Ed.). *Feminist approaches to science.* (pp. 57–76). New York: Pergammon.

Silva, M. C., & Rothbart, D. (1983). An analysis of changing trends in philosophies of science on nursing theory development and testing. *Advances in Nursing Science*, 6(3), 1–13.

Smith, D. (1990). *The conceptual practices of power: A feminist sociology of knowledge*. Toronto, Canada: University of Toronto Press.

Stainton, M. C. (1982). The birth of nursing science. *Canadian Nurse*, 78, 24–28.

Thompson, J. (1987). Critical scholarship: The critique of domination in nursing. *Advances in Nursing Science*, 10(1), 27–38.

Torrance, G. (1987). Socio-historical overview. In D. Coburn, C. D'Archy, G. Torrance, & P. New (Eds.). *Health care and Canadian Society: Sociological perspectives*. (pp. 6–32) Markham: Fitzhenry and Whiteside.

Watson, J. (1988). *Nursing: Human science and human care: A theory of nursing*. USA: National League of Nursing.

Webster, G., & Jacox, A. (1985). The liberation of nursing theory. In J. McCloskey & H. Grace (Eds.). *Current issues in nursing*. pp. 20–29. Boston, MA: Blackwell.

7

Debunking Myths in Nursing Theory and Research

PEGGY L. CHINN, RN, PhD, FAAN

This chapter examines myths that persist in the traditional male-defined scientific enterprise. Science per se is not rejected, but specific ways of confronting the myths are explored. The methods for debunking the myths derive from the concept of future search, wherein health and the values of nursing for the future direct the discovery of knowledge. The alternatives include a more ethical and responsible use of the methods of science as well as specific alternatives to science derived from Carper's (1978) patterns of knowing in nursing.

The nursing literature has reflected growing recognition of the limitations of the scientific method in addressing problems in nursing (Gorenberg, 1983; Munhall, 1982; Newman, 1979; Smith, M. C., 1984; Vredevoe, 1984; Webster, Jacox, & Baldwin, 1981). Taken together, the literature leaves the impression that we should perhaps forsake the scientific method; alternatives for acquiring knowledge in nursing are not adequately described, and the alternatives that are suggested are not clearly alternatives to the scientific method.

A fundamental issue that is lacking in most critiques of the scientific method is recognition that science is based on a male worldview and that the myths sustained by this partial worldview have perpetuated erroneous knowledge about the world. The purposes of this chapter are (a) to present an analysis of myths of science that arise from the partial male worldview, (b) to propose methods for debunking

these myths to attain a more whole science consistent with the essence of nursing, and (c) to propose alternative approaches to science where an alternative is indicated.

MYTHS

The concept of "myth" carries many meanings. Two dictionary definitions focus attention on the meanings that are relevant to the focus of this article: "a traditional story of ostensibly historical events that serves to unfold part of the worldview of a people, or explain a practice, belief, or natural phenomenon. . . ." and "an ill-founded belief held uncritically, especially by an interested group" (*Webster's New Collegiate Dictionary*, 1981).

Myths remain a powerful force in the creation of sociocultural patterns, and science and scientists are equally subject to their influence. Myths are not entirely false and in fact contain an element of reality. This is why they are so seductive and difficult to recognize. Since myths are based on a particular world-

Source: Chinn, P. L. (1985). Debunking myths in nursing theory and research. *IMAGE: Journal of Nurse Scholarship, 17* (2): 45-49. Reprinted with permission from Sigma Theta Tau International.

view, they function actually to shape and create reality. Until we examine myths critically, we are not able to sort out what is ill founded from that which is well founded, or whose interests are served.

Traditional science has created beliefs about reality that are taken to be "true." Science, for all practical purposes, rests on a white, upper-class, male view of the world (Spender, 1981). This view is not necessarily wrong or bad, but it is not universal. Regardless of the actual origins of the prevailing worldview or whether it arose from the maleness per se of its originators, the traits of this worldview are characterized as being male because of the remarkable consistency with such masculine concepts as power, control, instrumentation, technology, competition, rationality, logic, objectivity, hard data. Not only does this view rest on the superiority of male-assigned traits but it also disdains concepts that are consistent with that which is assigned as being "feminine"—soft data, subjectivity, feeling, emotion, intuition, and so forth. This arbitrary value assignment clearly does not serve the interests of nursing or the best interest of humanity. Spender (1980) spoke of the myth of the superiority of that which is masculine in language:

> The myth was made a long time ago and for centuries it has been fostered by women and men so that now it is deeply embedded in virtually every aspect of our existence. It is a myth which may be attacked but one which is not easy to eradicate, for all myths still have a hold over us long after they have been intellectually repudiated, and this one, which is fundamental to our social order, is particularly pervasive and particularly hard to dislodge. The fabric of our social organization has been woven to support and substantiate it and nothing less than a restructuring of our beliefs and values is necessary, if it is to be laid to rest. (pp. 1-2)

FUTURE SEARCH

Just as language is a powerful tool for conveying the prevailing worldview, an examination of new meanings for language can be used to create a shift. The word *research* is a useful starting point. The activities that happen under the name of research are often literally re-searching what has been done over and over again. Usually the hypotheses shift from project to project, but there is seldom any creativity in the conceptualizations or methods used primarily because credibility depends on doing the same thing (or close to it) in the same way. What this does is perpetuate the status quo—a past-oriented perspective.

Heide (1982) proposes that we shift our focus to future search. Future search requires that we envision the world as it could be, or as we want it to be—a healthy, productive, peaceful, enduring, nurturing environment and society. Once we have this vision, we can begin to discover knowledge that is required to create this world. As nursing scholars, we can end the perpetuation of a status quo that values illness more than health; we can enact what we know in our practice by focusing our scholarly energies in the direction of health for all. In short, we can be change agents (Smith, M. J., 1984).

Future-search methods that serve to debunk myths in nursing science rest on the following assumptions:

- Nursing's worldview is both reasonable and valuable. This worldview focuses on health, life, human interaction, and environmental integrity. Further, nursing values are intimately related to that which has been assigned a feminine value and as such contradicts many values of traditional science.
- The scientific method is useful for some questions but not for all questions.
- In conceptualizing methods of generating knowledge, it is not useful to think in terms

of dichotomies of "scientific" or "nonscientific." Other analogous concepts include "the received view" versus the "nonreceived view" (Webster, Jacox, & Baldwin, 1981) and "paradigm I logic" versus "paradigm II logic" (Tinkle & Beaton, 1983). These dichotomies imply that science remains the standard for judging all methods. Future search views science as one method, but not the standard for judging all methods.

- The appeal in the literature for alternative methods and logical systems are valid, and the types of knowledge that are required in nursing have been described (Carper, 1978). However, the methods are yet to be created, described and demonstrated to be useful.

THE MYTHS OF RE-SEARCH

There are several ways to approach a movement toward future search. The movement begins with debunking myths of the scientific enterprise. In considering the myths, I am not suggesting that we eliminate the concepts entirely; I am suggesting that we debunk these ideas as sacred truths, examine the dimensions of the idea that are partial or false, and move in a direction of wholeness consistent with our worldview.

Myth 1: The Myth of the Ultimate Truth

The myth of the ultimate truth leads us to think that truth is true because it is true. Scientific theory is supposed to represent reality, and reality is supposed to be truth. Truth, as it is conceptualized in the traditional scientific enterprise, is represented in the assumptions of theories and research. For the most part the assumptions are rarely recognized much less questioned. By subscribing to the assumptions

as "truth," we seek data that conform to our view and ignore contrary evidence that does not support the underlying assumption of what is true. We ignore as being idiosyncratic (insignificant) data that do not conform to our preconceived beliefs.

The method for debunking this myth is to identify and reverse existing assumptions. Once existing assumptions are reversed, contrary evidence can be sought that debunks the original assumption. In a world that is whole, with established scientific "truths" based on universal experience, all the evidence would be valued and integrated into our knowing. However, we do not live in such a world, and for now it is essential that we work diligently and deliberately to produce the evidence that we know contradicts much of what passes for truth about the world.

The work of Gilligan (1982) demonstrates the importance of questioning underlying "truths" and unstated assumptions. She studied with Kohlberg and learned his theory of moral development. Later, she realized there was important information that had not been disclosed in final reports of the research or integrated into the theory. Kohlberg's theory is based on all-male research. When the theory and tools derived from it were used with women, women were found not to achieve development beyond the third stage of a 10-stage process and were assumed to be inferior to men. Gilligan reexamined the theory and reversed the assumption that failing to be a "10" represents an inferiority. Using methods of traditional science but simply reversing the assumption of universality of the theory, she demonstrated contrary evidence required to debunk the myth of the universality of Kohlberg's theory, revealing that women are not inferior; the theory is inferior. In a very fundamental way, Kohlberg's theory does not withstand the test of universality, as Kohlberg has claimed. In the process of discovering contrary evidence, Gilligan also contributed knowledge that has begun to change how women are viewed—a hallmark of the future-search enterprise (see also Munhall, 1983).

Myth 2: The Myth of Objectivity

Traditional science prides itself on being "value free" and therefore objective and not subjective. Intellectually, some traditional scientists recognize that no science is value free; neither is it free from subjective influence. However, it is not the value-laden bias of the scientific enterprise that is the problem; it is the continuing failure to acknowledge and take seriously the nature of the values and subjective interpretations that are imposed on the so-called objective ideas, methods, and designs.

One of the dictionary meanings given for the word *objective* is particularly enlightening: "methods that eliminate the subjective by limiting choices to fixed alternatives requiring a minimum of creative interpretation (eg, tests of personality)" (*Webster's New Collegiate Dictionary*, 1981). Of course, the dictionary does not ask, Who determined the alternatives? What values influenced their choice of the "fixed alternatives?" Who decided that it was desirable to eliminate the "subjective" and "creative" in the testing of personality?

The most insidious technique used to perpetrate the myth of objectivity is the erasure, abdication, and obfuscation of responsibility, thereby obscuring the subjective influence. The scientific literature, including that in nursing, is abundant with such phrases as "research results show" (what research, what kind of research, by whom?), or "it is generally known that" (by whom?). This is a tradition that works well to obscure responsibility and should be a major ethical concern for all scientists of our day. It is both an individual and a collective problem.

The method for debunking the myth of objectivity is to name the responsible agent, to demystify the assumptions, the motives, the values, the processes that were used to arrive at the definition of what purported to be objective. We have a wonderful example in our own history of a nursing scholar who recognized this problem and took a strong stand opposing it. Writing in the *American Journal of Nursing* in 1915, Lavinia Dock stated:

> As a result of the European war, there are reappearances of ailments that were practically nonexistent. Gaseous gangrene, never seen in surgery now-a-days, has come again. . . . When we know how surely and certainly these diseases are caused by men's own acts and deeds, does it not seem as if we should say, "Man's actions have produced gas-gangrene and typhus;" instead of the flabby statement, "Typhus is prevalent; gas-gangrene is developing." Seeing such ruthless and dastardly energies at work, does one not understand Florence Nightingale's impatient contempt for the germ theory, and comprehend her insistence that it was the things people did that caused disease? (p. 666)

Exposing explicit responsibility exposes underlying assumptions and myths and creates a new view of reality. For example, Florence Nightingale experienced the horrors of war and the destruction of human life and health; she refused to accept that the unsanitary conditions that she witnessed were "natural." Her personal and subjective response to these conditions created an awareness of reality that was not generally accessible to other scholars of her day. Margaret Sanger grieved for the waste of human life and human potential that was created by the uncontrolled frequency of pregnancy, and she refused to assume that this condition was "natural." Her subjective, self-acknowledged response created the motive to seek the knowledge that would create health.

Myth 3: The Myth of the Perfect Method

The myth of the perfect method results in compulsive orderliness, repetitiveness, and a fixation on minute details. It encourages us toward mental laziness in envisioning alternative methods, alternative approaches, and alternative assumptions. We re-search and re-search to the point that we know less and less about more and more, failing to recognize the relevance or irrelevance of what we are studying. The perfect method, by definition, leads us on a path of examining small segments and parts of reality apart from the whole and is based on the assumption that a segmented analysis of the parts will yield knowledge of the whole.

The method for debunking this myth begins with the recognition that there is no one perfect method and that various methods must be used in relation to each question that is asked. Most important, this shift requires valuing alternative methods in a fundamental way. It requires refusing to apologize for what is presumed to be inadequate when contrasted with the "perfect method." It also requires that we cease to view alternative methods as merely a stepping stone to the "perfect method." The alternative methods, whether they are variations on the theme of the "'perfect method" or an entirely different approach (such as those I will describe in the following section), are to be used and developed for their own worth and value.

Nursing is faced with what might be called an imperative to debunk this myth arising from the nature of the work we do, what we have identified as important, and how we view our goals. In conceptualizing health, the client, the environment, and the nurse-client interactions, a clear holistic view has emerged. If we remain committed to this foundational view, then the traditional method, which requires studying parts or segments of things or people, is simply not adequate (Newman,

1979). A segmented, partial approach might serve to enlighten or might serve some limited pragmatic purpose; it might be preferable to adapt the traditional methods to complex problems rather than to do nothing; however, as new methods emerge, their future viability will depend on our conscious valuing of them, free from false judgment against the "standard" of the perfect method.

Myth 4: The Myth of Scientific Supremacy

The myth of scientific supremacy focuses on the religious-like quality of science as the means for delineating truth, knowledge, and reality—and as an end in and of itself. A critical component of this myth is the rejection of any other possibility for creating knowledge. Science, which is based on the notion of empirical validation, is thought to result in true knowledge; all other forms of knowledge are judged as being merely speculation, opinion, or not what can be conceptualized as knowledge. If this myth did not have a strong hold on us, we would long ago have begun serious work to develop other ways of knowing.

Science has served well to debunk myths perpetuated by the ancient philosophies and religions, and it is undoubtedly an effective way to obtain knowledge. However, science as the supreme end in and of itself has produced knowledge that has not turned out to be in the best human interest; indeed it has been used to create planetwide contamination and has brought us to the brink of worldwide destruction.

The method for debunking the myth of scientific supremacy is to insist on the integration of all patterns of knowing into the whole of knowing. The patterns of knowing described by Carper (see Chapter 1) derive from our own nursing literature and serve well as a basis for envisioning that which is possible. Any one patten of knowing used in isolation of the others is an incomplete, partial form of knowing. All patterns must be integrated to create what I would call Knowledge. Each pattern requires its own process of discovery and its own method for determining what is credible, as distinguished from isolated fantasy:

- Empirical knowledge is determined to be credible using empirical validation. This process requires verification—agreement that what is observed by one person in one situation is replicable in other instances by other observers. The evidence used to judge credibility is what we know as reliability and validity.
- Ethical knowledge is determined to be credible by the method of justification. The philosophic and logical premises surrounding an ethical dilemma are stated explicitly, and from these are derived logical evidence that justifies a decision, or a conclusion. Other observers do not have to agree with the decision, but the decision, the evidence that produces the decision, and the logic used must be judged to be responsible and just.
- Esthetics is judged to be credible through the method of criticism. Criticism as used in the arts is directed toward knowing, making explicit, exposing the meaning of the creative process/product. Consensus, or agreement between observers, related to meaning is not required but, for the criticism to function as a method for revealing credible esthetic meaning, consistency must exist between the expressions of the esthetic process and the criticism of it.
- Personal knowledge is determined to be credible through introspection. Introspection makes it possible to integrate and actualize that which is experienced in relation to others and the self. As introspection occurs, the authenticity of the self is revealed, and personal knowledge is actualized.

Myth 5: The Myth of Empirical Evidence

The myth of empirical evidence is the belief that "what is" is that which is observable through sensory experience, and whatever is not observable through sensory experience does not exist. Furthermore, whatever is observable is measurable; it is quantifiable. The fundamental usefulness of empirical validation of phenomena is not to be rejected, but the myth represents a good idea gone wild. The myth extends the value of empirical validation of phenomena to encompass the belief that, if something cannot be empirically validated, it does not exist or is not worth pursuing. Further, the myth sustains the tendency to proclaim that something either is or is not empirically accessible when in reality phenomena are relatively accessible to empirical knowing. Science has stimulated ideas that give rise to possibilities for empirical validation long before empirical validation is possible; we call this the discovery of instrumentation, or methods for empirical observation. As we have moved into areas of knowledge that are relatively inaccessible, we create methods that are increasingly indirect in relation to the phenomena, still naming the indirect measure "empirical evidence" to justify the scientific nature of our enterprise. Once this is done, we call the phenomenon empirically validated: It exists.

As we leap through these mental exercises, we fail to seriously confront the artifacts that are created in the process of "empirical validation." I am not arguing that highly abstract phenomena (eg, health or motive) cannot and should not be empirically validated; nor do I reject scholarly work in this direction; but I reject the assumption that empirical tools or observations are adequate to create comprehensive knowledge about these phenomena. I also question the assumption that empirical evidence itself will produce accurate knowledge.

The method for confronting the myth of empirical evidence is to recognize the limitations of empirical evidence in relation to developing knowledge and to value other ways of knowing related to the phenomena that we are exploring. As we recognize the limitations of empirical evidence, we can begin to untangle distortions that are created by artifacts of empirical validation. The untangling process will include improvements in our approaches to obtain empirical evidence as well as open possibilities for knowledge that do not derive from empirical evidence. I submit that our body of knowledge about a phenomenon such as "motive" in relation to health will ultimately require strong, sound empirical evidence free of artifacts. But the complex keys to understanding this and other phenomena do not reside solely within the scope of empirical validation. The key to understanding these complex phenomena requires integration of the methods of justification, criticism, and introspection as well.

Myth 6: The Myth of Higher Authority

The myth of higher authority governs the scientific enterprise in a number of ways. It perpetuates ethical, empirical, and moral dishonesty. Most scholarly work begins with a review of "authoritative" literature, and we use the authority of existing literature to justify everything we do. The halo effect that an idea or a belief acquires by being published is a remarkable transition that I can only perceive as being magic.

The very fact of being engaged in the academic/ scientific enterprise confers a societally sanctioned myth of authority. We are in a position to give or withhold information at will, to use, coerce, and manipulate people with little if any challenge to our authority. Even the language we use in research communicates authority—control, manipulation (of variables, conditions, numbers, people), inference, standardization, operationalization, subjects, instruments.

Being a scientist also confers the authority to assign value judgments and worth to phenomena, ideas, or things. The act of measuring produces dichotomous thinking, or hierarchical assignment of value. We speak of high and low, we rank order things and assign values to those things without questioning the meaning of the valuing or the contextual possibilities that might exist or be created by our valuing. This myth has made it possible for male scientists to assign the value of "the norm" to maleness. Simply assigning a value does not make a thing true or right, but assigning a value often creates the illusion of truth or rightness.

The method for debunking the myth of higher authority is to place ourselves in the position of the grassroots people with whom we work, or for whom our knowledge might have the most direct effect. In essence, this strategy is one of ethical justification, esthetic criticism, and personal introspection. We must reverse the myth that the scientific enterprise is by definition a higher authority and that the scientist by definition has rights or authorities that are different from those of any other individual. Once we make this shift in our thinking, we can examine how well our approaches, our methods, our conclusions are consistent with experiential reality.

Myth 7: The Myth of Significance

The myth of significance is most clearly recognized by examining the statistical concept of significance. When we are told that something is significant at the .01 level of probability, it assumes a halo effect of significance far beyond the strictly technical and statistical meaning of the term. The statistician and the researcher (we hope) know the limitations and restrictive meanings of the term *significance* in a statistical sense. However, scientists rarely adhere to the strict statistical meaning in interpreting their results. As long as the results reach statistical significance, the findings have meaning. If the results do not reach statistical significance, the findings must be explained and have little meaning. The "significance" of the results of studies is used to imply not the statistical concept but the more common language understanding of the term: that it is important. Rarely does anyone ask, Significant for what, for whom, in what context? We seldom ask for what purpose, or in whose interest, the scientific enterprise has been directed. These factors are critical in determining how much importance we attach to the results of our research—those that are statistically significant as well as those that are not.

The method for debunking the myth of significance is to apply the test of importance in relation to future-search purposes and goals regardless of the statistical findings. By shifting our attention to the importance of the research, we can detect ways in which the research may or may not contribute to knowledge that can create the kind of world in which we wish to live and work.

We will dis-cover many subtle ways in which our scientific enterprise limits the universality of the theories and the generalizability of the research. A statistically significant study that is based on white, male, middle-class values, that draws on a white, male, middle-class population (as in much nursing research), probably has little or no meaning, much less importance, for the majority of people in this world who are not white, middle-class, or male.

WHY DEBUNK MYTHS?

In conclusion, l want to acknowledge that there are pitfalls in taking a skeptical view of the status quo, even though scientists are by definition supposed to be skeptical. My interpretations of the myths of the scientific enterprise are deliberately severe to stimulate awareness of the actual behavioral practices of many scientists and the flaws in that which we take to be truth. I have not recommended the abandonment of science, but I do recommend that we equally credit the limitations of this method. By debunking the myths of science, we will find critical areas for new applications of that which is valuable in the scientific method and ways of integrating other patterns of knowing.

The fundamental question is not why we should question and challenge the myths of the scientific enterprise but why not? Why not conceptualize the purposes and the goals of our research and theory in terms of the world that we want to create? Why not seriously value other ways of knowing? Why not value nursing and health? Why not identify actions, behaviors, and assumptions that we know to be consistent with health and behave as scientists in ways that are consistent with our vision? I believe that we are already beginning to do this; and if we choose to, we will increasingly focus our energies in this direction.

Acknowledgments

This article was adapted from a presentation given at the Research Day sponsored by Sigma Theta Tau Alpha Nu Chapter, Villanova University, Villanova, Pennsylvania, November 2, 1984. The author wishes to acknowledge the contributions of Charlene Eldridge Wheeler in conceptualizing the myths; of Barbara Carper in critiquing the methods for determining credibility of ethical, esthetic, and personal knowledge; and of the members of the Nursing Theory Think Tank for discussion that prompted the development of this article.

REFERENCES

Carper, B. (1978). Fundamental patterns of knowing in nursing. *Advances in Nursing Science, 1*(1), 13-23. [Chapter 4 of this book]

Dock, L. (1915). Foreign department. *American Journal of Nursing, 15*(8), 666.

Gilligan, C. (1982). *In a different voice: Psychological theory and women's development.* Cambridge, MA: Harvard University Press.

Gorenberg, B. (1983). The research tradition of nursing: An emerging issue. *Nursing Research, 32*(6), 347-349.

Heide, W. S. (1982). *Feminism for the health of it.* Ann Arbor, Michigan, University Microfilms International, 1982. Also in preparation for publication (revised) by Margaretdaughters, Inc., P.O. Box 70, Buffalo, NY, 14222.

Munhall. P. L. (1982). Nursing philosophy and nursing research: In apposition or opposition? *Nursing Research, 31*(3), 176-177.

————. (1983). Methodological fallacies: A critical self-appraisal. *Advances in Nursing Science, 5*(4). 41-50.

Newman, M. (1979). *Theory development in nursing.* Philadelphia: F. A. Davis.

Smith, M. C. (1984). Research methodology: Epistemologic considerations. *Image: The Journal of Nursing Scholarship, 16*(2), 42-46.

Smith, M. J. (1984). Transformation: A key to shaping nursing. *Image: The Journal of Nursing Scholarship. 16*(1), 28-30.

Spender, D. (1980). *Man made language.* Boston: Routledge and Kegan Paul.

————. (1981). *Men's studies modified.* New York: Pergamon Press.

Tinkle, M. B., & Beaton, J. L. (1983). Toward a new view of Science: Implications for nursing research. *Advances in Nursing Science, 5*(2), 27-36.

Vredevoe, D. L. (1984). Curology: A basic science related to nursing. *Image: The Journal of Nursing Scholarship. 16*(3), 89-92.

Webster, G., Jacox, A. & Baldwin, B. (1981). Nursing theory and the ghost of the received view. In H. K. Grace & J. C. McCloskey (Eds.), *Current Issues in Nursing.* Boston: Blackwell Scientific Publications.

Webster's New Collegiate Dictionary. (1981). Springfield. MA: G.C. Merriam Co.

8

(Mis)Conceptions and Reconceptions about Traditional Science

KAREN L. SCHUMACHER, RN, MS

SUSAN R. GORTNER, RN, PhD, FAAN

"Traditional" science (ie, scientific work that has evolved from the natural sciences) is still said to rely on theory-neutral facts, quantitative data, and the search for universal laws. This depiction of science is incongruent with much contemporary thinking. This chapter examines three shifts in philosophy that are relevant for nursing science philosophy: the move from foundationalism to an understanding of the fallibility of science, the shift in emphasis from verification to justification of knowledge claims, and the examination of explanation by scientific realists. It is suggested that scientific realism may be a fruitful area of inquiry for philosophers of nursing science.

The past decade has witnessed significant commentary on the nature of nursing science and appropriate modes of inquiry, much of which has been published in *Advances in Nursing Science*. Part of the commentary has been directed toward philosophical foundations for nursing science that may be more consonant with the human state than with nature in general[1-7] and has resulted in publication of positions on Heideggerian/phenomenological philosophy,[8,9] critical social theory[10,11] and feminism.[12] In some essays, the approach to science that might be called "traditional" is portrayed as a static and monolithic entity, serving mostly as a foil against which to describe the philosophical position of the author(s).[13,14] As a result, the nursing literature lacks a systematic account of the philosophical underpinnings of the approach to science that evolved from the natural sciences.

This chapter seeks to balance the discourse about philosophical foundations for nursing science with a description of contemporary or postpositivistic thinking in the philosophy of science. Specifically, it identifies three misconceptions in the nursing critique of traditional science: the purported use of theory-neutral observations, the privilege granted quantitative data in warranting knowledge, and the search for universal laws. It argues that characterizing science in these ways is incongruent with contemporary philosophy of science and suggests some alternative ideas that may provide impetus for philosophical discourse around nursing science.

Before the discussion, however, a clarification of terminology is in order. Numerous terms are used to describe the philosophical basis for

Source: Schumacher, K. L., & Gortner, S. R. (1992). (Mis)conceptions and reconceptions about traditional science. *ANS, 14* (1): 1-11. Reprinted with permission from and copyright © 1992 Aspen Publishers, Inc.

what is referred to above as "traditional" science. *Empiricism, postempiricism, postpositivism, Cartesianism, objectivism, analytic empiricism,* and *naturalism* are terms used to denote a philosophy of science or an epistemological perspective associated with "scientific method," "empirical research," or simply "science." Even the term *logical positivism* continues to be used as a label[13,14] although logical positivism is generally considered to be dead as a philosophical movement.[6,15,16] While it cannot expect to clear up the terminological confusion, this essay will attempt to avoid falling prey to it. What is referred to as "traditional" science is the epistemological tradition that there is a world "out there" characterized to some extent by patterns and regularities; that it can be known, albeit imperfectly; and that knowing requires the mental discipline imposed by precision, logic, and attention to evidence. In this respect, "traditional" science is distinguished from personal opinion or private experience. This discussion uses the term *science* in the manner in which it is used by Ziman: "Science is public knowledge . . . a consensus of rational opinion over the widest possible field."[17(pp30,31)] In this respect, science is derived from a long intellectual tradition that began with attempts to know about the natural or physical world. However, no analogy is implied here between the physical world and human life. It is the use of disciplined reasoning and observation to discover and explain regularities in the world that makes science what it is. Although the phenomena of interest vary across scientific disciplines and may serve to establish disciplinary boundaries, the nature of scientific thinking has many similarities across disciplines.

FOUNDATIONALISM IN SCIENCE

One way in which "traditional" science has been characterized by some nursing scholars is in terms of its reliance on theory-neutral facts.[3,9] For example, Allen, Benner, and Diekelmann assert that "a statement can only be properly regarded as scientific if its truth or falsity can be ascertained by means of theory-neutral observations."[3(p25)] In this statement they implicitly refer to an epistemology that is foundationalist in that observation is seen as an indubitable source of knowledge. Empiricism in its classical sense was a philosophical doctrine that considered observation to be the foundation of knowledge.[18] Logical positivism was a twentieth-century variant of empiricism that combined an emphasis on observation as the source of knowledge with a logical analysis of the meaning of observation sentences.[19] Knowledge thus secured was considered infallible and led to the belief that certainty in science was possible.

The positivist doctrine that knowledge could be achieved with certainty by basing it on observations has been challenged on a number of fronts by postpositivistic philosophers of science. In nursing, the postpositivist refutation of the claim that there are theory-neutral observations or "brute facts" has been accurately described by Weekes[20] and Thompson.[4] The rejection of the positivistic notion that there are "basic statements" that constitute facts about the "immediately given" rests primarily on the distinction between sensory experience and the cognitive process of perception. As Kuhn put it: "As for a pure observation language, perhaps one will yet be devised. But three centuries after Descartes our hope for such an eventuality still depends exclusively upon a theory of perception and of the mind. And modern psychological experimentation is rapidly proliferating phenomena with which that theory can scarcely deal."[21(p126)] Hanson[22] gives a detailed argument against the notion of theory-neutral observations, showing that what one "observes" depends on perception rather than simply on retinal images. Furthermore, perception, or what stands out as relevant and significant, is a function of one's prior knowledge and experience, which in turn influences how one conceptually organizes sensory experience. If it were not so, we would be bombarded with chaotic, unintelligible sensory data.

Another problem with the idea of theory-neutral observations pertains to the use of instruments to aid the senses.[23-26] Many entities, while unobservable to the unaided human senses, can readily be observed with the aid of instruments. Thus, what must be considered unobservable and therefore theoretical at one point in history may become observable when an appropriate instrument is developed. For example, the cellular constituents of blood, unobservable before the invention of the microscope, are now considered observable. However, such observation presupposes a host of theories about the optics of the microscope as well as the appearance of the cells themselves. Thus, observation with the aid of an instrument can in no way be considered theory-neutral.

The idea that there is no theory-neutral observation language is now widely accepted by philosophers of science as diverse as Popper,[27] Kuhn,[21] Bernstein,[28] and Hanson.[22] The problems identified above have led Newton-Smith to propose that observation and theory, while essentially indistinguishable, may be, for practical purposes, thought of as a continuum ranging from the more observational to the more theoretical. The more observable an entity is, the easier it is to decide with confidence whether it applies, the less reliance on instruments is needed, and the easier it is to grasp the nature of the entity without learning a scientific theory.[25]

Two important (and widely accepted) conclusions resulted from the foregoing philosophical work on the nature of observation: there are no theory-neutral facts and there are no absolute knowledge sources. Thus, to claim that science is based on theory-neutral facts is to refer back to a philosophy of science that has been widely discredited. A more contemporary understanding of science is that articulated by Popper.[27] He proposed a fallibilistic conception of knowledge that is nonfoundational in that there are no ultimate sources of knowledge. Instead, science progresses through the elimination of error as successive theories are found to be false and replaced with better theories. Thus, science is a rational endeavor by virtue of its critical attitude, not by the certainty conferred by "brute facts."

THE WARRANTS FOR KNOWLEDGE

In the confusion following the demise of a foundational approach to philosophy of science, there is the risk of going to either of two extremes: radical skepticism or radical subjectivism.[28] However, neither of these extremes is necessary. In the aftermath of positivism, philosophers of science have turned their attention from the origins and foundation of knowledge to concern with the justification of knowledge claims.[18] In other words, a knowledge claim is judged on the merits of the evidence brought to bear on it. This point is essential for understanding contemporary philosophy of science. Its importance is based on the premise that scientific knowledge is public in nature, representing rational, informed, interconsensual opinion.[17,29] It is the justification of knowledge claims or "marshalling good reason in their behalf"[18(p17)] that separates science from private understanding and ideology. The assertion that knowledge claims in science must be warranted is a fundamental assumption in contemporary philosophy of science. However, to say that knowledge claims must be warranted is not to say that there is one privileged way of warranting them that applies equally to all knowledge claims. To establish a scientific knowledge claim, the scientist assembles evidence in its support. But what is the contemporary understanding of evidence?

Certainly observation continues to be an important element in the evidence brought to bear in support of a knowledge claim.[18,27,29,30] However, in the literature pertaining to the warrants for knowledge claims, one can detect a shift in language from the earlier exclusive use of the term *observation* to the more contemporary term *evidence*. It is useful to think of support for scientific theories in terms of evidence rather than observation alone, because "evidence" is a more inclusive term; it admits additional types of support for theories such as self-report by the subject, through either questionnaire or interview, as well as the use of reason. Further, it is not as encumbered with philosophical history as is the term *observation*. Implied is the assumption that the scientist has considerable latitude in deciding what evidence is needed to evaluate a particular knowledge claim.

Thinking broadly about evidence is important in nursing science, because it allows discourse to shift away from the truism that many phenomena cannot be reduced to sense data or observational terms. More fruitful are discussions about what constitutes "good evidence" for the existence and nature of a phenomenon. For example, family coping processes cannot be reduced to observable terms without losing much of what is inherent in the phenomenon. Such a loss of substantive information is unacceptable. On the other hand, it is not the case that "anything goes" when the scientist is investigating coping processes. The reasonable scientist would want to know what evidence about coping was brought to bear on the research question.

One of the most egregious assumptions about traditional science is that it constitutes a paradigm that disallows the use of qualitative data. This assumption tends to confound method with philosophical perspective and to promote the idea that using both linguistic and numerical data to address a research question violates fundamental philosophical assump-

tions of one perspective or the other. This assumption supports a "purist" position regarding appropriate data forms and limits the scope of inquiry.[10,31] While it may be the case that qualitative data are the sine qua non of phenomenological research, it is not true that data forms in "traditional" research have to be quantitative. Even though much scientific work within this framework is quantitative and even though some seemingly absurd efforts have been made to reduce mental phenomena to observable physiological parameters, there is no philosophical or historical basis for the supposed identification of traditional science with quantitative methods.[32,33] Research using inductive reasoning based on naturalistic observations and field notes has a respected place in modern science, going back at least as far as the nineteenth-century biologists. In field work or naturalistic research with persons it is reasonable and necessary to talk with them to elicit their experiences, subjective states, and meanings. The use of such data does not necessarily depart from the canons of traditional science.[34] It simply introduces a uniquely human form of data.

Although traditional science does not require the use of quantitative data, it does require that the scientist examine the evidence brought to bear on a particular question and ask whether it supports the claims of the scientist. One of the considerations in the examination of evidence is whether it is of sufficient scope to adequately address the phenomenon under study. While not identified specifically as such, the scope of scientific evidence has been an implied consideration in the concerns about appropriate data in nursing and other disciplines addressing social phenomena. Specifically, writings about qualitative and quantitative data, multimethod research, and triangulation are implicit efforts to increase the acceptable scope of evidence. Some writers, however, go beyond issues of the nature and scope of evidence and attempt to relate type of evidence to a specific scientific paradigm with the implication that that paradigm determines the type of evidence that is acceptable. Further, qualitative research is sometimes thought to constitute a paradigm rather than a type of evidence.[35]

The type of evidence used by the scientist (ie, numerical or linguistic data) should not be dependent on that paradigm, but rather on the phenomenon under investigation and the specific research question. This position is not novel, but reaffirms what Meleis has called a "passion for substance"[36] rather than philosophy or technique. Some research problems require evidence that is broad in scope in order to draw sound conclusions. In other investigations the need to achieve precision may require evidence that is more narrow in scope. Such decisions have no dogmatic "decision rules" to guide the investigator, nor is there anything in contemporary philosophy of science that requires them. Instead, they are left to the professional judgment of the scientist in the design of studies and to the community of scholars in judgment of investigational findings.

UNIVERSALITY

Traditional science has also been characterized in terms of its search for universal laws that predict and explain phenomena regardless of context.[3,9,37] For example, in describing what they refer to as Paradigm I science, Tinkle and Beaton claim that "this paradigm adopts the view that there is a body of facts and principles to be discovered and understood that are independent of any historical or social context. This search for truth seeks principles that are abstract, general, and universal."[3(p28)]

There are at least two issues inherent in the idea of universal laws. The first is the issue of universality itself, which is often held up as the antithesis of the contextual, historical understanding of human phenomena that nursing seeks. Traditional science is said to isolate phenomena from their contexts for investigation, the results of which are findings then considered "universal" rather than context dependent.

Recent philosophy of science suggests that the reality of universal laws may be as elusive as theory-neutral observations proved to be, even in the physical sciences. Addressing the problem of laws in physics, Cartwright[38] claims that true "laws" are scarce. She goes on to show that statements of lawful relationships usually are qualified by a *ceteris paribus* statement, which says that "all things being equal" such and such a relationship holds. Since all things are often not equal, it is up to the scientist to determine the conditions under which a certain pattern occurs and the conditions under which it changes. Such determinations are required in science in general and are not a special feature of the human sciences. Indeed, Cartwright notes that "I imagine that natural objects are much like people in societies. Their behavior is constrained by some specific laws and by a handful of general principles, but it is not determined in detail, even statistically."[38(p49)]

Even though the belief in universal laws may be misplaced, generalization of findings beyond the particular study sample is clearly valued in traditional approaches to science. If generalization were not allowed it would be difficult for clinicians to use the findings of research not conducted with their own patients. But as noted by Gortner, "all inference is context dependent in some sense."[6] Thus there must be some middle ground of generalization between universal law and the findings in a particular sample. Rather than thinking in terms of universal law, the reasonable scientist asks, To whom can these findings legitimately be generalized?

Although it is a misconception to say that contemporary science is by nature "acontextual," it is probably accurate to say that the way in which "context" is understood varies among investigators. Benner[8] describes person and context as inseparable and mutually constitutive, whereas in traditional science, person and situation variables are frequently isolated for study. While the importance of this distinction should not be discounted, it is an oversimplification to claim that traditional science always seeks universal relationships regardless of the situation. It is more fruitful to ask, What does the incorporation of context into a nursing investigation mean? Is it the inclusion of situational variables? Narrative description of the context from the perspectives of the participants? Both?

The second issue inherent in discussions of universal laws is that of causality and explanation. Statements of law in the classic manner described by Hempel[39,40] and Putnam[41] purport not only to make statements about regularities, but to explain them. In other words, laws deal with the "whys" of phenomena, not simply their occurrence. There is a long and complex tradition in philosophy on causation and explanation, which is beyond the scope of this article. Here we do not argue for a given form of explanation, but simply claim that the idea of causation is necessary in nursing science because of its relevance for clinical practice. Clinicians would be hampered indeed if they did not know the likely consequences of certain events (eg, states, behaviors) under given conditions.

The relevance of explanation for nursing science is based on the argument that causative states or processes are precisely where intervention should be aimed.[23] At the physiological level, the causative relationship between bed rest, diminished ventilation, and postoperative pneumonia has led to the intervention of early ambulation after surgery. At the social level, the lack of social support explains (partially) caregiver depression and has led to the intervention of support groups for caregivers. Illustrative examples like these suggest that causation is simply a matter of a linear relationship, which is not the case. Causation in human science is complex, multifaceted, and possibly multidirectional. However, these difficulties should not deter us from its consideration because it is necessary for clinically relevant science.

A current debate in philosophy of science that has received little attention in nursing may prove useful in thinking about explanation and causation. We refer to the debate between scientific realism and antirealism. The arguments presented shift discourse in philosophy of science away from questions like "How can science be rational if there are no absolute sources of knowledge?" to questions like "What is real?" and "What is the status of theoretical entities in science?"[23(p1)] One of the major distinctions between scientific realism and antirealism is the way in which theoretical entities are understood. (In the language of scientific realism, the term *theoretical entity* usually means unobservable entities, states, or processes.) The differing views on theoretical entities have implications for the respective positions on explanation and causality, as shown below.

The antirealists deny the existence of unobservable entities or processes and avoid issues of causality, claiming that scientific theories can describe and predict, but not explain.[23] To take this perspective it is necessary to maintain, to some extent, the distinction between observation and theory because, typically, antirealists assert that the notion of truth or falsity is relevant to observation even though it is not relevant to theory.[25,26,42] One of the most serious consequences of an antirealist construction of theories is that theories cannot explain.[23,25] Because the existence of any explanatory processes "behind" the observable phenomena is denied, science can legitimately only describe and predict observable entities. The logical positivists were antirealists who tried to disallow any discussion of theoretical entities in science, taking instead the extreme empirical position that what is real is observable. Since scientists regularly use theoretical terms (*electron* is the term often used as an example), the logical positivists modified their early position to that of instrumentalism. Instrumentalism is a type of antirealism that claims that theoretical terms are appropriately thought of as instruments, tools, or calculating devices, useful for systematizing and relating observations and for making predictions,[43] but that they do not refer to anything really existent. Since the logical positivists denied the existence of anything "behind" observables, they were opposed to discussions of causes and downplayed explanation.[23] It is the positivists' antirealism that makes their views inappropriate for nursing science. It is not possible in positivism to deal with the subjective aspects of persons, nor with perceived relational processes, nor with explanations without translating them into physiological states or behaviors.

On the other hand, scientific realists claim that unobservable (ie, theoretical) entities or processes have existence; moreover, it is these unobservable processes that often provide explanations for observable phenomena.[23,25,42] Thus, scientific realist discussions of causation focus on unobservable processes. There are three ingredients in scientific realism: ontological, epistemological, and causal.[23,25]

The ontological ingredient of scientific realism makes the claim that the unobservable entities represented by theoretical terms really exist. According to Boyd, the realist thinks of theoretical terms in scientific theories as

> putatively referring to expressions; that is, scientific theories should be interpreted 'realistically.' Scientific theories, interpreted realistically, are confirmable and in fact are often confirmed as approximately true. The reality which scientific theories describe is largely independent of our thoughts or theoretical commitments.[26(pp41-42)]

In other words, even though knowledge is always fallible, something like the phenomena postulated by science really exist. Thus, the realist claims that the scientist makes discoveries about the world as it really is.[42]

The epistemological ingredient of scientific realism relates to the notion of verisimilitude or "approximation to the truth."[25,27] Although the "truth" can never be fully established by virtue of the fallibility of all human knowledge, the idea of truth does not need to be abandoned. Rather, the scientist can employ the notion of truth as a regulative ideal, seeking to get closer to the truth by the successive development of better and better theories. In other words, we can, in principle, have warranted belief in theories.[23]

Finally, the causal ingredient of scientific realism relates to the explanatory power of theories. The theoretical or unobservable entities of a theory are causally responsible for, that is, they explain, observable phenomena.[23] If, as the positivists claimed, science can only describe and predict, it does not provide any guidance for intervention if something different from the predicted state is desired. For example, one could predict that mothers who engage actively in a career will be tired and stressed. But if intervention to change this situation for mothers is desired, a deeper understanding is required than prediction allows. The authors agree with Hacking's assertion that the relationship between unobservable theoretical entities and intervention is what makes scientific realism relevant for the practice of science. For the positivist, what is real is simply what can be observed. For the scientific realist, what affects us and what we can affect are also real, whether or not they can be observed.[23] Acknowledging this level of reality leads the scientist to deeper, more probing questions about it.

The interest here is in the causal and epistemological ingredients of scientific realism, because they support the claims that explanations are important in nursing science and practice and that the aim of the scientist is to discover better and better explanations (ie, closer approximations to the truth). However, the reader may well discern metaphysical overtones in the ontological question of whether what is unobservable exists, and a brief comment on these is appropriate. According to Hackling,[23] the current interest in antirealism and scientific realism among philosophers represents a shift in focus away from the rationality of science to consideration of what is "real." This shift raises metaphysical questions that philosophers of science have traditionally been reluctant to address. However, the way in which metaphysical questions are answered has implications for the claims of philosophers about what scientists can attempt to discover. The Enlightenment empiricists, especially Hume and Newton,[23] tried to dispense with the vague idea of "cause" and direct scientific inquiry to description and prediction through observation. The logical positivists were determined to rid science of metaphysics once and for all through their verification principle of meaning,[44] an attempt that failed because the verification principle was unverifiable by its own standards and therefore meaningless. Popper, a realist, argued with the logical positivists, claiming that metaphysical questions are important for science in that they often lead to deeper and more insightful inquiry.[45] The "metaphysical turn" in the philosophy of science of recent decades may be worth pursuing in nursing as we try to reconcile our perspective on human beings and human health with nursing science. Nursing scholars can explore scientific realism for the insights it may provide for a philosophy of nursing science. For now, we propose that scientific realism is relevant to nursing science in the following ways:

1. It supports the full range of nursing theory: descriptive, predictive, and explanatory.
2. It affirms the importance of including subjective client states in nursing theory and refutes the claim of the positivists that if it is not observable, it does not exist.
3. It adds the idea of the *substantive* content of explanations to discussions about *forms* of explanation.
4. It includes the notion of truth as a regulative ideal in science and claims that better theories are theories that are closer to the truth. In other words, some theories are better than others and the task of the scientist is to determine as well as possible which they are.

CONCLUSIONS

Traditional science along with its philosophical underpinnings is not the static and monolithic entity that it is sometimes portrayed as. As philosophy of science has become increasingly aligned with the practices of working scientists, its claims for science have become more moderate and qualified. Three significant developments in philosophy of science have occurred in the postpositivist era: the move from foundationalism to an understanding of the fallibility of science, the shift in emphasis from verification to justification of knowledge claims, and the recent examination of explanation by scientific realists. These developments are relevant for nursing science in that they are consonant with such nursing concerns as the appropriate warrants for knowledge, the generalization of research results, and explanation/causation. The issues addressed by scientific realism may be a fruitful area of philosophical inquiry for nurse scholars.

REFERENCES

1. Holmes CA. Alternatives to natural science foundations for nursing. *Int J Nurs Stud.* 1990; 27(3):187-198.
2. Munhall, PL. Nursing philosophy and nursing research: In apposition or opposition? *Nurs Res.* 1982;31(3); 176-181.
3. Allen D, Benner P, Diekelmann N. Three paradigms for nursing research: Methodological considerations. In: Chinn PL, ed. *Nursing Research Methodology: Issues and Explanation.* Rockville, Md: Aspen Publishers; 1986.
4. Thompson JL. Practical discourse on nursing: Going beyond empiricism and historicism. *ANS.* 1985;7(4):59-71.
5. Silva MC, Rothbart D. An analysis of changing trends in philosophies of science on nursing theory development and testing. *ANS.* 1984;6(2): 1-13.
6. Gortner SR. Knowledge in a practice discipline: Philosophy and pragmatics. In: *Nursing Research and Policy Formation: The Case of Prospective Payment.* Papers of the 1983 Scientific Session of the American Academy of Nursing. Kansas City, Mo: American Academy of Nursing; 1983.
7. Watson J. Nursing's scientific quest. *Nurs Outlook.* 1981;29(7):413-416.
8. Benner P. Quality of life: a phenomenological perspective on explanation, prediction, and understanding in nursing science. *ANS.* 1985; 8(1):1-14.
9. Leonard VW. A Heideggerian pheneomenlogic perspective on the concept of person. *ANS.* 1989;11(4):40-55.
10. Moccia P. A critique of compromise: Beyond the methods debate. *ANS.* 1988;10(4):1-9.
11. Stevens PE. A critical social reconceptualization of environment in nursing: Implications for methodology. *ANS.* 1989;11(4):56-68.
12. Bunting S, Campbell JC. Feminism and nursing: Historical perspectives. *ANS.* 1990;12(4):11-24.
13. Dzurec LC. The necessity for and evolution of multiple paradigms for nursing research: A poststructuralist perspective. *ANS.* 1989;11(4): 69-77.
14. Samecky MT. Historiography: A legitimate research methodology for nursing. *ANS.* 1990; 12(4):1-10.
15. Phillips DC. After the wake: Postpositivistic educational thought. *Educ Res.* 1983;12(5):4-12.
16. van Fraassen BC. *The Scientific Image.* Oxford, England: Clarendon Press; 1980.
17. Ziman J. What is science? In: Klemke ED, Hollinger R, Kline AD, eds. *Introductory Readings in the Philosophy of Science.* Buffalo, NY: Prometheus Books; 1980.
18. Phillips DC. *Philosophy, Science, and Social Inquiry.* Oxford, England: Pergamon Press; 1987.
19. Ayer AJ. Editor's introduction. In: Ayer AJ, ed. *Logical Positivism.* New York, NY: Free Press; 1959.
20. Weekes DP. Theory-free observation: Fact or fantasy? In: Chinn PL, ed. *Nursing Research Methodology: Issues and Explanation.* Rockville, Md: Aspen Publishers; 1986.
21. Kuhn TS. *The Structure of Scientific Revolutions.* 2nd ed. Chicago, Ill: University of Chicago Press; 1970.
22. Hanson NR. *Patterns of Discovery.* Cambridge, England: Cambridge University Press; 1958.
23. Hacking I. *Representing and Intervening.* Cambridge, England: Cambridge University Press; 1983.
24. Maxwell G. The ontological status of theoretical entities. In: Klemke ED, Hollinger R, Kline AD, eds. *Introductory Readings in the Philosophy of Science.* Buffalo, NY: Prometheus Books; 1980.
25. Newton-Smith WH. *The Rationality of Science.* London, England: Routledge & Kegan Paul; 1981.
26. Boyd, RN. The current status of scientific realism. In: Leplin J, ed. *Scientific Realism.* Berkeley, Calif: University of California Press; 1984.
27. Popper KR. *Conjectures and Refutations: The Growth of Scientific Knowledge.* New York, NY: Harper & Row; 1963.
28. Bernstein RJ. *Beyond Objectivism and Relativism: Science, Hermeneutics, and Praxis.* Philadelphia, Pa: University of Pennsylvania Press; 1988.
29. Gortner SR. Nursing values and science: Toward a science philosophy. *Image.* 1990;22(2):101-105.
30. Schultz PR, Meleis AI. Nursing epistemology: Traditions, insights, questions. *Image.* 1988;20(4): 217-221.
31. Phillips JR. Research blenders. *Nurs Sci Quart.* 1988;1:4-5.
32. Gortner SR. Nursing's syntax revisited: A critique. *Int J Nurs Stud.* In review.
33. Suppe F. Presented at the first symposium on knowledge development in nursing; September, 1990; Newport, RI.
34. Gortner SR, Schultz PR. Approaches to nursing science methods. *Image.* 1988;20(1):22-24.

35. Guba EC. The alternative paradigm dialog. In: Guba EG, ed. *The Paradigm Dialog*. Newbury Park, Calif: Sage; 1990.

36. Meleis AI. ReVisions in knowledge development: A passion for substance. *Sch Inq Nurs Pract*. 1987;1(1):5-19.

37. Tinkle MB, Beaton JL. Toward a new view of science: Implications for nursing research. *ANS*. 1983;5(2):27-36.

38. Cartwright N. *How the Laws of Physics Lie*. New York, NY: Oxford University Press; 1983.

39. Hempel C. *Philosophy of Natural Science*. Englewood Cliffs, NJ: Prentice Hall; 1966.

40. ————. *Aspects of Scientific Explanation*. New York; NY: Free Press; 1965.

41. Putnam H. The corroboration of theories. In: Hacking I, ed. *Scientific Revolutions*. New York, NY: Oxford University Press; 1981.

42. McMullin E. A case for scientific realism. In: Leplin J, ed. *Scientific Realism*. Berkeley, Calif: University of California Press; 1984.

43. Hesse M. Laws and theories. In Edwards P, ed. *The Encyclopaedia of Philosophy*. New York, NY: Macmillan; 1967.

44. Camap, R, Pap A, trans. The elimination of metaphysics through logical analysis of language. In: Ayer AJ, ed. *Logical Positivism*. New York, NY: Free Press; 1959.

45. Popper KR. Metaphysics and criticizability. In: Miller D, ed. *Popper Selections*. Princeton, NJ: Princeton University Press; 1985.

9

Nursing Science: Basic, Applied, or Practical? Implications for the Art of Nursing

JOY L. JOHNSON, RN, PhD

Nursing has long been described as both a science and an art. If the science of nursing is to be relevant to the art of nursing, then it must be conceptualized and pursued such that these two central components of nursing remain connected. Current conceptualizations of nursing science are examined in terms of the consequences that each conceptualization might have for the art of nursing. Pursuing nursing science as a basic science or an applied science disarticulates the science of nursing and the art of nursing. The author concludes that only if nursing science is conceptualized and pursued as a practical science will the science of nursing be consistently relevant to the art of nursing.

The nature of nursing science has been a subject of debate among nursing's scholars for over 25 years. Early debate focused on the question of whether nursing is a basic or an applied science. In recent years, a third alternative has been suggested, namely, that nursing is a practical science. Although some nurses have recently dismissed the entire issue regarding the nature of nursing science, arguing that pursuit of such an issue is either counterproductive or inconsequential, it is the opinion of this author that the proper resolution of this issue is essential to the advancement of the nursing discipline. As Schlotfeldt correctly stated, "There can be little doubt that one of the highest priorities for creating an appropriate future for nursing is that of identifying, structuring, and continuously advancing the knowledge that underlies the practices of professionals in the field."[1(p35)]

It is generally agreed that one important component of the nursing discipline is nursing science.[2] As such, the manner in which nursing science is conceptualized will determine the priorities for scientific nursing research and provide a measure for determining the relevance of various scientific research questions to the discipline. As Schwab correctly stated, "The conceptual structure of a discipline determines what we shall seek the truth about."[3(p205)] The way in which nursing science is conceptualized also has specific implications for nursing practice. To date, the practical consequences of holding any given position regarding the nature of nursing science have been largely ignored. However, because nurs-

Source: Johnson, J. L. (1991). Nursing science: Basic, applied, or practical? Implications for the art of nursing. *ANS, 14* (1): 7-16. Reprinted with permission from and copyright © 1991 Aspen Publishers, Inc.

ing is a practical discipline, it is essential that these consequences not be ignored but instead be examined in detail.

The way in which nursing science is conceptualized and pursued is of particular relevance to the art of nursing. Nursing is frequently referred to as both a science and an art. Yet, the relationship of these two aspects of nursing remains poorly understood. Peplau argued that the science and art of nursing are "interconnected if not inseparable."[4(p13)] Similarly, Greene[5] concluded that the science and art of nursing are complementary. Assuming that an essential relationship exists between nursing science and nursing art, it seems logical that the nature of this relationship will vary depending on how either the science or the art is defined. The purposes of this chapter are to argue that the science of nursing is best conceptualized and pursued as a practical science and to demonstrate that pursuing scientific nursing knowledge as a basic or applied science places the art of nursing in jeopardy.

EPISTEMOLOGICAL ASSUMPTIONS

Reasonable judgments about the merit of particular arguments cannot be made unless the terms used are clearly defined and the assumptions upon which the arguments rest are clearly set forth. Therefore, before proceeding with the main arguments of this chapter, it is essential that the assumptions upon which the author's analysis rests be described so that the reader can reasonably judge the arguments put forward. The following comments are confined to assumptions that are epistemological in nature. Other assumptions made by the author are articulated throughout the text.

First, it is assumed that the nature of nursing science is not simply a matter of personal preference or taste. Rather, it is assumed that the proper definition of nursing

science is a philosophic issue and that it is possible to pursue and to obtain knowledge about the nature of nursing science via philosophic inquiry. Just as scientific inquiry can yield knowledge about phenomena, philosophic inquiry, if properly pursued, is able to yield knowledge about phenomena. When philosophers reflect on, reason about, and judge objects of thought, they can and do obtain knowledge. The knowledge obtained is neither certain nor incorrigible. Neither philosophers nor scientists can claim that their endeavors yield knowledge that is beyond challenge. When judgments are compared against reality and validated as true, the philosopher can and does obtain knowledge, not mere opinion.[6] A clear distinction is therefore made between knowledge and mere opinion. For the purposes of this chapter, *knowledge* is defined as a probable truth that is responsible, reliable, well-founded, and reasonable. Mere *opinion*, on the other hand, is characterized as irresponsible, unreliable, unfounded, and unreasonable.[7]

The nature of nursing science is a controversial issue, in that contrary positions can be and have been explicated. Controversies can be fruitful in the pursuit of knowledge, in that they can prompt the careful consideration of contrary positions, which in turn can lead to beneficial insights and the discovery of new knowledge. However, rather than embracing controversies and attempting to resolve them, nurses have often accepted disagreement about contrary positions. In fact, a diversity of contrary positions has often been taken to be the endpoint of theoretical endeavors in nursing, rather than a starting point. For example, Schultz and Meleis argued that "it is inappropriate to use the language of truth in nursing or any other practice discipline that deals with complex human phenomena."[8(p220)] Instead, they argued that knowledge is a matter of context and perspective. Adam[9] called for a pluralism of theories in nursing, arguing that each theory will add to nursing's knowledge base. A diversity of positions is essential to the development of knowledge in any discipline. It is a discipline's diversity that prompts its members to reconsider positions, to change, and to continue to develop. Diversity itself, however, is not an appropriate end for the discipline of nursing. This chapter is based on the assumption that knowledge (in the sense of probable truth) is possible. If properly pursued, knowledge can be obtained about a variety of topics, including the nature of nursing science.

Nurses have demonstrated a reluctance to understand one another's positions and engage in rational debate about the nature of nursing science. Controversy is the starting point for all philosophic enterprises. By using the method of the dialectic (examining contrary positions, asking and pursuing answers to questions, examining common characteristics, and classifying characteristics), the assumptions underlying contrary positions as well as their implications can be examined and judged.[10] In this chapter, contrary positions regarding the nature of nursing science are taken as the starting point for analysis, rather than as an endpoint, and an attempt is made to examine the consequences of holding any one of four positions.

DEFINITIONS

For the purposes of this chapter, *science* is broadly defined as empirical knowledge that is grounded and tested in experience, specifically special experience.[7] *Special experience* refers to the experience we have as the result of investigative efforts. *Scientific knowledge* is, therefore, knowledge that is by nature general. Furthermore, it is assumed that the nature of the art of nursing has primacy over the nature of the science of nursing. In other words, explications regarding the nature of nursing science must presuppose the nature of nursing art.

This assumption is based on the argument that nursing science must ultimately serve the art of nursing and not the reverse.

Art is the name for any skill or technique and includes the useful, the liberal, and the fine arts. *Nursing art* is a useful art and can be broadly defined as the practical know-how that an individual nurse has in a particular situation, which is used to achieve a particular result.[11] Nursing art does not, therefore, refer to specific products, but rather, it refers to the ability to nurse well. Using this general definition of nursing art as a point of departure, conceptualizations of nursing science will be considered in terms of their consequences for nursing art.

NURSING SCIENCE

Currently, four positions regarding the nature of nursing science can be found in the nursing literature. It is held that nursing is a basic science, an applied science, or a practical science, or that nursing science consists of all three types of science. Serious consideration has not been given to the position that nursing is not a science. Accordingly, for the purposes of this chapter, it will be assumed that nursing is a science. Each of these four positions will be considered in turn.

Nursing Science as Basic

The basic sciences can be distinguished from other sciences on the basis of their goal or end. This mode of distinction is based on the fundamental difference between the theoretic and the practical intellect.[12,13] The operations of the intellect's cognitive power—the power to apprehend, judge, and reason and to understand and know—are theoretic if the end for which they are performed is knowledge. If knowledge is sought for the sake of carrying out a decision or executing a choice, then the intellectual operations are practical. As Wallace pointed out, "Theoretical knowledge has for its end the attainment of truth, and that alone, whereas practical knowledge seeks truth as a means to an end so as to order it to practice or operation."[11(p273)] The end of the basic sciences, therefore, is the attainment of knowledge and that alone, whereas the practical scientist is concerned with knowledge that leads to something doable or makeable. The work of the basic scientist is therefore solely analytic, in that its ultimate function is to analyze a conclusion backward to its proper principles.[11] The view that nursing is a basic science is supported by many nursing scholars. Although they have not always explicitly described nursing as a basic science per se, proponents of this view limit scientific inquiry in nursing to description and explanation.[14-17] For example, Moccia stated that the ultimate aim of nursing science is "the explanation and understanding of human phenomena."[15(p7)] Similarly, Gortner and Schultz state that "the goal of nursing science, as is true of other sciences, is to represent nature—in particular human nature—to understand it and explain it for the benefit of mankind."[14(p23)]

If nursing science is pursued as a basic science, nursing practice will be without the scientific understanding of nursing means, and nursing science will be composed entirely of description and explanation. Limiting nursing's scientific endeavors to description and explanation has dire consequences for the art of nursing, because it bars the possibility of scientific nursing theory that is predictive and prescriptive. In turn, the essential connection between nursing art and nursing science is severed. Without scientific knowledge of nursing means, the nurse is left to her or his own resources and to using trial and error to determine how descriptive knowledge should be applied in a particular situation; she or he lacks the necessary intellectual tools to nurse artfully. Just as painters must acknowledge

scientific principles and rules of color and proportion, so too the nurse artist must be guided by scientific rules and principles.

Basic scientific knowledge of human phenomena does not provide the nurse with the necessary knowledge to make decisions about the most effective course to follow in meeting a goal. For example, knowledge of the physiologic and anatomic factors that affect good ventilation in humans is not enough for the nurse who wants to effectively promote ventilation in a postoperative patient. The nurse must also have scientific knowledge of the specific means that can be used to enhance ventilation, such as deep breathing and coughing techniques or suctioning methods, as well as an understanding of how a nurse should position patients when attempting to maximize ventilation. Such scientific knowledge would consist of generalizations regarding what nurses ought to do to achieve particular nursing goals.

Some scholars have argued that nurses should not impose their own views on their clients and that scientists should avoid moral injunctions and limit knowledge claims to those which are purely descriptive. Moccia,[15] for example, argued that the use of knowledge that is predictive strips individuals of their potential for autonomous self-determination and reduces them to objects. Moccia's concern is one that many nurses share. How can science guide practice? Is it not immoral to impose a belief system on another individual? In part, these critical questions are built on a failure to recognize that the object of science is different from the object of art. As stated earlier, it is science that deals with generalizations, and it is art that deals with the application of these generalizations in a particular situation. In performing their art, nurses use both scientific knowledge of nursing interventions and their personal insights about what is required in the particular situation. Nursing science will never usurp the place of nursing art. In this light, the question that Schultz and Meleis raised—"Can the art of nursing yield as reliable and reproducible knowledge as the 'science' of nursing?"[8(p219)]—is clearly moot. This question is based on the false assumption that science and art are similar types of knowledge.

As poignant as the issues that Moccia[15] raises might be, one must also address the question of whether it is immoral to subject humans to a trial-and-error practice of nursing. The suggestion that nursing science remains basic gives the practitioner little choice but to proceed on a case-by-case basis, determining how scientific findings might be applied in each particular case. Nursing is by nature a human endeavor; nurses work with individuals to assist them in meeting particular human needs. The end of nursing, its justifying principle, is in the final analysis a moral one: the good of the person seeking care. In other words, nurses cannot avoid moral decisions.

Neither science of a basic nature nor the "creative use" of basic scientific knowledge will provide the tools necessary for the art of nursing. In practicing the art of nursing, the nurse must possess the knowledge of nursing means in conjunction with her or his knowledge of the particular situation at hand. To describe nursing science as basic is to sever the intimate link between nursing science and nursing art. Art and science are, consequently, left to function and develop in their own separate realms.

Some might argue that the realms of nursing art and nursing science should remain separate. That is, it might be contended that the art of nursing is best developed solely through experience using apprenticeship methods and that no essential connection exists between the art and science of nursing. If nursing art is attained solely through apprenticeship, however, it will be severely restricted. What will nurses who attain their art via apprenticeship do when they are confronted with situations that are entirely new? It is in these situations

that the apprenticeship approach fails, because the nurse does not have an understanding of the scientific nursing principles that guide her or his art. If nurses understand the scientific principles that guide their art, they will be better prepared to understand and analyze exceptional or new situations when they occur and, therefore, will better understand how the principles of practice can be modified.

Nursing Science as Applied

It has been proposed that conceptualizing nursing as an applied science corrects the inconsistencies and inadequacies of conceptualizing it as basic. The notion of an applied science is, to a certain extent, ambiguous. In the nursing literature, the term has been given a variety of meanings. Wallace's description of applied science[11] is useful in that it is clear and relatively simple. For this reason, Wallace's definition will serve as a basis for discussion. He suggested that an *applied science* is one that uses the knowledge of the basic sciences for some practical end.

In recent years, nurses have expressed great interest in deriving scientific theories that are applicable to nursing practice from the scientific theories of other disciplines. Meleis[18] argued that nurses' utilization of scientific theories from other disciplines is appropriate because theories are "resynthesized" using a nursing perspective. It is, without question, appropriate to utilize scientific theories from other disciplines in the development of scientific nursing knowledge. However, to conceptualize and pursue nursing science as an applied science, as Wallace[11] has defined it, is to limit the capacity of nurses to pursue and develop scientific knowledge that is directly relevant to the art of nursing. This limitation is primarily due to the fact that, if nursing is pursued as an applied science, advances in nursing science will be limited to the application of existing basic scientific theories. If nursing science is pursued as an applied science, nurses will be unable to directly pursue scientific nursing problems; instead, the science of nursing will rest with and ultimately be driven by the advancements of other disciplines, not by the needs arising from nursing practice.

If they are to be artful in their practice, nurses must have knowledge of scientific principles that dictate how specific ends can best be achieved in practice. If nursing art is to benefit, the nurse scientist must be free to pursue scientific knowledge that is directly relevant to practice. If nursing science is pursued as an applied science, the ultimate responsibility for developing the scientific principles that are the foundation of nursing art will rest with the basic scientific disciplines, not with nursing itself. Yet it is unlikely that the scientific knowledge essential for nursing practice will be developed by the other disciplines.

Questions about how best to achieve particular ends in nursing are the nursing discipline's unique concern. To allow the responsibility for knowledge development in the science of nursing to ultimately rest with other disciplines is to place the entire discipline of nursing in jeopardy. The art of nursing, in particular, is dependent on the development of scientific nursing knowledge that can guide it. Nurses cannot and should not depend on other disciplines to develop the scientific principles that are necessary for practice. If nurses pursue nursing science as an applied science, nurse scientists may be forced to wait indefinitely for the development of scientific principles that can be tested and applied to nursing practice. What basic scientist is currently studying the scientific principles that underlie mouth care for the comatose individual, the prevention of falls among the hospitalized elderly, or techniques for teaching an individual to care for his or her new ileostomy? Nursing scientists must be free to develop and test nursing interventions; their endeavors should not be unnecessarily constrained.

Nursing Science as Practical

The third conceptualization of nursing science to be considered is that of nursing as a practical science. This conceptualization of nursing science offers a solution to the limitations that are inherent in the other views, because it closely aligns the science of nursing with the art of nursing. While the basic sciences are concerned solely with understanding and proceed analytically, the practical sciences are concerned with the doable or makeable and proceed compositively. Practical scientists must also understand basic principles and causes, but their ultimate function is to apply these principles and causes to the construction of a composite singular. Practical sciences, unlike the basic sciences, are applicable to the performance of particular operations.[11]

The work of several nursing scholars can be seen as supporting the view that nursing science is a practical science. For example, although they did not use the term *practical science*, Wald and Leonard[19] claimed that nursing science must focus on the means to achieve particular changes. Dickoff and James[20] also argued that nursing science must ultimately focus on the practice of nursing. More recently, Orem[21] and Schlotfeldt[1] argued that the science of nursing must be practical: scientific inquiry in nursing must yield findings that are directly useful and relevant to nursing practice.

Although the aim of nursing practice is entirely practical, knowledge of specific practices must be based on knowledge of causes that may influence the attainment of the end being pursued.[20] Practical knowledge, therefore, presupposes theoretic knowledge. As Wallace stated, "Sciences are said to be practical because their knower intends operation, while they are also said to be theoretical because their knower intends truth and proceeds analytically, even though the science as such is concerned with something doable."[11(p277)]

When nursing science is conceptualized as a practical science, it is clear that nursing science's ultimate goal is to use knowledge of principles and causes in the development of specific nursing means that can achieve particular nursing ends and, thereby, the overall end of nursing. Accordingly, nurse scientists do not pursue knowledge for its own sake; their investigative efforts are dominated by the use that their discoveries will ultimately have for nursing practice.

When the science of nursing is conceptualized as practical, strong links are established between the art of nursing and the science of nursing, in that the scientific rules and principles of nursing practice can provide the basis for nursing art. As Adler[12] pointed out, in the ancient tradition, the opposite of art was empiricism, in that the artless individual was believed to proceed only by experience using a trial-and-error approach. "The empiric in medicine was one who lacked the art of healing because, lacking the relevant sciences, he worked by trial and error rather than by the light of fixed rules."[12(p157)] If the science of nursing is conceptualized as practical, it can provide the basis for the rules of nursing art. These rules must of course be possessed by the nurse as habits of operation. For example, artful nurses use the scientific principles of asepsis when dressing wounds; if they do not possess this knowledge as a habit, they would not be considered artful. If nurses ignore the rules of asepsis, they unnecessarily place their patients at risk and may fail to achieve their particular goals. When the principles of practice are known in a scientific way, the nurse will be best equipped to nurse artfully.

Nursing science alone does not ensure artful nursing, yet it is a necessary tool of the artful nurse. As Weidenbach[22] suggested, art involves the systematic application of both knowledge and skill in effecting a desired result. Scientific knowledge must be complemented by knowledge of the particular situation and skill if a nurse is to be artful. Flynn[23] indicated that the effective practitioner needed a balance of both science and art. The art of caring, she concluded, "is based on the skillful and humanistic application of scientific knowledge."[23(p17)]

Nursing Science as Basic, Applied, and Practical

Finally, some nurses have argued that nursing is a basic, an applied, *and* a practical science, while others have posited that the science of nursing consists of some other combination of these three conceptions. For example, Donaldson and Crowley[2] argued that scientific research that is basic, applied, and clinical is required for the discipline of nursing. Orem,[21] on the other hand, concluded that nursing science is both practical and applied. The argument that nursing consists of more than one type of science is generally used to support the position that nursing science consists of both practical and theoretic knowledge and to bolster the argument that it is appropriate for nurse scientists to "borrow" scientific theories from other disciplines and to apply these theories to nursing situations. To describe nursing science as basic, applied, and practical is, however, untenable because it leads to the conclusion that nursing science ultimately serves more than one end. What is at issue is not the types of knowledge required for nursing. Clearly, both practical and theoretic knowledge are necessary. The pivotal issue is the end that nursing science will ultimately serve. A unified science cannot at one and the same time have more than one overall end; if it does, it will be forever fragmented.

The proper ends of the basic and practical sciences are distinct. The practical sciences, unlike the basic sciences, are from the very outset directed toward operation.[24] The basic sciences, on the other hand, are directed solely toward the development of knowledge for its own sake. Nursing science cannot, therefore, be considered to be both practical and basic. This is not to say that theoretic knowledge is not essential to practical science. As discussed previously, practical science presupposes the existence of theoretic knowledge. Nursing as a practical science, therefore, includes within its unity knowledge of both the speculative and practical order.[24]

What of applied and practical sciences? Do they not serve the same end? Perhaps nursing science is best conceptualized as both practical and applied. One might argue that the applied and practical sciences both serve the same end. This conclusion is, however, erroneous. Consider how two nurse scientists, one using a practical perspective and the other an applied, would approach the same problem in nursing practice. The practical scientist would ask the question, "How can I develop a technique to solve this practical problem?" The applied nurse scientist would ask, "How can I apply existing scientific theory in such a way that I solve this practical problem?" Whereas the applied scientist is concerned only with attaining a practical end, the practical scientist is concerned with seeking knowledge to attain a practical end. The ends of these two forms of nursing science differ. The applied nurse scientist is interested solely in serving a practical end and is not concerned with knowledge development per se. The practical scientist, on the other hand, develops the knowledge necessary to achieve a particular end. The end served by the practical scientist is broader and is not constrained by the existence of basic science.[11] Because the applied and the practical sciences are radically different, nursing science cannot be considered to be both.

It is ill conceived to conceptualize nursing science as basic, applied, and practical. To do so is to accept that the science of nursing is not unified, but fragmented. If nursing science is pursued as a basic, an applied, and a practical

science, there will be no way to ensure that the science of nursing remains relevant to the art of nursing.

CONCLUSION

Current discussion in the nursing literature is focusing once again on the gap between nursing science and nursing practice. Nursing science, when pursued as an applied or basic science, will in the end fail to be consistently relevant to the art of nursing and, in turn, to nursing practice. Only if we correctly conceptualize nursing as a practical science will the science and art of nursing be properly connected. Nursing is clearly both a science and an art. To disarticulate these two aspects of nursing is to dismember nursing. If nursing science is to properly serve the goal of nursing, then it must be pursued as a practical science.

REFERENCES

1. Schlotfeldt RM. Structuring nursing knowledge: A priority for creating nursing's future. *Nurs Sci Q.* 1988;1:35-37.
2. Donaldson SK, Crowley DM. The discipline of nursing. *Nurs Outlook.* 1978;26:113-120.
3. Schwab JJ. The concept of the structure of the discipline. *Educ Rec.* 1962;43:197-205.
4. Peplau HE. The art and science of nursing: Similarities, differences and relationships. *Nurs Sci Q.* 1988;1:8-15.
5. Greene JA. Science, nursing and nursing science: A conceptual analysis. *ANS.* 1979;2(4): 57-64.
6. Adler MJ. *Ten Philosophical Mistakes.* New York, NY: Macmillan, 1985.
7. ———. *The Conditions of Philosophy: Its Checkered Past, Its Present Disorder, and Its Future Promise.* New York, NY: Antheneum, 1965.
8. Schultz PR, Meleis AI. Nursing epistemology: Traditions, insights, questions. *Image.* 1988;20: 217-221.
9. Adam E. Nursing theory: What it is and what it is not. *Nurs Papers.* 1987;19:5-13.

10. Adler MJ. *Dialectic*. London, England: Kegan Paul Trench & Trubner, 1927.
11. Wallace WA. *From a Realist Point of View: Essays on the Philosophy of Science*. 2nd ed. Washington, DC: University Press of America, 1983.
12. Adler MJ. *Poetry and Politics*. Pittsburgh: Duquesne, 1965.
13. Aristotle; Hardie RP, Gaye RK, trans. Physica. In: McKeon R, ed. *The Basic Works of Aristotle*. New York: Random House, 1941.
14. Gortner SR, Schultz PR. Approaches to nursing science methods. *Image*. 1988;20:22-24.
15. Moccia P. A critique of compromise: Beyond the methods debate. *ANS*. 1988;10(4):1-9.
16. Parse RR. *Man-Living-Heath: A Theory of Nursing*. New York, NY: Wiley, 1981.
17. Rogers ME. Nursing, science and art: A prospective. *Nurs Sci Q*. 1988;1:99-102.
18. Meleis AI. *Theoretical Nursing: Development and Progress*. Philadelphia, Pa: Lippincott, 1985.
19. Wald FS, Leonard RC. Towards development of nursing practice theory. *Nurs Res*. 1964;13:309-314.
20. Dickoff J, James P. A theory of theories: A position paper. *Nurs Res*. 1968;17:197-203.
21. Orem DE. The form of nursing science. *Nurs Sci Q*. 1988;1:75-79.
22. Weidenbach E. *Clinical Nursing: A Helping Art*. New York, NY: Springer, 1964.
23. Flynn PAR. *Holistic Health: The Art and Science of Care*. Bowie, Md: Prentice-Hall, 1980.
24. Maritain J; Phelan GB, trans. *The Degrees of Knowledge*. London, England: Geoffrey Bles, 1959.

10

What Constitutes Nursing Science?

JOHN R. PHILLIPS, RN, PhD

Science is an organized body of knowledge concerning human beings and their worlds; it encompasses "the attitudes and methods through which this body of knowledge is formed" (Chernow & Vallasi, 1993, p. 2452). Chernow and Vallasi (1993) also state that since scientific methods do not always guarantee scientific discovery, other factors such as intuition, experience, and good judgment "contribute to new developments in science" (p. 2452). In addition, a survey of the evolution of knowledge shows that abstract thinking is integral to the advancement of science. This broad view of science is essential in understanding the development of any particular science and its phenomena of concern.

This is especially true for nursing science with its unique body of knowledge. Controversy arises, however, when attempts are made to identify this body of knowledge, where some nurses make little distinction between nursing knowledge and the knowledge of other sciences, such as medicine. Too, some nursing models and theories still include knowledge from other sciences that has not been transposed into a nursing perspective. Furthermore, it must be determined how or if these nursing models and theories can be used to generate *nursing* knowledge that constitutes nursing science.

Some nurses may say this is a moot point, and probably not worthy of further pursuit. However, one needs to realize that it is nursing science that gives direction to the further generation of nursing knowledge, and it is nursing science that provides the knowledge for all aspects of nursing. Moreover, it is through the art of nursing, "the imaginative and creative use of knowledge" (Rogers, 1988, p. 100), that nurses can know and understand the health care needs of people. How adequately can this be achieved if nursing science is not constituted with nursing knowledge?

Fawcett (1993, 1995) in her metaparadigm of nursing has helped to provide an understanding of what constitutes nursing science. Her analysis and evaluation of nursing models and theories make it clear that there is a particular perspective of the metaparadigm concepts for each of the nursing models and theories. For example, the definitions of person, environment, health, and nursing are different for each model and theory. Since each nursing model and theory has a different philosophical and theoretical foundation, nurses who use them have different realities of nursing. How are these differences related to what constitutes nursing science?

Parse (1987) and Newman (1992) in their paradigms of nursing and Fawcett (1993) in her worldviews of nursing address these differences and provide for further understanding of what constitutes nursing science. The

Source: Phillips, J. R. (1996) What Constitutes Nursing Science? *Nursing Science Quarterly.* 9(2):48–49. Reprinted with permission by Chestnut House Publications

use of these paradigms and worldviews reveals that some nursing models and theories are composed of conflicting philosophical and theoretical foundations. Too, some nursing models and theories overlap more than one paradigm or worldview. If a nursing model or theory lacks coherence within its philosophical and theoretical foundation and overlaps more than one paradigm or worldview, then a close examination of it is needed to determine whether it constitutes nursing science. Will a time come when particular nursing models or theories will no longer be appropriate to constitute nursing science?

Nursing models and theories provide multiple diverse and divergent nursing realities. These realities foster creative ideas and insights that are essential to the methods that are used to discover knowledge. It is time, however, to evaluate how the various scientific methods contribute to the development of nursing science. Realizing, for example, that statistics is only one language of science, nurses can no longer be satisfied with only the traditional scientific methods that often give a cloudy vision of what nursing science is. Nurses must emerge from the womb of other sciences so as to give birth to scientific methods that give a clear vision of what nursing is and can be, knowing that today there is only an inkling of the future of nursing science.

Nurses can design these new methods through a creative synthesis of the various aspects of science and the human processes such as intuition and lived experiences. Some of our current nursing scientific methods already provide for imaginative, abstract, and logical reasoning processes that are required to discover knowledge to develop nursing science. Such scientific methods will give unity to nursing science through the diversity of nursing models and theories. This assumption is acceptable when Moody's (1990) quote of Bronowski is considered: "Science is nothing else than the search to discover unity in the wild variety of nature or . . . in the variety of our experiences" (p. 18).

A cumulative body of knowledge that is flexible and open to change flows from the unitary nature of nursing science. The wholeness of this knowledge provides further understanding of the ambiguity and uncertainty found in the multiple realities of nursing models and theories. This understanding will reveal the rigid and static nature of knowledge from other sciences, which in many instances is outdated and not from a nursing perspective. However, as nurses develop knowledge through the use of nursing models and theories, they must remain in doubt and be open to changes in it (Wilson, 1985). This is essential if nurses are to advance a nursing science that provides the knowledge for the changing art of nursing, where there is concern for the wholeness of people.

Questions of what constitutes nursing science have revealed an evolving phenomenon in nursing. The revelation is that facts alone do not constitute nursing science, however important they may be; it is the pattern of knowledge that gives unity to nursing science. As the pattern is revealed, nurses are being challenged to relook at what constitutes nursing science. Needless to say, the focus on the pattern of knowledge brings a profound provocation to create a new vision of nursing science, a vision that will eventually sever the umbilical cord of subjugation to the knowledge of other sciences. This new vision may save some of the nursing models and theories from becoming obsolete, even extinct.

The recognition and use of the pattern of knowledge is moving nursing science to the forefront of science in general. This new, prominent position enables nurses to respond to the public's desire for quality health care, where the concern is the healing of the whole person. In such an arena of health care, nurses will not compete with other health care providers since they will be using nursing knowledge for the practice of nursing, rather than knowledge from other sciences, particularly medicine. Can we say that the "gap" between theory and practice will disappear as nurses continue to use nursing models and theories that constitute the nursing science for their practice?

Yes, nursing models and theories do constitute nursing science. Nurses must not accept the perennial denigration of nursing models and theories and the call to abandon them for the knowledge from other sciences. If nurses do, nursing will become a wasteland filled with "illiterate nurses" where all of humanity will suffer in immeasurable ways.

Nursing models and theories are the savior of nursing science, and nurses' ravenous use of them will bring redemption from a wasteland composed of knowledge from other sciences. This is the power that nursing models and theories give nurses in determining what constitutes nursing science, its knowledge, and its scientific methods. As nurses continue to use nursing models and theories, nursing science will no longer be invisible in the world of science.

REFERENCES

Chernow, B. A., & Vallasi, G. A. (1993). *The Columbia encyclopedia* (5th ed.). New York: Columbia University Press.

Fawcett, J. (1993). *Analysis and evaluation of nursing theories*. Philadelphia: Davis.

Fawcett, J. (1995). *Analysis and evaluation of conceptual models of nursing* (3rd ed.). Philadelphia: Davis.

Moody, L. E. (1990). *Advancing nursing science through research, volume 1*. Newbury Park, CA: Sage.

Newman, M. A. (1992). Prevailing paradigms in nursing. *Nursing Outlook, 40*, 10–13, 32.

Parse, R. R. (1987). *Nursing science: Major paradigms, theories, and critiques*. Philadelphia: Saunders.

Rogers, M. E. (1988). Nursing science and art: A prospective. *Nursing Science Quarterly, 1*, 99–102.

Wilson, H. S. (1985). *Research in nursing*. Menlo Park, CA: Addison-Wesley.

11

Nursing Science in the Global Community

SHAKÉ KETEFIAN, RN, EdD, FAAN RICHARD W. REDMAN, RN, PhD

Knowledge development and research are generally embedded in cultural values and perspectives. This article examines the development of knowledge in nursing in a global context and addresses the degree to which Western values and the social environment in the United States shape nursing theory development. Three perspectives illustrate the influence of U.S. values and contextual factors. Questions are raised about the relevance of knowledge to other cultural or national contexts. Recommendations are made for nursing inquiry that makes knowledge more applicable to the global community. [Keywords: Knowledge development; International nursing]

For many years, nurses from other countries have been enrolled in U.S. graduate programs. Colling and Liu (1995) report a 10% increase in international students attending U.S. graduate programs in nursing in the past decade. In their survey of international students, these authors identified 239 students from 49 countries. In many parts of the world, U.S. nursing appears to be highly regarded.

As the diversity and ethnic mix of the U.S. population has increased, global awareness has also increased. In the past decade, many institutions and nurses have become involved in international activities such as consultation, collaborative research, and exchange visitor arrangements.

Yet, despite the increase in international activities, the nature of nursing theory, research, education, and practice has not changed appreciably to be globally relevant.

The degree to which parochialism may have played a role in explaining the slow pace of change in this regard has not been fully examined.

Boyacigiller and Adler (1991) examined the degree to which Western parochialism and ethnocentrism are embedded in the concepts of organizational theory. These authors reviewed the research literature in management science from three perspectives: (a) the influence of post World War II America and its environment on organizational theory development; (b) the volume of international articles published in American management journals; and (c) the degree to which American beliefs and values have shaped organizational theory development. Their assessment, overall, was that organizational theories are parochial and many do not acknowledge awareness of non-U.S. contexts, models, or values. Many Americans have shaped theories central to organizational and human behavior with the assumption that these beliefs have universal applicability. Free will (versus deter-

Source: Ketefian, S., Redman, R. (1997) Nursing Science in the Global Community. IMAGE: *Journal of Nursing Scholarship* 29(1):11–15. Reprinted with permission by Sigma Theta Tau International

minism) and individualism (versus collectivism) are just two examples of how Western values have shaped research and theory in organizational science. The authors call for the development of organizational sciences in which universal, intercultural theories are clearly explicit.

Following the approach taken by Boyacigiller and Adler (1991), we describe three perspectives in our examination: (a) contextual—the influence of the U.S. social environment on nursing theory development; (b) quantitative—the rapid expansion of U.S. doctoral programs in nursing, the shaping of nursing journals by U.S. nurse scientists, and the degree of international scientific representation in these journals; and (c) qualitative—the degree to which U.S. values have shaped nursing theory development. The status of multicultural knowledge development in the United States is then presented followed by selected recommendations. Given the magnitude of the topic, no attempt is made to be comprehensive. Rather, the ideas presented represent select perspectives and observations of the authors who are educators in the United States, but who have had extensive international experience. The views presented here are intended to serve as catalysts for further discussion.

PERSPECTIVES

Contextual Perspective

The influence of social forces on American nursing can be examined from several perspectives. These include (a) social trends and values and how they shape nursing knowledge development, (b) the influence of technology and reimbursement systems on nomenclature in nursing, and (c) the development of nursing education and research infrastructures as social phenomena. Each is de-

scribed briefly to illustrate the contextual influences.

Many recent U.S. social movements have had considerable effect on nursing theory. One example is the emphasis on health promotion and risk reduction. The social emphasis on behavior related to diet, exercise, and other types of health-promoting behaviors have influenced the shaping of public policy as well as the education of health professionals. To a considerable degree, they have also shaped the direction of nursing science and research. Another example is the way in which the emergence of the women's movement has shaped the thinking of a whole generation of women and has led to the development of new public policies in education, employment, health, and other domains. Recognition that women's health problems should be given priority has led to research by health professionals, including nurses, resulting in a body of scientific knowledge in this domain.

The Nursing Interventions Classification (NIC) work at Iowa (McCloskey & Bulechek, 1994) is another example of a social force influencing nursing knowledge development. NIC has been developed as a comprehensive classification of treatments that nurses perform in an attempt to create a standardized language of both nurse- and physician-initiated nursing interventions. Interest in developing this taxonomy can be traced in part to the need for nurses to develop a universal language. Catalytic social forces such as the rapid technologic development of literature data bases, clinical information systems in practice settings, and the need for taxonomies that are compatible with reimbursement systems have resulted in the need for standardized nursing nomenclature. This development has profound implications for nursing practice and knowledge development internationally. The degree to which U.S. nursing interventions are shaping the rapid development of "universal" taxonomies and languages that reflect nursing practice throughout the world is a pressing question. In addition, there is considerable interest in using taxonomies such as NIC to redefine nursing knowledge inductively. Again, the degree to which U.S. nursing interventions and practices reflect nursing practice in other countries is a question of critical importance internationally.

Social values and contextual influence also relate to the quality of nursing care. Definitions of nursing care quality vary, ranging from using the proper amount of resources to accomplish nursing goals to meeting patients' requirements. Assessing the quality of nursing care, whether focused on the appropriateness of a given intervention to a patient's needs or the selection of alternatives as a function of resources available illustrates how context-dependent quality can be. The expectations of a client, the socially defined role of the nurse, and the technology available can vary considerably. Furthermore, the importance of each of these variables in the quality equation can vary, depending on the context, and in turn drive the research questions and methodologies. Thus, the manner in which the pressing questions of the discipline are framed are very likely to reflect the values, philosophy, and practices of the culture and society in which they are asked.

Explorations of theory in nursing began in the 1960s. Since then, in an effort to define what is distinctive about nursing science and theory, nurse scholars and theorists have widely debated their ideas. Many of these ideas have been characterized as metatheories or conceptual frameworks. In the past decade, the nursing literature has reflected a shift in thinking. Now many investigators favor working with propositions and theories characterized as middle-range theories rather than with conceptual frameworks because middle-range theories provide the basis for generating testable hypotheses related to particular nursing phenomena and to particular patient populations.

Expansion of doctoral programs along with the magnitude and refinement of nursing research over the past several decades has been impressive. Thus, it can be argued that such advances in U.S. nursing have rightfully placed it in an enviable position vis-à-vis international peers.

The scope and orientation of much of nursing research is American without global characteristics. Frequently, research findings are presented and received by international colleagues as though the work is applicable to other national and cultural contexts. In addressing such issues, Zwanger (1987) states that American nurses are recognized as leaders in doctoral education in the world and that,

> They are . . . the oracles of the international academic nursing community. As a consequence, in many instances, their ambiguous tendencies, unclarified ideas, and conceptions are accepted as bona fide facts (pp. 33–34).

Zwanger draws on the Israeli experience in stating that some of those who complete their degree in the United States wish to transplant American ideas to their native land. She then describes the inappropriateness of doing so, which in some cases results in failure to function effectively in one's home settings. She makes a case for U.S. doctoral faculty to "pay attention to global content and international nursing issues," emphasize comparative studies, and assist international students to gear their doctoral research to problems in their own countries.

Quantitative Perspective

The International Council of Nurses now represents 110 national associations as members, with a total of 1 million nurses (Splane & Splane, 1994). Of 110 schools worldwide offering doctoral degrees in nursing, 62 are in the United States and 48 in all other countries combined. Moreover, according to anecdotal data, an indeterminate number of non-U.S. educational programs are programs where nurses have the opportunity to obtain doctoral degrees in fields other than nursing.

A limited number of international exchanges of students and faculty has occurred over the years (Fenton, 1994), although exchange has gained momentum recently. Yet, such opportunities are not made available to students by many institutions; further, international exchanges typically occur during undergraduate study rather than graduate study. At the doctoral level, during the 1970s, many institutions either abandoned a second language requirement altogether or began accepting a computer language in its stead. A recent American Academy of Nursing publication (1995) identifies five graduate programs in nursing in the United States with a cross-cultural focus, some of which include international nursing. Thus, in most cases, doctoral students' exposure to the world beyond the United States might come when they have the opportunity to study with international students as peers.

Examination of the growth in journal publication and in doctoral education gives readers another perspective on the growth in nursing knowledge and science. The major journal for reporting research in nursing, *Nursing Research*, was established in 1952 by the *American Journal of Nursing* Company; later it was followed by the publication of *Research in Nursing and Health* in 1977, and *Advances in Nursing Science* in 1978. Since that time, many journals have been established that report research in nursing, nursing theory, and nursing practice. As specialty organizations grew, so did journals concerned with the practice and research of their clinical area of practice. In the early days of *Nursing Research*, it was not uncommon to see papers authored by social scientists, reporting on studies concerned with *nurses* rather than with *nursing*.

Ketefian and Redman (1994) reported that the first doctoral programs in nursing were established in 1933 (Teachers College, Columbia University), and 1934 (New York University), both offering the Doctor of Education degree. In the next 25 years, only two more programs were established. Growth in doctoral programs since then has been exponential. Of the 62 institutions in the United States offering doctoral degrees in nursing 75% offer the PhD, the remainder offer a DNS, DNSc, or EdD. As to the nature of these programs, Grace (1978) and Murphy (1981) have described the development of doctoral programs in three phases: Phase I (inception to 1959) is characterized by focusing on education *for* nurses for functional roles; Phase II (1960–69) is characterized by a focus on education *for* nurses in a second discipline, referred to as nurse scientist training; Phase III (1970 to the present) is characterized by a focus on education *in* and *of* nursing.

A review of the content of U.S. journals suggests that many report on international issues, some have articles co-authored by nurses from overseas, and others have a regular international column. But the effect of these developments, while significant, is not major. Many libraries now subscribe to international journals; yet class assignments do not often include readings from these journals. A few journals now have international representatives on their review boards.

Qualitative Perspective

The Code for Nurses (ANA, 1985) represents embodiment of the values of American Nursing. The preamble reads, in part:

> When making clinical judgments, nurses base their decisions on consideration of consequences and of universal moral principles, both of which prescribe and justify nursing actions. The most funda-

mental of these principles is respect for persons. Other principles stemming from this basic principle are autonomy (self-determination), beneficence (doing good), nonmaleficence (avoiding harm), veracity (truth-telling), confidentiality (respecting privileged information), fidelity (keeping promises), and justice (treating people fairly)" (p. i).

The values in the code, and others emanating from them, find expression in nursing theories and conceptual frameworks developed by U.S. scholars. Indeed, they permeate the nursing literature. These values are at times explicit and at other times implicit.

Why are value assumptions important? Values have important effects on people, communities, and societies; the primary concern of nursing is people—individually or in the aggregate. An understanding of behavior and the values that underlie behavior, becomes a critical starting point for designing and implementing nursing interventions. Value assumptions underlying U.S. nursing are profoundly influenced by American culture, social mores, and the biases of the people who produce this literature. Yet, a reading of U.S. literature suggests that the ideas therein are claimed to be either acultural or universal.

Most nursing theories and nursing research are developed and implemented in the United States, and therefore, can be said to be influenced by the social and cultural context of this country. In the next section, we offer specific examples of the influence of culturally-specific values and assumptions—and present comparisons or contrasts gleaned from the literature.

Graduate and Higher Education in Nursing. In the United States, it is assumed that academic study is "good" and necessary for nursing education and that higher educa-

tion (at college and university level) is even better. However, in many countries these are not assumptions; the terms often have different meanings.

Hockey (1987) draws on her knowledge and experience in European countries, and states that in some countries "higher education" refers to academic study beyond that required for qualification for practice. In addition, she explains that typically with higher education come leadership positions, even though some nurses do not wish to assume such positions. Thus she poses the dilemma in ethical terms: Is "higher education" necessary for nursing? In another poignant example from the Austrian experience, she reveals that nurse training begins at age 15, and notes that "nursing autonomy assumes a different meaning" under these circumstances (p. 77).

Another author from the same conference describes the experience of Norway and its dilemmas which highlight value conflicts and value differences of a significant magnitude for that country. The main dilemma posed by Haugen Bunch (1987) is whether Norwegian nurses should study in the United States or in Norway. Each choice is described as having significant consequences for Norwegian nursing. She describes the choices as (a) studying social and natural sciences, (b) developing nursing science, or (c) blending the two. At the University of Bergen (Norway), where an Institute of Caring Sciences was established in 1979, many believe that caring is not subject to scientific inquiry, that nursing cannot be both holistic and scientific, that science may compromise the nursing discipline, that nursing can use relevant scientific principles from other disciplines, and that there is no need for a separate nursing science. Thus, if nurses study in Norway, with its tutorial educational model, their role models will not be nurses and they will learn the traditions of other disciplines rather than of nursing. If, on the other hand, they study in the United States, they will be socialized in nursing's scientific tradition and will have nurse role models. Haugen Bunch warns that for those educated in the U.S. there will be the danger of bringing back to Norway "undigested American knowledge that is presented as 'Norwegian truisms'—forgetting the need for value clarification so that the knowledge will fit Norwegian culture and traditions" (p. 103). Throughout her presentation she emphasizes the importance of adapting and testing theories and concepts before, "being applied and integrated to the Norwegian culture" (p. 103).

Nursing Science and Japan.   According to a Japanese nurse who did graduate work in the United States, Japanese nurses have imported nursing knowledge and literature since the end of the 19th century. The works of many American authors and theorists have been translated into Japanese by exchange nurses and by those who came to the U.S. for master's and doctoral degrees (Minami, 1987). Minami claims that many of these nurses "were not aware of the differences between the Japanese and American cultures or social context" (p. 66), and claimed that nursing was universal. She describes fundamental differences in the cultural milieu of the two countries that make concepts developed in one country inapplicable or irrelevant in the other. She also describes dilemmas faced by American-educated Japanese nurses in functioning in their home settings. Communication differences, for example, exist in eight areas: physical proximity; self disclosure; trust in words; boundary in human relationships; commitment and contract; dependency and independence; autonomy and independence; and confrontation (p. 70). She says that Americans communicate with language while Japanese communicate with empathy; and she provides examples. These differences are characterized by Boyacigiller and Adler (1991) as high-context or low-context cultures. The external environment, the situation, and non-verbal behavior determine communication in high-context cultures like the Japanese, and subtlety, facial expression, relationship, and timing are valued. In low-context cultures like the USA, meaning comes from the spoken word and legal contracts are valued.

Multicultural Knowledge Development in the United States

Rapid change in the demographic composition of the U.S. population has occurred within the past several decades. Some demographers estimate that by the twenty-first century, one-third to one-half of the population will be other than Euro-Caucasian. Thus a reversal is anticipated whereby groups that were minorities will collectively become the majority. The importance of a change of such magnitude is immense. An appreciation for diversity and for the varying needs of people who are different—with regard to any number of characteristics—is needed. Nowhere is this appreciation more compelling than in health care and nursing.

A small group of nurse investigators has been developing research and theory that is culturally sensitive. In a recent American Academy of Nursing monograph (AAN, 1995), a group of authors define culturally-competent care as that which "takes into account issues related to diversity, marginalization, and vulnerability due to culture, race, gender, and sexual orientation" (p. 4). In their assessment of the state of knowledge development in this area, the authors identify the dearth of principles to guide selection of culturally sensitive research questions and selection of culturally appropriate methodologies. Many nursing programs do not offer content relevant to this area and fewer still require doctoral students to enroll in seminars about cross-cultural nursing.

The authors of the AAN monograph (1995) identify two metatheories and studies based on them that have shown promise of generating knowledge that is culturally sensitive. One theory is Leininger's (1985), wherein she posits that care, as the essence of nursing, is universal across cultures, although its forms and expressions may vary. The authors cite a number of nursing studies in which Leininger's theory helped researchers generate knowledge related to cultural care. The other metatheory cited is the "self-care deficit theory" (Orem, 1991). This theory enables study of self-care practices used by diverse social groups. Its relevance for populations in a number of European countries—as well as Mexico and Thailand—is being studied by a network of collaborators (AAN, 1995).

In addition to the two metatheories, others are being developed that are referred to as "situation specific theories" (AAN, 1995). Examples are studies of Middle Eastern immigrants (Lipson, Reizian, & Meleis, 1987; Meleis, 1981; Meleis & Jonsen, 1983), patterns of health-seeking behaviors among Arab children (May, 1985), and post-partum transition among Arab women (El Sayed, 1986). The authors contend that, collectively, such studies can be synthesized to provide conceptualizations of patterns of responses to health-illness transitions, thus enabling development of a situation-specific theory in a particular population (AAN, 1995, p. 10).

Methodological concerns in the conduct of research with ethnically and racially diverse groups have received increasing attention as well. The U.S. Department of Health and Human Services (1990) has recently stipulated that ethnically and racially different groups be included as research subjects. Porter and Villarruel (1993) provide a cogent analysis of research issues and propose a set of guidelines to be considered for the design of research. Consideration of appropriate sensitivity is reflected in conceptualizing and conducting research, including each step of the research process and investigator activities. It is implied that unless these design considerations are present and deliberatively addressed, the relevance and applicability of the outcome of the research to diverse populations would be questionable.

Other Knowledge Development Strategies. Over the years, nurses in many countries have identified their inability to describe nursing practice, client populations, or geographic areas as a serious constraint (Clark, 1994). To meet this need, and to contribute to knowledge development for nursing, various classification systems have been developed. The Nursing Minimum Data Set was developed by Werley in the late 1960s (Werley & Lang, 1988) and in turn spurred other developments.

In the early 1980s, a classification of nursing diagnoses was proposed by the North American Nursing Diagnosis Association, where the phenomenon of concern is patient status (McLane, 1987). More recently, the Nursing Interventions Classification (NIC) project was developed. The use of nursing diagnoses and NIC are becoming widespread in the United States and internationally. Such standardization has many advantages: it helps expand nursing's knowledge base, provides a common language to communicate the functions of nursing, provides shared understanding of nursing practice across national and cultural boundaries, and highlights the distinctive contribution nursing makes toward solving health problems. The International Council of Nurses currently has a project in progress with these goals in mind (Clark, 1994). Although we do not know how the different knowledge development strategies will evolve, significant developments are providing the basis on which to build continuing work by nurse scholars in doctoral programs around the world.

Next Steps

Some authors discuss the urgent need to develop nursing knowledge relevant to the health of the global community (Meleis, 1993). A Western perspective generally pervades organizing concepts and frameworks in nursing and thus is a dominating influence in knowledge development and research. Meleis expressed concern that U.S. nursing doctoral programs may be producing nurse scientists who do not challenge Western perspectives, particularly in terms of definitions and assumptions related to nursing phenomena.

In 1997 we are at a critical juncture for American nursing science. Given the global society in which we live, nursing science now faces the challenge of moving to its next phase of development, which we call "becoming globally relevant." This movement entails a variety of activities and changes in the way we do science, a responsibility that should be shared by scientists in the U.S. and internationally. We need to test nursing models, propositions, and hypotheses in several countries; include relevant content in educational programs; provide opportunities for doctoral students to develop nursing research internships abroad; involve international scholars in editorial review boards; increase the representation of international authors in U.S. journals and vice versa; encourage international students to focus their dissertations on topics pertinent to their countries; integrate collaborative international research in the ongoing work of scientists in leading nursing institutions throughout the world, and expand the criteria for promotion and tenure to include such activity.

We hope the questions raised in this essay will be viewed as opportunities by the global nursing community. If future discussions result in recognition of the challenges facing nursing knowledge development and doctoral education throughout the world, then our purpose will have been served.

REFERENCES

American Academy of Nursing. (1995). *Diversity, marginalization, and culturally-competent health care: Issues in knowledge development*. Washington, DC: Author.

American Nurses Association. (1985). *Code for nurses with interpretive statements*. Kansas City, MO: Author.

Boyacigiller, N.A., & Adler, N.J. (1991). The parochial dinosaur: Organizational science in a global context. *Academy of Management Science, 16(2)*, 262–290.

Clark, J. (1994). The international classification of nursing. In J. McCloskey, & H.K. Grace (Eds.). *Current issues in nursing* (4th ed.) (143–147). St. Louis, MO: Mosby-Year Book.

Colling, J.C., & Liu, Y.C. (1995). International nurses' experiences seeking graduate education in the United States. *Journal of Nursing Education, 34(4)*, 162–166.

El Sayed, Y.A. (1986). *The successive-unsettled transitions of migration and their impact on postpartum concerns of Arab immigrant women*. Unpublished doctoral dissertation, University of California, San Francisco.

Fenton, M.V. (1994). Development of models of international exchange to upgrade nursing education. In J. McCloskey, & H.K. Grace (Eds.). *Current issues in nursing* (4th ed.) 202–206. St. Louis, MO: Mosby-Year Book.

Grace, H. (1978). The development of doctoral education in nursing: An historical perspective. *Journal of Nursing Education, 17(4)*, 17–27.

Haugen Bunch, E. (1987). International perspectives and implications for doctoral education in nursing: Norwegian perspective. In *International perspectives and implications for doctoral education in nursing* (97–105). Portland, OR: Oregon Health Sciences University School of Nursing.

Hockey, L. (1987). Ethical issues in higher education in nursing. In *International perspectives and implications for doctoral education in nursing* (75–85). Portland, OR: Oregon Health Sciences University School of Nursing.

Ketefian, S., & Redman, R.W. (1994). The changing face of graduate education. In J. McCloskey, &

H.K. Grace (Eds.). *Current issues in nursing* (4th ed.) (188–195). St. Louis, MO: Mosby-Year Book.

Leininger, M.M. (1985). Ethnography and ethnonursing: Models and modes of qualitative data analysis. In M.M. Leininger (Ed.). *Qualitative methods in nursing*. New York: Grune & Stratton.

Lipson, J.G., Reizian, A., & Meleis, A.I. (1987). Arab-American patients: A medical record review. *Social Science and Medicine, 24(2)*, 101–107.

May, K.M. (1985). *Arab-American immigrant parents' social networks and health care of children*. Unpublished doctoral dissertation, University of California, San Francisco.

McCloskey, J.C., & Bulechek, G.M. (1994). Standardizing the language for nursing treatments: An overview of the issues. *Nursing Outlook, 42(2)*, 45–63.

McLane, A.M. (1987). *Classification of nursing diagnoses: Proceedings of the seventh conference*. St. Louis, MO: Mosby-Year Book.

Meleis, A.I. (1981). The Arab-American in the Western health care system. *American Journal of Nursing, 6*, 1180–1183.

Meleis, A.I., & Jonsen, A. (1983). Ethical crises and cultural differences. *The Western Journal of Medicine, 138(6)*, 889–893.

Meleis, A.I. (1993). A passion for substance revisited: Global transitions and international commitments. In *Proceedings of the 1993 Annual forum on doctoral nursing education* (5–22). St. Paul, MN, University of Minnesota School of Nursing.

Minami, H. (1987). Reflections of the cultural and social milieu on the development of nursing science in Japan. In *International perspectives and implications for doctoral education in nursing* (63–74). Portland, OR: Oregon Health Sciences University School of Nursing.

Murphy, J.F. (1981). Doctoral education in, of, and for nursing: An historical analysis. *Nursing Outlook, 29(11)*, 645–649.

Orem, D.E. (1991). *Nursing: Concepts of practice* (4th ed.). New York: McGraw-Hill.

Porter, C.P., & Villarruel, A.M. (1993). Nursing research with African American and Hispanic people: Guidelines for action. *Nursing Outlook, 41(2)*, 59–67.

Splane, V.H., & Splane, R.B. (1994). International nursing leaders. In J. McCloskey & H.K. Grace (Eds.). *Current issues in nursing* (4th ed.) (49–56). St. Louis, MO: Mosby-Year Book.

US Department of Health and Human Services. (1990). *Healthy people 2000: National health promotion and disease prevention objectives. Superintendent of documents*. Washington, D.C.: US Government Printing Office.

Werley, H.H., & Lang, N.M. (Eds.). (1988). *Identification of the nursing minimum data set*. New York: Springer.

Zwanger, L. (1987). International perspectives and implications for doctoral education in nursing: The Israeli case. In *International perspectives and implications for doctoral education in nursing* (17–43). Portland, Or: Oregon Health Sciences University School of Nursing.

Part III

NURSING'S METAPARADIGM: CONCEPTUALIZATIONS OF CLIENT AND ENVIRONMENT

A discipline's specialized body of knowledge includes its philosophy, theories, and frameworks or models; major concepts of the discipline reflect its scope of knowledge. Nursing's scope of knowledge is represented in the nursing metaparadigm, which consists of four major concepts: person/client, health, environment, and nursing. These concepts were generally accepted in the 1970s and are the major building blocks for nursing theories and models. Although these four concepts were viewed as essential to grand nursing models and theories, each nurse theorist defined these concepts differently, according to her own philosophical perspective and assumptions about persons, health, environment, and nursing. Although some argue that the nursing discipline needs to establish a major model or theory to guide practice and research, other behavioral disciplines base their practice on numerous theories and models. Also, some nurse scholars insist that nurses be purists and use only nursing theories, while others believe that theories from nursing and other disciplines are complementary and can be adapted and integrated to provide holistic nursing practice. Although these different views may confuse some nurses, others believe these dialogues stimulate thinking and will advance the science of nursing. The following chapters present several nurse scholars' different perspectives on the nursing metaparadigm and meanings of client and environment.

In 1978, Jacqueline Fawcett was the first author to describe the nursing metaparadigm as consisting of four major concepts, which were eventually accepted by the nursing discipline. In her chapter, "On the Requirements for a Metaparadigm: An Invitation to Dialogue," she begins with a description of the requirements for any discipline's metaparadigm. Next, Fawcett presents different concepts introduced by other nurse scholars and provides rational explanations as to the limitations of these concepts in nursing's metaparadigm. She invites scholars to critique her treatise, and one of several responses concludes this chapter. Violet Malinski's response refers to Kuhn's definition of a metaparadigm and others' interpretation of Kuhn's work. Malinski further challenges Fawcett's paper on the basis of changes in nurse scholars' worldviews, which occurred as nurses moved from the empirical, reductionistic, cause-effect linear view of human-environment interactions to a probablistic, interactive, non-linear worldview of simultaneous human-environment interactions, labeled "humanistic nursing science."

The vast majority of nursing models, theories, and articles refer to the recipient of care as a person or client. Few nursing models designate the family or community as client, although they may refer to the client within the context of the family or community. In her chapter, "Clarifying the Concept of "Client" for Health-Care Policy Formulation: Ethical Implications," Phyllis Schultz describes why nurses must consider the broader implications of the clients' aggregate population. She effectively presents steps for ethical decision making to support minority aggregate groups when faced with a scarcity of resources in contemporary health delivery systems.

Environment, as a metaparadigm concept in nursing models and theories, has been defined in various ways. Some nurse theorists never define it; others describe environment as internal and external factors that influence the individual, and some theorists view it as the reciprocal client-environment interaction. More recently, some nurse scholars have expanded the definition of environment to include the effect of social, political, and economic factors that influence clients' health. Patricia Butterfield, in her chapter, "Thinking Upstream: Nurturing a Conceptual Understanding of the Societal Context of Health Behavior," encourages nurses to consider these broad contextual factors that contribute to both individual and aggregate client health problems. She admonishes nurses to become more politically active in their communities if they truly want to promote health rather than merely treating individuals with health problems.

In the 1990s, Dorothy Kleffel began exploring various perspectives for defining the meaning of environment. In her article, "Environment Paradigms: Moving Toward an Ecocentric Perspective," she examines the traditional view of the client's immediate surroundings, mentions the effects of regional disasters, and describes how broad global effects of worldwide hunger, ozone depletion, human overpopulation, and other relevant changes have a global affect on humans' health. Kleffel analyzes the effects of three environmental paradigms—egocentric, homocentric, and ecocentric—on humans' health worldwide and encourages nurses to consider an ecocentric perspective that would encompass global environmental health for all peoples.

12

On the Requirements for a Metaparadigm: An Invitation to Dialogue

JACQUELINE FAWCETT, RN, PhD, FAAN

VIOLET M. MALINSKI, RN, PhD

The purpose of this article is to present four requirements for the metaparadigm of any discipline and to extend an invitation to the scholars of all disciplines to engage in dialogue about the appropriateness and utility of the four requirements. [Keywords: Metaparadigm, Paradigm]

COMMENTARY: Jacqueline Fawcett

DEFINITION AND FUNCTIONS OF A METAPARADIGM

The metaparadigm of any discipline is made up of global concepts that identify the phenomena of interest to a discipline and global propositions that state the relationships among those phenomena (Kuhn, 1977). The metaparadigm is the most abstract component in the structural hierarchy of knowledge of any discipline and "acts as an encapsulating unit, or framework, within which the more restricted . . . structures develop" (Eckberg & Hill, 1979, p. 927). Those more restricted structures include the major philosophical orientations or worldviews of a discipline, as well

as the conceptual models and theories that guide research and other scholarly activities and the empirical indicators that operationalize theoretical concepts.

The metaparadigm represents "the broadest consensus within a discipline. It provides the general parameters of the field and gives scientists [and clinicians] a broad orientation from which to work" (Hardy, 1978, p. 38). Thus, the functions of a metaparadigm are to summarize the intellectual and social missions of a discipline and place a boundary on the subject matter of that discipline (Kim, 1989).

FOUR REQUIREMENTS FOR A METAPARADIGM

The definition and functions of a metaparadigm led the author to the identification of four requirements that are appropriate for the metaparadigm of any discipline. First, a metaparadigm must *identify a domain that is distinctive from the domains of other disciplines.* That re-

Source: Fawcett J., Malinski V. (1996). On the requirements for a metaparadigm: An invitation to dialogue. *Nursing Science Quarterly*, 9(3):94–97, 100–101. Reprinted with permission by Chestnut House Publications

quirement is fulfilled only when the concepts and propositions represent a unique perspective for inquiry and practice. Second, a metaparadigm must *encompass all phenomena of interest to the discipline in a parsimonious manner*. That requirement is fulfilled only if the concepts and propositions are global and if there are no redundancies in concepts or propositions. Third, a metaparadigm must *be perspective-neutral*. That requirement is fulfilled only if the concepts and propositions do not represent a specific perspective, that is, a specific paradigm or conceptual model, or a combination of perspectives. Fourth, a metaparadigm must *be international in scope and substance*. That requirement, which is a corollary of the third requirement, is fulfilled only if the concepts and propositions do not reflect particular national, cultural, or ethnic beliefs and values.

The specification of the four requirements for a metaparadigm provide criteria that can be used to judge the status of any proposal for metaparadigm concepts and propositions. As an example, the author will judge the extent to which her conceptualization of the metaparadigm of nursing and some of the subsequent challenges to that conceptualization meet the four requirements.

THE METAPARADIGM OF NURSING

The author first identified the central concepts of nursing in 1978 and formalized them, along with four relational propositions, as the metaparadigm of nursing in 1984 (Fawcett, 1978, 1984). The concepts are person, environment, health, and nursing. "Person" refers to the recipient of nursing, including individuals, families, communities, and other groups; "environment" refers to the person's significant others and physical surroundings, as well as to the setting in which nursing occurs, which can

range from the person's home to clinical agencies to society as a whole. "Health" is the person's state of well-being, which can range from high-level wellness to terminal illness. Finally, "nursing" refers to the definition of nursing, the *actions taken by nurses on behalf of or in conjunction with the person, and the goals or outcomes of nursing actions*. Nursing actions *typically are viewed as a systematic process of assessment, labeling, planning, intervention, and evaluation*.

The metaparadigm concepts are linked in four propositions that are identified in the writings of Donaldson and Crowley (1978) and Gortner (1980). The first proposition links the person and health; it states that the discipline of nursing is concerned with the principles and laws that govern the life-process, well-being, and optimal functioning of human beings, sick or well.

The second proposition emphasizes the interaction between the person and the environment; it states that the discipline of nursing is concerned with the patterning of human behavior in interaction with the environment in normal life events and critical life situations. The third proposition links health and nursing; it declares that the discipline of nursing is concerned with the nursing actions or processes by which positive changes in health status are effected. The fourth proposition links the person, the environment, and health; it asserts that the discipline of nursing is concerned with the wholeness or health of human beings, recognizing that they are in continuous interaction with their environments.

The author's conceptualization of the metaparadigm of nursing meets the four requirements for any metaparadigm cited above. In particular, the four metaparadigm concepts are generally regarded as the central or domain concepts of nursing (Flaskerud & Halloran, 1980; Jennings, 1987; Wagner, 1986). In addition, the metaparadigm propositions provide a unique perspective of the concepts that helps to distinguish nursing from other disciplines. The first three propositions represent recurrent themes identified in the writings of Florence Nightingale and many other nursing scholars and clinicians of the 19th and 20th centuries. Donaldson and Crowley (1978) commented that "these themes suggest boundaries of an area for systematic [i]nquiry and theory development with potential for making the nature of the discipline of nursing more explicit than it is at present" (p. 113). The fourth proposition, according to Donaldson and Crowley (1978), "evolves from the practical aim of optimizing of human environments for health" (p. 119).

Taken together, the four concepts and four propositions identify the unique focus of the discipline of nursing and encompass all relevant phenomena in a parsimonious manner. Furthermore, the concepts and propositions are perspective-neutral because they do not reflect a specific paradigm or conceptual model. Moreover, the metaparadigm concepts and propositions do not reflect the beliefs and values of any one country or culture and, therefore, are international in scope and substance.

Proposals for Alternative Metaparadigm Concepts and Propositions

This conceptualization of the metaparadigm of nursing certainly should not be regarded as premature closure on explication of phenomena of interest to the discipline of nursing. Indeed, it is anticipated that modifications in the metaparadigm concepts and propositions will be offered as the discipline of nursing evolves. To date, however, the various proposals for alternatives to the four metaparadigm concepts and propositions have not fulfilled one or more of the requirements for a metaparadigm.

One suggested modification in the conceptualization of the metaparadigm of nursing is that the term client replace person (Newman, 1983). Client, however, reflects a particular view of the person (patient would be still another particular view), and, therefore, is not a perspective-neutral concept. Consequently, the suggested modification does not fulfill the third requirement for a metaparadigm.

Another proposed modification is the elimination of the concept nursing from the metaparadigm. Conway (1985) claimed that "nursing" represents the discipline or the profession and is not an appropriate metaparadigm concept because it creates a tautology. Similarly, Meleis (1991) commented, "It would be an instance of tautological conceptualizing to define nursing by all the concepts and then include nursing as one of the concepts" (p. 101). Inasmuch as the metaparadigm concept nursing stands for nursing activities or actions, the author does not think that a tautology was, in fact, created.

Furthermore, inasmuch as Conway (1985) did not offer a substitute metaparadigm concept to represent the actions or activities of nurses, her proposal to eliminate nursing from the metaparadigm does not encompass all phenomena of interest to the discipline of nursing. Moreover, Conway offered no justification for the uniqueness of a discipline dealing only with the person, environment, and health. Her proposal, therefore, does not fulfill the first and second requirements for a metaparadigm.

Still another modification in the metaparadigm is the exclusion of the concept health. Kim (1987) identified four domains of nursing knowledge: the client domain, the client-nurse domain, the practice domain, and the environment domain. Kim's failure to explicitly identify health in her proposal creates a void in an otherwise informative explication of the discipline of nursing. Her view of the domains of nursing knowledge, therefore, does not fulfill the second requirement for a metaparadigm.

Another modification focuses on the addition of metaparadigm concepts. Meleis (1991) maintains that the domain of nursing knowledge encompasses seven central concepts: nursing client, transitions, interaction, nursing process, environment, nursing therapeutics, and health. The inclusion of nursing process, nursing therapeutics, and interactions in Meleis's proposal represents a redundancy that can be avoided by use of the single concept, nursing. Moreover, the inclusion of transitions reflects a particular perspective of human life. Thus, Meleis's proposal for the central concepts of nursing, although meritorious, does not meet the second and third requirements for a metaparadigm.

Four other suggested modifications in the author's conceptualization of the metaparadigm of nursing are more radical than rewording, adding, or eliminating a concept. One radical proposal calls for a new metaparadigm proposition that would replace the four propositions of the author's conceptualization. Newman, Sime, and Corcoran-Perry (1991) claim that the focus of the discipline of nursing is summarized in the following statement: "Nursing is the study of caring in the human health experience" (p. 3). Despite those authors' claims to the contrary, their proposition represents just one frame of reference for nursing and for health. In fact, Newman and her colleagues (1991) ended their paper by maintaining that caring in the human health experience can be most fully elaborated only through a unitary-transformative perspective. Moreover, although the authors offered their proposition as a single statement that integrated "concepts commonly identified with nursing at the metaparadigm level" (p. 3), and although they identified the metaparadigm concepts as person, environment, health, and nursing, their proposition does not include environment.

In an attempt to clarify their position, Newman, Sime, and Corcoran-Perry (1992) later stated, "We view the concept of environment as inherent in and inseparable from the integrated focus of caring in the human health experience" (p. vii). Despite that clarification, the substitute proposition does not meet the second and third requirements for a metaparadigm because it is neither sufficiently comprehensive nor perspective-neutral.

Another radical proposal comes from Malloch et al., (1992), who suggest a revision of the Newman, Sime, and Corcoran-Perry (1991) statement. Their focus statement is: "Nursing is the study and practice of caring within contexts of the human health experience" (p. vi). Malloch and her colleagues maintain that their statement extends the focus of the discipline to nursing practice and incorporates the environment by the use of the term "contexts." They note that environment "includes, but is not limited to, culture, community, and ecology" (p. vi). Moreover, they claim that the use of the term caring brings unity to the metaparadigm concepts of person, environment, health, and nursing. Apparently, they do not regard caring as a particular perspective of nursing. Although this substitute proposition is sufficiently comprehensive, it does not meet the third requirement for a metaparadigm because it is not perspective-neutral.

Still another radical proposal calls for the substitution of a proposition asserting the centrality of caring to the discipline of nursing. Leininger (1990) claimed that "human care/caring [is] the central phenomenon and essence of nursing" (p. 19), and Watson (1990) maintained that "human caring needs to be explicitly incorporated into nursing's metaparadigm" (p. 21). Even more to the point, Leininger (1991) maintained that "care is the essence of nursing and the central, dominant, and unifying focus of nursing" (p. 35).

Both Leininger and Watson have failed to acknowledge that, although the term caring is included in several conceptualizations of the discipline of nursing (Morse, Solberg, Neander, Bottorff, & Johnson, 1990), it is not a dominant theme in every conceptualization and, therefore, does not represent a discipline-wide viewpoint. In fact, caring reflects a particular view of nursing and a particular kind of nursing (Eriksson, 1989). Furthermore, as Swanson (1991) pointed out, although there may be "characteristic behavior patterns that are universal expressions of nurse caring . . . caring is not uniquely a nursing phenomenon" (p. 165). Caring behaviors, moreover, may not be generalizable across national and cultural boundaries (Mandelbaum, 1991). And, as Rogers (1992) asserted, "As such, caring does not identify nurses any more than it identifies workers from another field. Everyone needs to care" (p. 33). Consequently, the proposal to substitute caring for nursing in the metaparadigm does not meet the first, third, and fourth requirements for a metaparadigm.

The fourth radical proposal comes from Meleis and Trangenstein (1994), who maintain that "facilitating transitions is a focus for the discipline of nursing" and that "the mission of nursing . . . [is] facilitating and dealing with people who are undergoing transitions" (p. 255). They go on to describe a conceptual framework that has transitions as its central concept. Inasmuch as Meleis and Trangenstein explicitly identify their work as a conceptual framework, and inasmuch as transitions represent just one way in which to view "the process and outcome of complex person-environment interactions" (p. 256), their proposal is not perspective-neutral. Thus, at best it does not meet the third requirement for a metaparadigm.

AN INVITATION TO DIALOGUE

The author concludes by extending an invitation to the scholars of all disciplines to debate the appropriateness of the four requirements for a metaparadigm presented here. In particular, discussion is invited on the soundness and logic of the four requirements, as well as their utility as criteria to judge proposals for the metaparadigm concepts and propositions of any discipline.

REFERENCES

Conway, M. E. (1985). Toward greater specificity in defining nursing's metaparadigm. *Advances in Nursing Science, 7*(4), 73–81.

Donaldson, S. K., & Crowley, D. M. (1978). The discipline of nursing. *Nursing Outlook, 26,* 113–120.

Eckberg, D. L., & Hill, L., Jr. (1979). The paradigm concept and sociology: A critical review. *American Sociological Review, 44,* 925–937.

Eriksson, K. (1989). Caring paradigms. A study of the origins and the development of caring paradigms among nursing students. *Scandinavian Journal of Caring Science, 3,* 169–176.

Fawcett, J. (1978). The "what" of theory development. In *Theory development: What, why, how?* (pp. 17–33). New York: National League for Nursing.

Fawcett, J. (1984). The metaparadigm of nursing. Current status and future refinements. *Image: The Journal of Nursing Scholarship, 16,* 84–87.

Flaskerud, J. H., & Halloran, E. J. (1980). Areas of agreement in nursing theory development. *Advances in Nursing Science, 3*(1), 1–7.

Gortner, S. R. (1980). Nursing science in transition. *Nursing Research, 29,* 180–183.

Hardy, M. E. (1978). Perspectives on nursing theory. *Advances in Nursing Science, 1*(1), 37–48.

Jennings, B. M. (1987). Nursing theory development: Successes and challenges. *Journal of Advanced Nursing, 12,* 63–69.

Kim, H. S. (1987). Structuring the nursing knowledge system: A typology of four domains. *Scholarly Inquiry for Nursing Practice, 1,* 99–110.

Kim, H. S. (1989). Theoretical thinking in nursing: Problems and prospects. *Recent Advances in Nursing, 24,* 106–122.

Kuhn, T. S. (1977). Second thoughts on paradigms. In F. Suppe (Ed.), *The structure of scientific theories* (2nd ed., pp. 459–517). Chicago: University of Illinois Press.

Leininger, M. M. (1990). Historic and epistemologic dimensions of care and caring with future directions. In J. S. Stevenson & T. Tripp-Reimer (Eds.),

Knowledge about care and caring: State of the art and future developments (pp. 19–31). Kansas City, MO: American Academy of Nursing.

Leininger, M. M. (1991). The theory of culture care diversity and universality. In M. M. Leininger (Ed.), *Culture care diversity and universality: A theory of nursing* (pp. 5–65). New York: National League for Nursing.

Malloch, K., Martinez, R., Nelson, L., Predeger, B., Speakman, L., Steinbinder, A., & Tracy, J. (1992). To the editor [Letter]. *Advances in Nursing Science, 15*(2), vi–vii.

Mandelbaum, J. (1991). Why there cannot be an international theory of nursing. *International Nursing Review, 38,* 53–55, 48.

Meleis, A. I. (1991). *Theoretical nursing: Development and progress* (2nd ed.), Philadelphia: Lippincott.

Meleis, A. I., & Trangenstein, P. A. (1994). Facilitating transitions: Redefinition of the nursing mission. *Nursing Outlook, 42,* 255–259.

Morse, J. M., Solberg, S. M., Neander, W. L., Bottorff, J. L., & Johnson, J. L. (1990). Concepts of caring and caring as a concept. *Advances in Nursing Science, 13*(1), 1–14.

Newman, M. A. (1983). The continuing revolution: A history of nursing science. In N. L. Chaska (Ed.), *The nursing profession: A time to speak* (pp. 385–393). New York: McGraw Hill.

Newman, M. A., Sime, A. M., & Corcoran-Perry, S. A. (1991). The focus of the discipline of nursing. *Advances in Nursing Science, 14*(1), 1–6.

Newman, M. A., Sime, A. M., & Corcoran-Perry, S. A. (1992). Authors' reply [Letter to the Editor]. *Advances in Nursing Science, 14*(3), vi–vii.

Rogers, M. E. (1992). Nursing science and the space age. *Nursing Science Quarterly, 5,* 27–34.

Swanson, K. M. (1991). Empirical development of a middle range theory of caring. *Nursing Research, 40,* 161–165.

Wagner, J. D. (1986). Nurse scholars' perceptions of nursing's metaparadigm. *Dissertation Abstracts International, 47,* 1932B.

Watson, J. (1990). Caring knowledge and informed moral passion. *Advances in Nursing Science, 13*(1), 15–24.

RESPONSE: Violet M. Malinski

Fawcett presents a scholarly argument for her delineation of the metaparadigm of nursing and the requirements that she believes support its validity. As a first step in dialogue, this author proposes an examination of the basic idea of the metaparadigm itself. Perhaps it is time to drop the metaparadigm entirely. The desire to identify some grand, unifying schema for all of nursing is no longer warranted. Nursing is showing itself to be more diverse than homogeneous. If there is indeed a unifying metaparadigm that presents global concepts and propositions that identify nursing, it must be so broad and general as to be relatively meaningless in terms of defining the scope of nursing and providing direction for all of its members. This is a problem posed by Fawcett's second requirement, as well.

One major problem with the idea of a metaparadigm stems from the confusion over Kuhn's (1970) work that is readily apparent in the literature. Masterman (1970) identified 21 different interpretations given by Kuhn himself in the first edition of *The Structure of Scientific Revolutions.* They can be clustered into three groups, one of which represents the idea of the metaparadigm, a pre-theoretical structure reflecting consensus on a common perspective acknowledged by the discipline.

Hardy (1978) used Kuhn's ideas regarding the development of scientific knowledge to classify nursing as preparadigm science. She described the metaparadigm as the "total world view within a discipline" (p. 38), representing the broadest consensus regarding the focus and boundaries of any given discipline. Hardy interpreted Kuhn's (1970) work as supporting two types of paradigms: this broad, abstract metaparadigm plus exemplars, paradigms more restricted in scope. According to Hardy, a discipline may have more than one exemplar paradigm existing under the umbrella of the metaparadigm. Kuhn (1977), however, maintained that he had intended his discussion of paradigms as exemplars to be understood in the sense of standard examples (exemplars) of problems and solutions, a more limited interpretation than Hardy's. Problems with attempts to use Kuhn's ideas as a guide arise because of the multiple interpretations possible. He himself lamented the "excessive plasticity" of the word "paradigm" in later work (Kuhn, 1977, p. 10). As a replacement, he suggested the term "disciplinary matrix" be used to represent the shared elements serving as a common framework for communication and judgments by a cohort of professionals.

Riegel et al., (1992) used this idea of a disciplinary matrix to present a generative philosophy of science for nursing. They also suggested that members of a discipline share a worldview which is based on its matrix, or structure and content. What then happens when novel, creative ideas emerge that do not fit this worldview and are not embraced by the majority? "Data judged by most members as anomalous may be seen as innovative and provocative by a sub-group who moves the discipline in a new direction" (Riegel et al., 1992, p. 119). Such movement has the potential to generate a new or different-focused discipline. One unanswered question for these authors is whether one discipline can "reside within or overlap with another" (Riegel et al., 1992, p. 119).

Thus the metaparadigm is intended to represent a broad consensus—the majority view. What happens to the minority who may, indeed, be striving to move the discipline in a new direction? Nursing theories and models representing the simultaneity (Parse, 1987) or unitary-transformative (Newman, Sime, & Corcoran-Perry, 1991) worldviews represent a different focus in nursing.

Using Kuhn's definition of a paradigm as a worldview that guides inquiry, Parse (1987) identified two competing conceptualizations or worldviews in nursing. She cited this as a positive development reflecting the growth of nursing as a scientific discipline. The simultaneity and totality worldviews are different, however, "Theories are grounded in the belief system of the paradigm, which means that the definitions of the concepts of the theories are congruent with beliefs set forth in the para-

digm" (Parse, 1987, p. 2). The totality worldview represents the traditional, majority perspective of nursing, whereas the simultaneity worldview represents an emerging, minority perspective.

Peplau (1987) echoed Parse's view that competing paradigms had, indeed, emerged. Like Parse, Peplau (1987) welcomed them and the "intense conflict, argument, discussion, and comparisons of performance in research" (p. 22) that should emerge to challenge the adherents of each. Peplau (1987) cited Donaldson and Crowley's 1978 work as an example of an effort to synthesize common themes across the works of many nurse scholars. She acknowledged Fawcett's effort to develop the metaparadigm concepts from Donaldson and Crowley's themes as well as other nursing literature. However, Peplau (1987) questions whether this effort represents nursing's need for cohesion "or suggests a unified field theory of nursing, and, therefore, a lack of distinct, different, self-contained knowledge in the paradigms thus merged. . . ." (p. 22).

This attempt at consensus and merger is reflected in Fawcett's third criterion that a metaparadigm be perspective-neutral. However, the metaparadigm is not perspective-neutral but reflective of the dominant view in nursing. For example, the metaparadigm concept "nursing" is used by Fawcett (1996) to reflect "actions taken by nurses on behalf of or in conjunction with the person, and the goals or outcomes of nursing actions . . . typically . . . viewed as a systematic process of assessment, labeling, planning, intervention, and evaluation" (p. 95). This reflects those theories and models that fit the totality worldview but not the simultaneity one. This distinction needs to be acknowledged, not glossed over. A view of the person as participating in change through freely choosing is not amenable to a nursing process used to identify interventions designed to achieve positive outcomes and an evaluation based on the degree of success in attaining these outcomes (Cody & Mitchell, 1992). The identification of nursing as a human science further suggests that the discipline must draw on a base different from the natural sciences. " 'Biological' manifestations are not ignored but are subsumed within the experience of the person. . . ." (Cody & Mitchell, 1992, p. 61).

Such a shift was inaugurated with the nursing science of Martha Rogers (1970). Traditionally nursing has articulated a systems view of the holistic person interacting with the environment. Added to this was a belief in prediction and the value of objective methods in research (Newman, 1994). Cowling (1993) clearly articulated the differences between systems thinking and unitary thinking, ushered in by Rogers. Nursing has evolved beyond the pre-paradigm stage identified by Hardy (1978) and is now struggling with the meaning of a paradigm shift (Newman, 1994). Although Newman et al., (1991) maintained that the unitary-transformative perspective, their name for this shift in worldviews, is essential for nursing, it is still the minority view in nursing.

In recognition of these differences, if the metaparadigm is retained as a viable structure then perhaps there are two metaparadigms that need to be identified. Fawcett's conceptualization may encompass the totality theorists. For the simultaneity theorists, Sarter's (1988) foundational attempt to identify common philosophical themes may provide the starting point.

Sarter examined the work of Rogers, Parse, Newman, and Watson (including a critique of the latter's work showing where she diverges from the other three), and described the following pattern of themes: process, evolutionary change (human consciousness, not physical evolution), health as evolution, self-transcendence, openness, pattern, and space and time as nonlinear, fluid, and relative. Although Sarter stated her intent as con-

tributing to a single metaparadigm of nursing, it is clear that such themes do not describe the ideas of totality theorists such as Orem, Roy, and Neuman. Perhaps Sarter's initial attempt could be pursued with the intent to delineate a second metaparadigm serving as an umbrella for a second disciplinary group in nursing. Suppe (1977) offered physics as an example of a discipline with co-existing disciplinary matrixes, one based on relativity theory, one on classical mechanics. He challenged Kuhn's interpretation of a shared disciplinary matrix, proposing that in reality this would mean "all disciplinary groups will consist of a single individual" (Suppe, 1977, p. 498).

This reflects a different interpretation of the metaparadigm. Rather than a preexisting umbrella structure whose concepts and propositions would be reflected in all subsequent models and theories developed in the discipline, the metaparadigm(s) would be synthesized from the paradigms, and the models and theories falling under them. Rather than a static structure, fixed by the historical evolution of the discipline, it would be a constantly evolving one, changing with changes in the discipline. Perhaps nursing needs this type of radical shift in definition to get out from under the historical baggage still weighing down its members. In a short television review of a play on Broadway called "Sacrilege," the nun who aspires to priesthood explains her situation to the priest along the lines of: Imagine you were educated to be a doctor and were told you could only be a nurse? In 1996 and beyond, struggling through the meaning of the radical paradigm shift behind a true nursing science underwriting a practice autonomous from medicine merits a different metaparadigm.

Assuming the metaparadigm is retained, Fawcett's discussion of proposed alternative concepts and propositions shows that it is too early to accept any one delineation as definitive. Some of the suggestions deserve further exploration. For example, "client" does represent a particular view, as does "patient," but it is a view consistent with nursing's philosophical beliefs about the uniqueness and autonomy of human beings. Perhaps "client" is more inclusive than "person," more readily suggesting that nurses can be speaking of one individual, groups of individuals, or a community as a whole. Although particular caring behaviors will not generalize across all cultures, the existence of caring behaviors will. They will be actualized as appropriate within any given culture. Arguments can be made for the suitability of various proposals. They attest to the fact that nursing is not static but is continually evolving and changing.

Fawcett's criteria and invitation to dialogue represent an important contribution to this process. Those who are pursuing alternatives should be encouraged to move forward, continuing the dialogue.

REFERENCES

Cody, W. K., & Mitchell, G. J. (1992). Parse's theory as a model for practice: The cutting edge. *Advances in Nursing Science, 15*(2), 52–65.

Cowling, W. R., III. (1993). Unitary knowing in nursing practice. *Nursing Science Quarterly, 6*, 201–207.

Fawcett, J. (1996). On the requirements for a metaparadigm: An invitation to dialogue: Commentary. *Nursing Science Quarterly, 9*, 94–97.

Hardy, M. E. (1978). Perspective on nursing theory. *Advances in Nursing Science, 1*(1), 37–48.

Kuhn, T. S. (1970). *The structure of scientific revolutions, 2nd ed.* Chicago: The University of Chicago Press.

Kuhn, T. S. (1977). Second thoughts on paradigms. In F. Suppe (Ed.), *The structure of scientific theories, 2nd ed.* (pp. 459–482). Chicago: University of Illinois Press.

Masterman, M. (1970). The nature of paradigm. In I. Lakatos & A. Musgrave (Eds.), *Criticism and the growth of knowledge* (pp. 59–89). London: Cambridge Press.

Newman, M. A. (1994). Theory for nursing practice. *Nursing Science Quarterly, 7*, 153–157.

Newman, M. A., Sime, A. M., & Corcoran-Perry, S. A. (1991). The focus of the discipline of nursing. *Advances in Nursing Science, 14*(1), 1–6.

Parse, R. R. (1987). Paradigms and theories. In R. R. Parse (Ed.), *Nursing science: Major paradigms, theories, and critiques* (pp. 1–11). Philadelphia: Saunders.

Peplau, H. E. (1987). Nursing science: A historical perspective. In R. R. Parse (Ed.), *Nursing science: Major paradigms, theories, and critiques* (pp. 13–29). Philadelphia: Saunders.

Riegel, B., Omery, A., Calvillo, E., Elsayed, N.G., Lee, P., Shuler, P. & Siegel, B.E. (1992). Moving beyond: A generative philosophy of science. *Image Journal of Nursing Scholarship, 24*, 115–119.

Rogers, M. E. (1970). *An introduction to the theoretical basis of nursing.* Philadelphia: Davis.

Sarter, B. (1988). Philosophical sources of nursing theory. *Nursing Science Quarterly, 1*, 52–59.

Suppe, F. (1977). Exemplars, theories and disciplinary matrixes. In F. Suppe (Ed.), *The structure of scientific theories, 2nd ed.* (pp. 483–499). Chicago: University of Illinois Press.

13

Clarifying the Concept of "Client" for Health-Care Policy Formulation: Ethical Implications

PHYLLIS R. SCHULTZ, RN, MN, PhD

Health-care professionals continue to focus their ethical decision making on problems and dilemmas of individual clients, often ignoring health and illness patterns in populations and organizational and community dimensions of ethical alternatives. Such a focus leads to choices that may not reflect the preferences or shared values of the community; it leads to choices that limit or ignore a search for the common good in favor of preserving what is good for individuals.

CLARIFYING "CLIENT"

One reason ethical decision making from an aggregate, organizational, and community perspective has been hampered in its development and adoption by health-care practitioners is the continuing emphasis in health-care delivery on the individual person, while neglecting the family, work group, community, or societal conditions and forces that may account for health problems. As a result of defining the client as a single person, or at most a single family, there is a corollary tendency to focus on ethical dilemmas that apply only to individuals in particular cases (e.g., to

discontinue life-saving efforts or not, to treat or not). Built into this individualist approach is the implicit notion that these decisions have little or no impact on provider organizations or the community, that is, the outcome only affects those who are directly involved. The facts deny this notion, however. If a decision is made to treat a particular severely deformed newborn, the cost of that treatment is such that the subsequent scarcity of resources to which a provider organization has access, or the lack of resources within the community generally, will force a decision to not treat others. This type of situation can be defined as an "ethical dilemma of the aggregate," the former as an "ethical dilemma of the individual."

For dilemmas of the aggregate to be attended to equally, the definition of *client* must be reconceptualized to include "more than one"[1]; the new definition must include aggregates of individuals *and* such collective entities as families, groups, formal and informal organizations, communities of locality, and communities of affinity. This is a tall order, for, as Archer has noted, "to shift from focusing on an individual or a [single] family as the client to focusing on an aggregate or community as the client requires a considerable adjustment in one's thinking."[2(p36)] Despite the fact that for many years there has been a viewpoint in the health-care literature advocating such an ad-

Source: Schultz, P. R. (1987). Clarifying the concept of "client" for health care policy formulation: Ethical implications. *Family and Community Health, 10* (1): 73-82. Reprinted with permission from and copyright © 1987 Aspen Publishers, Inc.

justment in thinking,[3-7] the prevailing attitude and focus among most health-care professionals is toward individuals.

A limited review of the literature reveals that the term *aggregate* is often used synonymously with the terms *groups, groups-at-risk, subpopulations,* and *populations.* These terms are used in redirecting the focus to families, groups, organizations, and communities as the "client."[3] These terms reflect that *group* is used in two ways in the health literature: (1) as a collectivity of single individuals in which a numerical or statistical count of the individuals defines the aggregate, and (2) as an interactional unit or system in which the whole is more than the sum of the individual persons. Sampson and Marthas[8] offer some helpful distinctions between these two usages. The term *group* refers to

> associations between two or more persons who are in some kind of interdependent relationship to one another. . . . [By contrast, an aggregate is only] a collectivity of persons who share some characteristic in common. . . . Of course, when that shared characteristic becomes relevant to the members' definitions of themselves and others, then we have the beginnings of a group.[8(p22)]

Thus, identification and interdependence among members of an aggregate are dimensions of interactional units that distinguish them from mere statistical collectivities. These distinguishing definitions provide some clues as to how members of community health and organizational disciplines can redefine the term *client* to reflect their practice.

In nursing, for example, attempts to define the term *client* as more than a single individual focus on "the aggregate,"[2-5] "the community,"[2,6,7] and "the organization."[9-11] To be congruent with the basic assumptions and defining concepts of nursing as a discipline,

however, the concepts of health, environment, and interaction must be a part of any definition of client.[12] Therefore, for the purpose of defining the term *client* as more than one in nursing, an aggregate is a collectivity of individual human beings with a health- or illness-related personal or environmental characteristic in common.[2-4] The aggregate may vary in size from a few to an entire population. At some point, the individuals in the aggregate may define themselves in relation to the collective, interact with each other, and become interdependent to some degree. When and if this occurs, the social interactional unit that emerges is more than the sum of the individuals. Thus two distinctive phenomena can be identified—interactional units (ie, families, groups, organizations, communities) and aggregates that are part of the structural components of such units—each with properties and dimensions. For example, a metropolitan tertiary-care hospital is a type of interactional unit. Persons with chronic obstructive lung disease who receive their care and treatment from that hospital and identify the hospital as their care source are one type of aggregate that comprise its structure. The members of this aggregate may become interactive if they identify the hospital as their care source, or begin to participate with their caregivers and each other in support or therapeutic groups. The above reasoning can be summarized with the following argument: (1) Interaction is basic to the practice of nursing,[12] and (2) aggregates, by definition, are not interactional;[8,13] therefore, (3) interactional units (ie, families, groups, organizations, or communities) with which aggregates are associated are the appropriate focus of practice when "client" is more than one.

It is not appropriate to neglect aggregates, however. Rather, assessing the health-related dimensions of the aggregates associated with interactional units is as essential to the nursing care of families, groups, or communities as assessing the physical, psychologic, social, cultural, and spiritual dimensions of the person is to nursing care of the individual. It is through an understanding of the health-related dimensions of aggregates in addition to the structures and processes of the interactional units associated with them that nursing programs of care can be designed and implemented when the client is more than one. Such programs of care can be understood to be a type of nursing treatment modality when the client is redefined in this manner.[1] This reasoning may apply to other health-care disciplines, such as community psychology, health administration, health education, medicine, nutrition, and social work, as well as nursing.

Two points can be summarized from the position developed above: (1) Community health nurse clinicians and nurse administrators (and perhaps other community health providers) have interactional units as clients and (2) to care properly for these types of clients requires attending to the statistical aggregates associated with them as well as to the properties and dimensions of the interactional units themselves.

IMPLICATIONS FOR ETHICAL DECISION MAKING

Ethical decision making is a reasoning process that "ends in the choice of a morally justifiable action to be taken in a given situation."[14(p89)] When ethical decision making is cast within the perspective of a reconceptualization of the client as interactional units and their associated aggregates, steps in the process can be elaborated to facilitate a resolution to what has been called the dilemmas of the aggregate. Thompson and Thompson[14] have described a model for bioethical decision making that is useful as an organizing framework.

However, it is important to note that heretofore the framework has been used most commonly to assist health-care professionals or families to resolve dilemmas of individuals. The purpose in using the model here is to explicate the ethical decision-making processes for dealing with dilemmas that involve more than single individuals. It includes 10 steps of which only the first six are explicated below to assist with the resolution of dilemmas of the aggregate. As a context for applying the Thompson and Thompson model, the following example must be considered.

A tertiary-care hospital in a large metropolitan community is faced with increasing numbers of persons seeking hospitalization who are unable to pay and are uninsured. (It is estimated that the number of such persons throughout the United States was greater than 35 million in 1986.[15]) Concurrently, the hospital is experiencing a scarcity of resources due to the economic depression in the United States, public policies to curtail health-care costs, and decreases in charitable contributions. The hospital's raison d'etre is to care for the ill and injured who request care. However, to protect the hospital's viability, such care must be paid for in one of three ways: direct payment by the individuals; third-party payment, such as insurance; or charitable contributions targeted for such care. This is a dilemma because it is a "situation of ambiguity and conflict with equally unattractive alternatives for choice, decision making, and action."[16(p38)] This is not just a dilemma of whether to care for particular individuals. It is an ethical dilemma of the aggregate because the individuals involved are "unknown persons in possible future peril";[17(p81)] namely, those individuals who will be denied care in the future if the hospital establishes a policy of limiting the number of persons who will receive uncompensated care.

With reference to the reconceptualization of the client, both the aggregate of uninsured persons and the interactional units with which they are associated (e.g., the hospital or its community) must be taken into account in the formulation of a policy from an ethical perspective.

The First Step

The first step in ethical decision making in health care as defined by Thompson and Thompson is, "Review the situation to determine health problems, decisions needed, ethical components, and key individuals."[14(p99)] If a health-care organization is the interactional unit of focus (ie, the client), members can be identified who can proceed with the decision-making process by following the four parts of this first step.

Determining Health Problems

To determine health problems, information that describes the aggregate must be reviewed by asking the following questions: How many uninsured, unable-to-pay persons are provided service annually? What are their demographic characteristics? What percentage of potential total revenues does their care represent? What types of health problems do they have? How do their lengths of stay and problems compare with persons who can pay? These questions reflect an orientation to the aggregate and the associated interactional unit (ie, the hospital). By contrast, an orientation to a dilemma of the individual would generate questions such as the following: How serious is the condition? What other resources does the individual have? How costly is the care likely to be and could a payment plan be worked out?

Identifying the Proper Decision

To determine the nature of the decision that is needed, the following questions must be answered: Does an organizational policy need to be formulated? If so, will it take the form of a statement of the number of such persons that will be served in a given time period?

Identifying Ethical Components

Once the nature of the decision has been identified, the components of such a decision must be clarified. Aroskar noted that allocation of scarce resources "falls into the area of distributive justice—a most difficult point of social concern for individuals and communities [and health-care organizations]."[16(p38)] She reviewed four possible ethical positions that could undergird the development of such a policy: egoistic, deontologic, utilitarian, and fairness. For example, if organization decision makers took an egoistic position, they would develop a policy that would be to the best advantage of their institution (eg, a policy that would maintain the financial viability of the institution and protect the investment of the stockholders).

If a deontologic position were taken, advantage or the consequences of the policy would be superseded by rules of "right behavior" (eg, a health-care organization is obligated to provide care regardless of the consequences, regardless of whether providing uncompensated care threatens the financial viability of the institution).

The utilitarian position is generally stated as "the greatest good and the least amount of harm for the greatest number of persons,"[16(p39)] which could result in a policy that provided at least some care (eg, emergency care) for all, but stopped short of full treatment of the problems. This can be viewed as a more "community-oriented ethic,"[16] but it remains an unresolved issue in American health care.[17]

The "justice as fairness" position is based on the principle that "inequalities are allowed only to improve the condition of the least advantaged in the community."[16(p40)] This means that a policy would be developed by organizational decision makers that would permit some inequalities of status and treatment in order to provide care to the poorest and sickest of the uninsured. These are some of the ethical alternatives that are available to organization decision makers.

Determining Key Individuals

The fourth part of the first step[14] is to determine who are the key individuals within the organization who will implement the decision and the policy. The policy must create the conditions within which moral action and caring by individuals can flourish.[18] This means the policy must be one that does not put individual health-care providers in a conflictive situation with their personal and professional value commitments. Health-care organization policy (or lack thereof) can place the burden of rejecting someone for care on the shoulders of individual care providers, which puts them in a conflictive situation; or, if formulated from the perspective presented here, it can create the condition in which the caregivers can act according to their moral principles. This is most likely to occur if the policy is formulated according to the steps discussed below.

The Second Step

The second step suggested by Thompson and Thompson is to "gather additional information to clarify the situation."[14(p99)] Additional information to be gathered may be to learn what other health-care organizations within the community are doing with regard to the uninsured. To what extent are all provider organizations within the community faced with the same dilemma? Is the organizational dilemma a community dilemma? Again, to ask these kinds of questions is to take an interactional unit and aggregate perspective in contrast to gathering additional information about particular uninsured individuals. Also, it opens the way to thinking about "the common good" for the community and for society at large rather than merely preserving the self-interest of particular individuals or particular health-care organizations.[19]

It is the idea that individuals and organizations are members of what Beauchamp has called a "body politic."[19(p29)] He stated, "Common citizenship, despite diversity and divergence of interests, presumes an underlying shared set of loyalties and obligations to support the ends of the political community, among which public health and safety are central."[19(p19)] This idea leads to consideration of the community as the client, in addition to the health-care organization.

Some additional information to be gathered as part of the second step concerns whether there is a point of view about care of the uninsured emerging in the community. To what extent is the community aware that health-care provider organizations are facing this dilemma? Is there a forum in which the issues involved can be discussed? Is there a need for a community policy that will create the conditions in which moral action and caring by organizations as well as individuals can flourish?

The Third Step

At the third step, members of the organization or community are directed to "identify the ethical issues in the situation."[14(p99)] Questions to be asked by members of the provider organization or the community include the following: Is the shared value of members of the provider organization or the community one that supports the preservation of individual autonomy in preference to beneficence or justice? Are profits for stockholders more important than providing care to the community?

The Fourth Step

The task at the fourth step is to "define personal and professional moral positions."[14(p99)] The personal and moral positions of several types of organizational and community members must be identified and discussed. To what extent will the position and policy taken by the provider organization violate professional ethical codes? Nurses and physicians, for example, are bound by their respective professional codes to care for individuals in need. If an organizational policy is formulated to limit the numbers of persons who cannot pay, how can such conflict be resolved when individual practitioners must confront particular uninsured persons who present for care?

Fry specifically identified this type of dilemma as characteristic of community health nursing practice.[20] She stated, "Accountability in community health nursing may mean being answerable for how the health of aggregate groups has been promoted, protected and/or met rather than being answerable for how the health of individuals has been promoted, protected and/or met."[20(p178)] Today, however, this prescription is not limited to nurses nor to the community health domain as traditionally defined. This same dilemma is faced by healthcare workers of all specialties in most healthcare settings because of the pressures to try to care for persons with finite and limited organizational and community resources.

The Fifth and Sixth Steps

The fifth and sixth steps involve identifying moral positions of key individuals involved, especially identifying conflicting moral positions, if any.[14(p99)] The moral positions of those organizational members who must articulate the policy to the public and implement it in the organization must be considered. Identifying potential moral-value conflicts with the policy in advance can prevent the undermining of the policy or the demoralization of those involved in its implementation.

Here there may be differences among various professional groups or individual members. For example, Gilligan[21] and Noddings[18] suggest that there may be a feminine perspective (largely expressed by, but not necessarily limited to, women) involved in the resolution of dilemmas such as the one being discussed. This idea is relevant here. Nursing is one health discipline whose members are mostly women and the proportion of women among health educators, social workers, nutritionists, and community psychologists is high. Also, the number of women in medicine is increasing. Gilligan found that the women she had interviewed made sense of moral dilemmas in terms of care, responsibility, and relationships rather than by rights and rules.[21] Whereas the traditional "conception of morality as justice ties development to the logic of equality and reciprocity,"[21(p73)] the feminine ethics of caring gives "subjectivity its proper place" in relationships[18(p6)] and insists on "the reconstruction of the dilemma in its contextual particularity."[21(p100)]

The universality of this conception of morality is not in rules of conduct that hold in every case but in the response to human pain and suffering called forth by the dilemma. Women know that ultimately they are responsible and will be held accountable for the caring that is the consequence of any choice or policy. So, Gilligan[21] observes, their initial consideration in moral problem solving is one of survival of the self so that whatever caring is to occur can be realized. The second consideration of women is to learn enough about the realities of the dilemma to ensure that the most good and least harm is identified in the alternative actions. Their third consideration is that the most adequate guide to the resolution of conflicts is a "reflective understanding of care."[21(p105)] Noddings, whose development of the caring approach to ethics follows the same general pattern as the one just sketched, stresses the importance that the "one caring" be genuinely "engrossed" and "present" to the others who are parties to the dilemma.[18(p16)]

THE CHALLENGE OF THE THOMPSON AND THOMPSON MODEL

The caring perspective on ethical decision making, to which point the explication of the Thompson and Thompson model has progressed, is important for reasons already indicated, but it also carries a challenge to policy makers. If caring, as elaborated by Gilligan and Noddings, is intended to focus on particular individuals in concrete contexts, how can such an ethical outlook be reconciled with a commitment to clients who are merely statistical, abstractly designated entities? In the course of following the steps outlined above, members of an organization or community can work through a wide spectrum of considerations, from the descriptive statistical realities of the aggregate of persons unable to pay to the pain, anxiety, and suffering of particular individuals, their families, and the professionals in the situation who must give or deny the care. From a feminine perspective (not just from an entrepreneurial perspective), it makes sense for the managers or board of directors of a healthcare provider organization to raise the question of its survival. If the burden of caring for those unable to pay becomes too great, the organization will fail and what care was available will no longer be available.

What is critical to the resolution of dilemmas of the aggregate, however, is the open discussion and dialogue within the organization and the community so that the full context of the dilemma can be revealed. In the full revealing of the context lies the hope for discovering fair, least harmful alternatives that can provide the conditions within which moral action can occur. This is the potential of complementing a focus on individuals, their immediate families, and their immediate professional caregivers with an aggregate, organizational, and community perspective.

CONCLUSION

In *Habits of the Heart*, Bellah et al.[22] explored whether American society can resolve the tension between individual interest and the public good. They noted, "In a free republic, it is the task of the citizen, whether ruler or ruled, to cultivate civic virtue in order to mitigate [this] tension and render it manageable."[22(p270)] In the dilemmas that confront the citizenry in family and community health and across the entire spectrum of health care, such virtue must be cultivated by attending both to dilemmas of the individual and to dilemmas of the aggregate.

REFERENCES

1. Schultz PR: When "person/client" is more than one. Expanding a foundational concept. Unpublished manuscript, Denver, Colorado, 1986.
2. Archer SE, Fleshman RP: *Community Health Nursing*, ed 2. Monterey, Calif, Wadsworth, 1985.
3. Williams, CA: Community nursing—what is it? *NO* 1977;25:250-255.
4. Williams, CA: Population-focused practice, in Stanhope M, Lancaster J (eds): *Community Health Nursing: Process and Practice for Promoting Health*. St. Louis, Mosby, 1984.
5. Williams, CA: Population-focused community health nursing and nursing administration: A new synthesis, in McCloskey JC, Grace HK (eds): *Current Issues in Nursing*, ed 2. Boston, Blackwell Scientific, 1985.
6. Clemen SA, Eigsti DG, McGuire SL: *Comprehensive Family and Community Health Nursing*, New York, McGraw-Hill, 1981.
7. Goeppinger J: Community as client: Using the nursing process to promote health, in Stanhope M, Lancaster J (eds): *Community Health Nursing: Process and Practice for Promoting Health*. St. Louis, Mosby, 1984.
8. Sampson EE, Marthas MS: *Group Process for the Health Professions*. New York, Wiley, 1977.
9. Beyers M: Getting on top of organizational change, part 3: The corporate nurse executive. *J Nurs Adm* 1984;14(December):32-37.

10. Chaska NL: Theories of nursing and organizations: Generating integrated models for administrative practice, in Chaska NL (ed): *The Nursing Profession: A Time to Speak*. New York, McGraw-Hill, 1983.

11. Stevens BJ: Applying nursing theory in nursing administration, in Chaska NL (ed): *The Nursing Profession: A Time to Speak*. New York, McGraw-Hill, 1983.

12. Meleis AI: Theoretical development and domain concepts, in Moccia, P: *New Approaches to Theory Development*. New York, National League for Nursing, 1986.

13. Crozier M: The relationship between micro and macrosociology. *Human Relations* 1972;25(3):239-251.

14. Thompson JE, Thompson HO: *Bioethical Decision Making for Nurses*, ed 2. Norwalk, CT, Appleton-Century-Crofts, 1985.

15. Sidel V: The fabric of public health: 1985 presidential address. *Am J Public Health* 1986;76(4):373-379.

16. Aroskar MA: Ethical issues in community health nursing. *Nurs Clin North Am* 1979;14(1):35-44.

17. Childress JF: *Priorities in Biomedical Ethics*. Philadelphia, Westminster, 1981.

18. Noddings N: *Caring: A Feminine Approach to Ethics & Moral Education*. Berkeley, University of California Press, 1984.

19. Beauchamp DE: Community: The neglected tradition of public health. *Hastings Cent Rep* 1985;15(December):28-36.

20. Fry ST: Dilemma in community health ethics. *NO* 1983;31(3):176-179.

21. Gilligan C: *In a Different Voice: Psychological Theory and Women's Development*. Cambridge, Mass, Harvard University Press, 1982.

22. Bellah RN, Madsen R, Sullivan WM, et al: *Habits of the Heart*. New York, Harper & Row, 1985.

14

Thinking Upstream: Nurturing a Conceptual Understanding of the Societal Context of Health Behavior

PATRICIA G. BUTTERFIELD, RN, MS

This chapter addresses the issue of overreliance on theories that define nursing in terms of a one-to-one relationship at the expense of theoretical perspectives that emphasize the societal context of health. When individuals are perceived as the focus of nursing action, the nurse is likely to propose intervention strategies aimed at either changing the behaviors of the individual or modifying the individual's perceptions of the world. When nurses understand the social, political, economic influences that shape the health of a society, they are more likely to recognize social action as a nursing role and work on behalf of populations.

Despite acknowledgment that an understanding of population health is essential in professional nursing, descriptions of one-to-one relationships predominate in the literature read by most nurses. Such portrayals often emphasize the evolution of the relationship between nurse and client with minimal attention to forces outside the relationship that have been paramount in shaping the client's health behaviors. Yet for most people their cultural heritage, social roles, and economic situations have a far more profound influence on health behaviors than do interactions with any health-care professional. Examination of nursing problems from a "think small" perspective[1(p504)] fosters inadequate consideration of these social, environmental, and political determinants of health. This perspective results not only in a restricted range of intervention possibilities for the nurse, but also in a distorted impression of clients' behaviors. An understanding of the complex social, political, and economic forces that shape people's lives is necessary for nurses to promote health in individuals and groups. If nurses are not given an opportunity to appreciate the gestalt of populations and societies, they will be unable to develop a basis for analyzing problems.

This chapter addresses the issue of overreliance on theories that define nursing primarily in terms of a one-to-one relationship and the inherent conflict between these theories and the goal of enabling nurses to promote health through population-based interventions.

Source: Butterfield, P. G. (1990). Thinking upstream: Nurturing a conceptual understanding of the societal context of health behavior. *ANS, 12* (2): 1-8. Reprinted with permission from and copyright © 1990 Aspen Publishers, Inc.

NURSING'S ROLE IN PUSHING UPSTREAM

In his description of the frustrations of medical practice, McKinlay[2] uses the image of a swiftly flowing river to represent illness. In this analogy, physicians are so caught up in rescuing victims from the river that they have no time to look upstream to see who is pushing their patients into the perilous waters. The author uses this example to demonstrate the ultimate futility of "downstream endeavors,"[2(p9)] which are characterized by short-term, individual-based interventions, and he challenges health-care providers to focus more of their energies "upstream, where the real problems lie."[2(p9)] Upstream endeavors focus on modifying economic, political, and environmental factors that have been shown to be the precursors of poor health throughout the world. Although the analogy cites medical practice, it also aptly describes the dilemmas of a considerable portion of nursing practice. And while nursing has a rich historical record of providing preventive and population-based care, the current American health system, which emphasizes episodic and individual-based care, has done woefully little to stem the tide of chronic illness, to which 70 percent of the American population succumbs.

What is the cost of a continued emphasis on a microscopic perspective? How does a theoretical focus on the individual preclude understanding of a larger perspective? Dreher[1] maintains that a conservative scope of practice often uses psychologic theories to explain patterns of health and health care. In this mode of practice, low compliance, broken appointments, and reluctance to participate in care are all attributed to motivation or attitude problems on the part of the client. Nurses are charged with the responsibility of altering client attitudes toward health, rather than altering the system itself, "even though such negative attitudes may well be a realistic appraisal of health care."[1(p505)] Greater emphasis is paid to the psychologic symptoms of poor health than to socioeconomic causes; "indeed the symptoms are being taken as its causes."[1(p505)] The nurse who views the world from such a perspective does not entertain the possibility of working to alter the system itself or empowering clients to do so.

Involvement in social reform is considered to be within the realm of nursing practice.[3] Dreher[1] acknowledges the historical role of public health nurses in facilitating social change and notes that social involvement and activism are expected of nurses in this area of practice. The American Nurses' Association (ANA) Social Policy Statement delineates, among other social concerns, the "provision for the public health through use of preventive and environmental measures and increased assumption of responsibility by individuals, families, and other groups"[3(p4)] and addresses nursing's role in response to those concerns. However, in her review of the document, White[4] notes an incongruence between nursing's social concerns, which clearly transcend individual-based practice, and the description of nursing as "a practice in which interpersonal closeness of the professional kind develops and aids the investigation and discussion of problems, as nurse and patient (or family or group) seek jointly to resolve those concerns."[3(p19)] White[4] also notes the document's neglect of the population focus and possibilities for modifying the environment. Clearly, nursing has yet to reconcile many of the differences between operationalization of a population-centered practice and policies that define nursing primarily in terms of individual-focused care.

Three theoretic approaches will be contrasted below to demonstrate how they may lead the nurse to draw different conclusions not only about the reasons for client behavior, but also about the range of interventions available to the nurse.

THE DOWNSTREAM VIEW: THE INDIVIDUAL AS THE LOCUS OF CHANGE

The health belief model evolved from the premise that the world of the perceiver determines what he or she will do. The social psychologists[5,6] who outlined this model were strongly influenced by Lewin and the view that a person's daily activities are guided by processes of attraction to positive valences and avoidance of negative valences. From these inceptions evolved a model that purports to explain why people do or do not engage in a preventive health action in response to a specific disease threat. The model places the burden of action exclusively on the client; only those clients who have distorted or negative perceptions of the specified disease or recommended health action will fail to act. In practice, this model focuses the nurse's energies on interventions designed to modify the client's distorted perceptions. Although the process of promoting behavior change may be masked under the premise of mutually defined goals, passive acceptance of the nurse's advice is the desired outcome of the relationship.

Although the health belief model was not designed to specify intervention strategies, it can lead the nurse to deduce that client problems can be solved merely by altering the client's belief system. The model addresses the concept of "perceived benefits versus perceived barriers/costs associated with taking a health action."[6(p563)] Nurses may easily interpret this situation as a need to modify the client's perceptions of benefits and barriers. For example, clients with problems accessing adequate health care might receive counseling aimed at helping them see these barriers in a new light; the model does not include the possibility that the nurse may become involved in activities that promote equal access to all in need.

True to its historical roots, the model offers an explanation of health behaviors that, in many ways, is similar to a mechanical system. From the health belief model, one easily concludes that compliance can be induced by using model variables as catalysts to stimulate action. For example, an intervention study based on health belief model precepts sought to increase follow-up in hypertensive clients by increasing the clients' awareness of their susceptibility to hypertension and of its danger.[7] Clients received education, over the telephone or in the emergency department, that was designed to increase their perception of the benefits of follow-up. According to these authors, the interventions resulted in a dramatic increase in compliance. However, they noted several client groups that failed to respond to the intervention, most notably a small group of clients who had no available child care. Although this study demonstrates the predictive power of health belief model concepts, it also exemplifies the limitations of the model. The health belief model may be effective in promoting behavioral change through the alteration of clients' perspectives, but it does not acknowledge responsibility for the health-care professional to reduce or ameliorate client barriers.

In fact, some of the proponents of the health belief model readily acknowledge the limitations of the model and caution users against generalizing it beyond the domain of the individual psyche. In their review of 10 years of research with the model, Janz and Becker[8] remind researchers that the model can only account for the variance in health behaviors that is explained by the attitudes and beliefs of an individual. Melnyk's[9] recent review of the concept of barriers reinforces the notion that, because the health belief model is based on subjective perceptions, research that adopts this theoretic basis must take care to include the subjects', rather than the researchers', perceptions of barriers. Janz and Becker[8] address the influence of other factors such as habituation and nonhealth reasons on making positive changes in health behavior, and they acknowledge the influence of environmental and economic factors that prohibit individuals from undertaking a more healthy way of life.

The health belief model is but a prototype for the type of theoretic perspective that has dominated nursing education and thus nursing practice. The model's strength—its narrow scope—is also its limitation: One is not drawn outside it to those forces that shape the characteristics that the model describes.

THE UPSTREAM VIEW: SOCIETY AS THE LOCUS OF CHANGE

Milio's Framework for Prevention

Milio's framework for prevention[10] provides a thought-provoking complement to the health belief model and a mechanism for directing attention upstream and examining opportunities for nursing intervention at the population level. Milio moves the focus of attention upstream by pointing out that it is the range of available health choices, rather than the choices made at any one time, that is paramount in shaping the overall health status of a society. She maintains that the range of choices widely available to individuals is shaped, to a large degree, by policy decisions in both governmental and private organizations. Rather than concentrate efforts on imparting information to change patterns of individual behavior, she advocates national-level policy making as the most effective means of favorably affecting the health of most Americans.

Milio[10] proposes that health deficits often result from an imbalance between a population's health needs and its health-sustaining re-sources, with affluent societies afflicted by the diseases associated with excess (obesity, alcoholism) and the poor afflicted by diseases that result from inadequate or unsafe food, shelter, and water. In this context, the poor in affluent societies may experience the least desirable combination of factors. Milio notes that although socioeconomic realities deprive many Americans of a health-sustaining environment, "cigarettes, sucrose, pollutants, and tensions are readily available to the poor."[10(p436)]

The range of health-promoting or health-damaging choices available to individuals is affected by their personal resources and their societal resources. Personal resources include one's awareness, knowledge, and beliefs, including those of one's family and friends, as well as money, time, and the urgency of other priorities. Societal resources are strongly influenced by community and national locale and include the availability and cost of health services, environmental protection, safe shelter, and the penalties or rewards given for failure to select the given options.

Milio notes the fallacy of the commonly held assumption in health education that knowing health-generating behaviors implies acting in accordance with that knowledge, and she cites the lifestyles of health professionals in support of her argument. She proposes that "most human beings, professional or nonprofessional, provider or consumer, make the easiest choices available to them most of the time."[10(p435)] Therefore, health-promoting choices must be more readily available and less costly than health-damaging options if individuals are to be healthy and a society is to improve its health status.

The opportunities for a society to make healthy choices have been a central theme throughout Milio's work. In a recent book she elaborated on this theme:

Personal behavior patterns are not simply "free" choices about "lifestyle," isolated from their personal and economic context. Lifestyles are, rather, patterns of choices made from the alternatives that are available to people according to their socioeconomic circumstances and the ease with which they are able to choose certain ones over others.[11(p76)]

Milio is critical of many traditional approaches to health education that emphasize knowledge acquisition and consequently expect behavior change. In addressing the role of public health in primary care, Milio voices concern that "health damage accumulates in societies too, vitiating their vitality . . . [and charges nurses to redirect energies] so as to foster conditions that help people to retain a self-sustaining physiological and social balance."[12(pp188,189)]

One cannot help but note the similarities between Milio's health resources and the concepts in the health belief model. The health belief model is more comprehensive than Milio's framework in examining the internal dynamics of health decision making. However, Milio offers a different set of insights into the arena of health behaviors by proposing that many low-income individuals are acting within the constraints of their limited resources. Furthermore, she goes beyond the individual focus and addresses changes in the health of populations as a result of shifts in decision making by significant numbers of people within a population.

Critical Social Theory

Just as Milio uses societal awareness as an aid to understanding health behaviors, critical social theory employs similar means to expose social inequities that prohibit people from reaching their full potential. This theoretic approach is based on the belief that life is structured by social meanings that are determined, rather one-sidedly, through social domination.[13] In contrast to the assumptions of analytic empiricism, critical theory maintains that standards of truth are socially determined and that no form of scientific inquiry is value free.[13,15] Proponents of this theoretic approach posit that social discourse that is not distorted from power imbalances will stimulate the evolution of a more rational society. The interests of truth are served only when people are able to voice their beliefs without fear of authority or retribution.[13]

Allen[14] discusses how nursing practice can be enriched by enabling clients to remove the conscious and unconscious constraints in their everyday lives. He states that women and the economically impoverished are especially vulnerable to being labeled by pseudodiseases that are rooted in social formations, such as hysteria and depression. Health-care providers often frame such problems only within the context of the individual or, at best, the family. But critical social theory can enable a nurse to reframe such an interpretation to gain an understanding of the historical play of social forces that have limited the choices truly available to the involved parties. Through exploration of the societal forces, traditions, and roles that have created the meanings of health and illness, clients may be freed of the isolation and alienation that accompany individual problem ownership.

At the collective level, Waitzkin asserts that the current emphasis on lifestyle diverts attention from important sources of illness in the capitalist industrial environment; "it also puts the burden of health squarely on the individual rather than seeking collective solutions to health problems."[16(p664)] Salmon[17] supports this position by noting that the basic tenets of Western medicine promote the delineation of individual factors of health and illness, while obscuring the exploration of their social and economic roots. He states that critical social theory "can aid in uncovering larger dimensions impacting health that are usually unseen or misrepresented by ideological biases. Thus, the social reality of health conditions can be both understood and changed."[17(p75)]

Because the theory holds that each person is responsible for creating social conditions in which all members of society are able to speak freely, the nurse is challenged, as an individual and as a member of the profession, to expose power imbalances that prohibit people from achieving their full potential. Nurses versed in critical theory are equipped to see beyond the perpetuation of status quo ideas and may be able to generate unique ideas that are unencumbered by previous stereotypes.[14]

Other Examples of Upstream Thinking

Recent nursing literature provides several other examples of upstream thinking. In a thought-provoking commentary on an intervention program for middle-aged women experiencing subclinical depression, Davis[18] (cited in Gordon and Ledray) notes a lack of congruence between the study's portrayal of depression as a problem with societal roots and its instruction in coping strategies as the intervention program. While recognizing the merits of the intervention program, she comments that, "if our principal task as progressive nurses is to develop and utilize interventions that will ameliorate these social problems, then the emphasis in nursing education and practice might well be on those social actions that aim to change basic social factors such as ageism and sexism."[18(p277)]

Chopoorian[19] takes a different tack, emphasizing the concept of environment and suggesting that nurses develop a consciousness of the social, political, and economic aspects of environment. She maintains that a static portrayal of the environment precludes nurses from acting as advocates for people who lack adequate housing and health care and live in intolerable circumstances. She charges nurses to move beyond a psychosocial conceptualization of the environment into a sociopolitical-economic conceptualization. Through this reconceptualization, nurses will see that human responses to health and illnesses "are related to the structure of the social world, the economic and political policies that govern that structure, and the human, social relationships that are produced by the structure and the policies."[19(p46)]

THE NEED FOR ALTERNATIVE PERSPECTIVES

The danger of the conservative perspective lies not within its content, but rather in the omission of other, larger theories that enable nurses to view situations from both a microscopic and a macroscopic perspective. In discussing the dilemmas of "studying health behavior as an individual phenomena [sic], rather than in the context of a broader social change phenomena [sic]," Cummings[20(p93)] reminds us that the approaches are complementary, and both are necessary to a comprehensive understanding of health promotion. The strengths and utility of each theoretic approach are most clearly revealed through an understanding of alternative approaches.

Nursing needs conceptual foundations that enable its practitioners to understand health problems manifested at community, national, and international levels as well as those at the individual and family levels. The continued bias in favor of individual-focused theories robs nurses of an understanding of the richness and complexity of forces that shape the behavior of populations. The omission of theories that relate nursing to the social context of behavior may leave nurses with a minimal understanding of their responsibilities to facilitate change at this level and without the tools to promote such change in an effective and systematic manner.

Maglacas[21] provides a global perspective on the health conditions of societies throughout the world and draws attention to the gaps in service access between the rich and the poor. She then charges nurses within each society and culture to act in response to the inequities in health within that society. If nurses are to be able to enact change at the societal level, they need to be provided with theoretic frameworks that are consistent with such ends and with theoretic perspectives in which social, economic, and political forces are given equal weight with the interpersonal aspects of nursing. Through these means, nurses gain insight into the social precursors of poor health and restricted opportunities and learn rationales for engaging in social action. By tipping the scales of nursing back toward consideration of theories that address health from a societal perspective, nurses can receive not only a richness of understanding but also the means by which to enact this kind of change.

REFERENCES

1. Dreher MC. The conflict of conservatism in public health nursing education. *Nurs Outlook.* 1982;30:504-509.
2. McKinlay JB. A case for refocussing upstream: The political economy of illness. In: Jaco EG, ed. *Patients, Physicians, and Illness.* 3rd ed. New York, NY: Free Press; 1979:9-25.
3. American Nurses' Association. *Nursing: A Social Policy Statement.* Kansas City, Mo: American Nurses' Association; 1980.
4. White CM. A critique of the ANA social policy statement. *Nurs Outlook.* 1984;32:328-331.
5. Rosenstock IM. Historical origins of the health belief model. In: Becker MH, ed. *The Health Belief Model and Personal Health Behavior.* Thorofare, NJ: Charles B. Slack; 1974:1-8.
6. Becker MH, Maiman LA. Models of health-related behavior. In: Mechanic D, ed. *Handbook of Health, Health Care, and the Health Professions.* New York, NY: Free Press; 1983:539-568.
7. Jones PK, Jones SL, Katz J. Improving follow-up among hypertensive patients using a health belief model intervention. *Arch Intern Med.* 1987; 147:1557-1560.
8. Janz NK, Becker MH. The health belief model: A decade later. *Health Educ Q.* 1984;11:1-47.
9. Melnyk KM. Barriers: A critical review of recent literature. *Nurs Res.* 1988;37:196-201.
10. Milio N. A framework for prevention: Changing health-damaging to health-generating life patterns. *Am J Public Health.* 1976;66:435-439.
11. Milio N. *Promoting Health Through Public Policy.* Philadelphia, Penn: F.A. Davis; 1981.
12. Milio N. *Primary Care and the Public's Health.* Lexington, Mass: Lexington Books; 1983.
13. Allen D, Diekelmann N, Bennet P. Three paradigms for nursing research. In: Chinn P, ed. *Nursing Research Methodology: Issues & Implementation.* Rockville, Md: Aspen Publishers; 1986:23-28.
14. Allen DG. Nursing research and social control: Alternate models of science that emphasize understanding and emancipation. *Image: The Journal of Nursing Scholarship.* 1985;17:58-64.
15. Allen DG. Critical social theory as a model for analyzing ethical issues in family and community health. *Fam Commun Health.* 1987;10:63-72.
16. Waitzkin H. A Marxist view of health and health care. In: Mechanic D, ed. *Handbook of Health, Health Care, and the Health Professions.* New York, NY: Free Press; 1983:657-682.
17. Salmon JW. Dilemmas in studying social change versus individual change: Considerations from political economy. In: Duffy ME, Pender NJ, eds. *Conceptual Issues in Health Promotion—A Report of Proceedings of a Wingspread Conference.* Indianapolis, Ind: Sigma Theta Tau; 1987:70-81.
18. Davis AJ. Cited by Gordon VC, Ledray LE. Growth-support intervention for the treatment of depression in women of middle years. *West J Nurs Res.* 1986;8:263-283.

19. Chopoorian TJ. Reconceptualizing the environment. In: Moccia P, ed. *New Approaches to Theory Development*. New York, NY: National League for Nursing; 1986: 39-54. Publication 15-1992.

20. Cummings KM. Dilemmas in studying health as an individual phenomenon. In: Duffy ME, Pender NJ, eds. *Conceptual Issues in Health Promotion—A Report of Proceedings of a Wingspread Conference*. Indianapolis, Ind: Sigma Theta Tau; 1987:91-96.

21. Maglacas AM. Health for all: Nursing's role. *Nurs Outlook*. 1988;36:66-71.

15

Environmental Paradigms: Moving Toward an Ecocentric Perspective

DOROTHY KLEFFEL, RN, MPH, DNSc

This article examines a taxonomy of three environmental paradigms. The egocentric paradigm is grounded in the person and is based on the assumption that what is good for the individual is good for society. The homocentric paradigm is grounded in society and reflects the utilitarian ethic of the greatest good for the greatest number of people. The ecocentric paradigm is grounded in the cosmos, and the environment is considered whole, living, and interconnected. Historically, nurses have adhered primarily to the egocentric paradigm and to a lesser extent to the homocentric paradigm. However, because the world has become a global community, contemporary nurse scholars are shifting to the ecocentric paradigm. [Keywords: Ecocentric, Environment, Paradigm, Philosophy]

The environmental focus of nursing has traditionally been centered on clients' immediate surroundings in the hospital or other institution, home, or community. This circumscribed environmental worldview of nursing is undergoing change as nurses become aware of the adverse effects of environmental disasters and degradation on human health. Regional catastrophic environmental events like the Bhopal chemical leak, the Chernobyl nuclear disaster, and the Exxon Valdez oil spill have had immediate and lasting consequences. Global dimensions of the decline of the planet's environment include worldwide temperature rise, ozone depletion, destruction of the world's forests, human overpopulation, depleted fish popu-

lations, soil erosion, worldwide hunger, homelessness, and massive species extinction.[1,2] These are not isolated environmental problems that can be addressed by individual effort; they require the coordinated effort of people across the entire planet. Nurses are beginning to understand the scope of environmental threats that threaten everything that exists, living and nonliving. Nurses' enhanced consciousness of the environment has caused the profession to question its current assumptions about the environmental domain of nursing knowledge.

Nursing scholars are becoming cognizant that the existing environmental paradigm does not provide the knowledge and theoretical base to account for environmental conditions that compromise health promotion and interfere with optimum health. Nurses in general do not understand the interrelations between social, political, and economic struc-

Source: Kleffel, D. (1996). Environmental paradigms: Moving toward an ecocentric perspective *Adv Nurs Sci*, 18 (4): 1–10. Reprinted with permission by from and copyright © 1996 Aspen Publishers, Inc.

tures and the origins of health and illnesses.[3] Nursing theory does not adequately describe the concept of the environment. Almost all nursing research conducted in the domain of environment involves only the immediate milieu of the client, family, or nurse.[4] Nursing's care theories do not allow for nonhuman interchange of care or caring because of their anthropocentricity. Anthropocentrism results in the subjugation of nonhuman nature, which jeopardizes the quality of the physical world and causes other forms of oppression and domination.[5]

These critiques of nursing's environmental assumptions indicate that the profession is experiencing an environmental paradigm shift. A *paradigm* is the body of values, commitments, beliefs, and knowledge shared by members of a profession. Research guidelines, questions, and methodology emanate from the paradigm. When new knowledge is discovered that no longer fits the paradigm, or when the paradigm no longer provides model problems and solutions, an anomaly exists. When anomalies become so numerous and significant that they can no longer be ignored, investigations are initiated by the profession. Theories are explored and rejected until a new paradigm emerges that leads to a new basis for practice.[6]

Contemporary nursing scholars are exploring a variety of new environmental ideas and theories as the profession changes its environmental worldview. To contribute to this dialogue, I examine a taxonomy of three environmental paradigms—egocentric, homocentric, and ecocentric—that summarize the assumptions of Western culture regarding the natural world since the 17th century.[7,8] I propose the inclusion of the ecocentric environmental perspective into a central position in nursing's body of knowledge. This mainstreaming of a global view would encourage and support nurses to act with others in averting worldwide environmental disaster.

EGOCENTRIC APPROACH

The egocentric approach is grounded at the personal level and assumes that what is best for the individual is best for society. It is concerned with liberty, rights, and independent action of the individual. It is the dominant Western worldview. Its philosophical foundation is individualistic and mechanistic and includes the thought of Plato, mainstream Christianity, Descartes, Hegel, George Berkeley, Hobbes, Locke, Adam Smith, Malthus, and Garrett Hardin.[8] The egocentric approach is a mechanistic paradigm and assumes that matter is composed of atomic parts, the whole is equal to the sum of the parts, causation is a matter of external action on inactive parts, quantitative change is more important than qualitative change, and there is dualistic separation of mind–body and matter–spirit.[7] In the egocentric approach, the individual is the focus of change.

Most practicing nurses adhere to the egocentric worldview. Their approach is individualistic. They regard the environment as the immediate surroundings or circumstances of the individual or as an interactional field that individuals adapt to, adjust to, or control.[3] The environment is defined in relation to the individual person rather than in terms of its own essence and intrinsic value.

Because the egocentric approach has been the dominant perspective in the Western world, many nurse theorists incorporated those ideas into their theories. An example of a nurse theorist who adhered to the egocentric paradigm was Roy.[9] She defined the environment as all internal and external conditions, circumstances, and influences surrounding and affecting the development and behavior of individuals and groups. Stimuli emanate from the environment and are categorized as focal (immediately confronting the person), contextual (all other stimuli present), and residual (beliefs and attitudes that impinge on the situation). The purpose of nursing is to enhance the adaptation of the patient to environmental stimuli. Roy[10] believed that the science of nursing focuses on human life processes as the core knowledge to be developed. Roy's theory is considered egocentric because of its emphasis on individual adaptation to the environment and on human beings to the exclusion of the rest of nature.

Egocentrism has been the guiding ethic of private entrepreneurs and corporations whose goal is maximization of profit from the development of natural resources. The egocentric approach is limited because of its assumption that the individual good is the highest good that will ultimately benefit society as a whole and that humans are fundamentally different from other creatures, which they are to dominate and control.[7]

HOMOCENTRIC APPROACH

The homocentric approach is the utilitarian ethic and is grounded at the social level.[7,8] Social justice, rather than individual progress, is the key value. Decisions are made based on the common good, which is the greatest good for the largest number of people. Humans are considered stewards and caretakers of the natural world. The philosophical foundations of homocentrism are both materialism and positivism. Its assumptions are that humans have a cultural heritage in addition to their genetic inheritance that results in their being qualitatively different from animals, that the determinants of human affairs are social rather than individual, and that culture is a cumulative progress that can continue indefinitely. All social problems are viewed as ultimately solvable. Exponents of the homocentric approach include John S. Mill and Jeremy Bentham

(utilitarian theorists), Barry Commoner (socialist ecology), Karl Marx and Mao Tse Tung (political theorists), and Jørgen Randers and Donella and Dennis Meadows (limits-to-growth theorists).

The body of knowledge derived from epidemiology serves as an information base for the practice of public health nursing. Public health nurses use epidemiology in diagnosing, planning, treating, and evaluating community health problems. The nurse who interacts with individual clients and families uses the information for assessing, planning, intervening, and evaluating at the community level.[11] Epidemiology is considered homocentric because of its emphasis on the health of populations rather than individuals.

In the homocentric view, the environment is the focus of change rather than the individual. The homocentric approach to the environment is basically anthropocentric in that humans are to manage nature for the benefit of humans. The management of nature for the intrinsic benefit of other species is not considered in this paradigm.[7]

ECOCENTRIC APPROACH

The ecocentric approach is grounded in the cosmos. The whole environment, including inanimate elements such as rocks and minerals, along with animate animals and plants, is assigned intrinsic value. It is rooted in holistic rather than mechanistic metaphysics. It assumes that everything is connected to everything else, that the whole is greater than the sum of its parts, that meaning is dependent on context, that biological and social systems are open, and that humans and nonhumans are one within the same organic system. Exponents of the ecocentric approach include most traditional Eastern systems of thought, traditional Native American philosophies, Thoreau, Gary Snyder, Theodore Rozak, Aldo Leopold,

Rachel Carson, Fritjof Capra, deep ecology, the holographic model, and ecofeminism.[7,8]

Within the ecocentric paradigm are four contemporary nursing theorists. Sarter[12] compared the philosophical perspectives of fellow nursing theorists Rogers, Neuman, Watson, and Parse and found common shared holistic themes of process, evolution of consciousness, self-transcendence, open systems, harmony, relativity of space and time, pattern, and holism. *Process* is the evolutionary change of human consciousness; *self-transcendence* is the method of the evolution of human consciousness through higher and higher levels toward unity with the universe. *Open systems* are the dynamic and continuous interactions between the person and the world and are essential for the evolution of human consciousness. *Harmony* is considered to exist both within the person and between the person and the environment. Space and time are considered nonlinear, relative, and fluid, with the past and future merging into the present. *Pattern* is information that represents the whole. Pattern recognition is nursing action that looks for patterns representing the whole rather than parts of the whole. Sarter noted that each of these theorists has been influenced, either directly or indirectly, by Eastern philosophies. She believed that the foundation of a commonly held nursing worldview has been laid.

Watson[13] has continued to develop her ecocentric perspectives, moving toward a unitary–transformative viewpoint. This model has eliminated the subject–object and mind–body duality. It acknowledges unity and integrality between humans and the environment; thus conceptualized, human beings and their worlds are not separated.

Other modern nursing scholars also adhere to the ecocentric paradigm. Schuster[14] advocated for a conscious choice of earth dwelling through self-identification and interconnectedness with all beings, which lead one naturally to care for the world in day-to-day living.

It is a way of being in the world that allows for all of creation, not just humans, to emerge.

Kleffel,[15] during a qualitative research study, identified 17 distinguished scholars whose work has addressed broad environmental dimensions related to nursing. All except two explicitly reflected the ecocentric paradigm and perceived the environment to be alive, whole, interconnected, and interacting. These scholars add strength to the idea of the united nursing worldview described by Sarter.[12]

The ecocentric approach has some philosophical difficulties. The central problem is finding a philosophically adequate justification for the intrinsic value of nonhuman nature. In mainstream Western thought, only humans have intrinsic worth, while the rest of nature has instrumental value as a resource for humans. It is not considered wrong to kill the last of a species or use the last mineral if human survival is at stake.[7]

ECOCENTRISM IN THE WORLD'S TRADITIONS

The egocentric paradigm has been the dominant worldview of most practicing nurses working in hospitals and other health institutions and is ascribed to by the greatest number of nurses in the profession. The homocentric perspective has influenced far fewer nurses, traditionally those practicing in the field of public health nursing, although there are signs of a shifting of the profession toward the homocentric approach in the form of aggregate and population-based nursing.[16] The ecocentric view is only beginning to inform the profession and has not yet achieved significant prominence in nursing scholarship or practice.

Embracing an ecocentric viewpoint has exhilarating potential for transforming nursing scholarship and practice beyond its traditional boundaries. We are now living in a global culture that is united by economic interdependence, international air transportation, and worldwide communications networks. Contemporary environmental degradation and disasters that adversely affect humans have moved into the global arena. Actions stem from worldviews, and the worldview of nursing has been mostly egocentric. Moving to the ecocentric paradigm will encourage nurses to address worldwide environmental problems that affect the health of everything that exists.

Solving global environmental problems will entail international efforts from a variety of disciplines and from many cultures. Such an approach will entail collaborative problem solving by people with differing traditions and cultural backgrounds. To work together, a common global environmental worldview that can incorporate these diverse perspectives is needed. The ecocentric paradigm, which is compatible with elements of Native American traditional ideas, Eastern philosophies, and contemporary Western thought, holds great promise for a unified worldview to which all humans can subscribe.

Native American Tradition

There are difficulties in universalizing the Native American belief system because it comprises so many different cultures. However, some generalizations can be made.[17] The Native American attitude was to regard all entities in the environment as having consciousness, reason, and volition as intense and complete as humans. These entities included the earth itself, the sky, the winds, rocks, streams, trees, insects, birds, and animals. This pervasive spirit in everything was considered a part of the Great Spirit, which fostered the perception of humans and nature as being unified and akin. The Native American's social circle or community included all nonhuman natural entities as well as other humans.

The consequences of the Native American inspirited worldview of nature produced a harmony between them and their environment that restrained their killing of animals and gathering of plants to what was necessary for survival. Although there were occasional examples of destruction of nature during periods of enormous cultural stress, the overall and usual effort was conservation of resources. The Native American cultural traditions were not altruistic; they considered it in their own self-interest to defer to nature, which they believed would withhold its sustenance or actively retaliate if provoked.[17]

Eastern Systems of Thought

Similar themes of a unified, living, conscious, and interacting world are found in almost all Eastern systems of thought. With the exception of Islam, these systems are antihierarchal and anthropocentric. Although Islam maintains that humans are dominant over nature, a view similar to the Judeo-Christian tradition, it instructs its adherents to prevent environmental deterioration because the world is God's creation.[18] Other Eastern philosophies emphasize harmony and balance. All aspects of the environment interact, with the parts being within the whole and the whole being within the parts. Humans are a part of the whole and admonished to live in equilibrium with all other parts of the planet.[19]

Some examples of Eastern thought include the law of Karma of the Advita Vedanta, which binds humans together in continuity with the natural world.[20] The *wu wei* of Taoism is an awareness that allows one to maximize creative possibilities of oneself as a dimension of the environment.[21] The *Chi* of Chinese thought is a vital force that is the basic structure of the cosmos and exists in all things. Nature is the result of fusion and merging of vital forces to form the "great harmony."[22]

A popular image for portraying the manner in which things exist is described from the *Hua-yen* school of Buddhism.[23] From the great god Indra there hangs a marvelous net that stretches out infinitely in all directions. There is a jewel in each eye of the net. Since the net is infinite in dimension, the jewels are infinite in number. When one jewel is selected and carefully looked at, all of the other jewels in the net are reflected. In addition, each of the jewels reflected is also reflecting all of the other jewels, so that an infinite reflecting process occurs.

This image symbolizes the cosmos, in which there is an infinitely repeated interrelationship among all of the members of the cosmos. Thus, the part and the whole are one and the same, for what we identify as a part is merely an abstraction from a unitary whole. There is no part-and-whole duality as in Western thought. This totalistic world is a living body in which each cell derives its life from the other cells and in return gives life to the others.

Western Approaches

The ecocentric environmental themes found in Eastern and traditional Native American worldviews originated in ancient times. Several modern Western ecocentric environmental approaches reflect these ideas. The science of ecology, along with relativity and quantum theory, is creating a postmodern scientific worldview. This emerging worldview is in congruence with the traditional and indigenous environmental paradigms of preindustrial cultures.[24] Naess criticized traditional ecology (an egocentric approach), which he dubbed "shallow ecology,"[25(p95)] as being concerned only with pollution control and resource conservation in the interests of people in developed countries. He argued that there are deeper concerns (hence the phrase "deep ecology," also called "radical environmental-ism") that touch on the principles of diversity, complexity, autonomy, decentralization, symbiosis, egalitarianism, and classlessness. Deep ecology derives its essence from some Eastern and Native American ideas as well as from feminism, John Muir, and other naturalist literature.[26]

The modern Gaia hypothesis is reminiscent of the ancient living organic theory. This view of the environment was proposed by Lovelock,[27,28] an atmospheric chemist. Lovelock saw the evolution of the species of living organisms as being so closely coupled with the evolution of their physical and chemical environment that together they constitute a single and indivisible evolutionary process. No clear distinction is made between living and nonliving material. The planet's organisms act together as a unity to regulate the global environment by adjusting the rates at which gases are produced and removed from the atmosphere. Lovelock warned that the earth's ability to self-regulate is affected by natural or human activity, which could force the climate into a new and different stable state that would result in the elimination of all living organisms.

The idea of the planet's stable state in the modern Gaia hypothesis reflects the idea of harmony in ancient Taoist thought. In both notions, the balance of the environment of the planet must be maintained, or ecological disaster will result.

Bohm,[29] a physicist and one of the early pioneers of the holographic model, believed that the universe is organized along holographic principles. Everything in the universe is part of a continuum, a seamless extension of everything else. There are no separate parts, just as a geyser in a fountain is not separated from the water from which it flows. However, the universe is not an undifferentiated mass. Things can have their own unique qualities and still be part of an undivided whole. Similarly, consciousness is present in all matter in various degrees. The universe cannot be divided into living and nonliving things. All things are interconnected; like a hologram, every portion of the universe contains the whole.

There are similarities of imagery between the holographic model and Indra's net. The giant hologram and Indra's net symbolize the cosmos. All parts of the hologram are interconnected; each jewel in Indra's net is connected with every other jewel. The parts of the hologram and each jewel of Indra's net reflect the whole. The whole of the hologram and the whole of Indra's net reflect each part or jewel. Bohm believed that fragmentation is the cause of most present-day problems. Applied to the environment, one portion of the planet cannot be harmed without resulting damage to the entire planet.

Another modern Western ecocentric view is ecofeminism. Ecofeminism is a theory that women and the environment are interconnected as both share and have been subjected to the same patriarchal domination.[30] A failure to understand these connections will result in the continued exploitation of both women and environment at the theory, policy, and practice levels. Ecofeminists recognize the interconnectedness of women and the environment and recognize the necessity of uniting feminism and ecology. However, feminist theory is not environmentally sensitive. Deep ecology and the Gaia hypothesis share themes of unity and wholeness to which ecofeminists can subscribe; however, both are oriented toward a patriarchal culture. Ecofeminists hold the view that the connections between the twin dominations of women and nature require a feminist theory and practice informed by an ecological perspective and an environmentalism informed by a feminist perspective.[31]

Ecofeminism is against domination of all kinds, including ageism, sexism, and the exploitation of nature. It is contextual and rela-

tional and includes consideration of nonhuman relationships with each other, humans, and the community. Ecofeminism identifies human nature within the historical context. It is antireductionist and pluralistic, centralizing on diversity of humans and nonhumans, yet affirming that humans are a part of the ecological community. Ecofeminism provides a central place for values that are typically underrepresented or ignored in our society such as care, love, friendship, and appropriate trust. Ecofeminism views theory building, objectivity, and knowledge as historically and contextually situated and as changing over time.[31,32]

IMPLEMENTING THE ECOCENTRIC PARADIGM

Understanding that the environment is alive, whole, interconnected, and interacting and that humans are one with the environment will encourage nurses to practice in an environmentally sensitive manner in whatever setting they work. Nurses working in local settings will understand the relationships between organizational resource use and the worldwide environment. Using the adage "think globally, act locally," they will act within their sphere by doing such things as calling for institutional audits of their work environment, taking client environmental histories, counseling clients regarding the effects of ozone depletion on the incidence of skin cancers and cataracts, reducing the use of toxic materials, purchasing recycled materials and supplies, using products with environmentally friendly packaging, saving water, managing waste safely, using both sides of the paper when copying reports and forms, using reusable products, reducing the use of disposable items, buying rechargeable batteries,[33] and questioning animal experimentation.[34]

Moving to the ecocentric paradigm will mean extending the concept of the nursing client to include the planetary environment. Some nurses will choose to work in the global environmental arena and address international environmental causes of illnesses. For instance, the alarming increase of breast cancer worldwide is an area where nurses could make a difference. In the United States the risk of breast cancer has increased from 1 in 20 in 1960 to 1 in 8 today. Other industrial countries have similar rates. The incidence in developing countries is also rising, but at a slower rate. Risk factors and lifestyle account for only 20% to 30% of breast cancer cases. Some experts believe that pollutants and chemicals that duplicate or interfere with the effects of estrogen are a possible cause. They point to the fact that in Israel, breast cancer mortality in premenopausal women declined by 30 percent following regulations to reduce levels of DDT and carcinogenic pesticides in dietary fat.[35] Other experts believe that low-level radiation and synthetic chemicals such as chlorines are responsible for the increase in breast cancer in women.[36]

Mainstream medicine and science have ignored the possible environmental causes of breast cancer, focusing on the identification of women with risk factors, early case finding through breast self-examination, routine mammograms, and changing lifestyles (smoking cessation, exercise, and lowering dietary fat intake). By contrast, groups like the Women's Environment and Development Organization and Greenpeace are advocating for public attention to the possible links between the environment and breast cancer.[37] Nurses have followed medicine's lead by emphasizing compliance with breast self-examination, counseling women with risk factors associated with breast cancer, and providing education regarding healthy lifestyles. However, they have not directed their attention toward the relationships between breast cancer and the environment, which are being ignored by most research organizations. Using a global, multidisciplinary perspective, nurses could network with other researchers throughout the world to coordinate investigative efforts to identify environmental causes of breast cancer.

Emerging strains of recurring infectious diseases is another area where nurses could make a difference. AIDS, Lyme disease, the Hanta virus, the deadly Ebola virus, the recurrence of plague in India, and the increases in cholera, tuberculosis, and malaria worldwide are examples of conditions related to environmental alterations, climate changes, rapid international travel, and other human activity.[38] Although these diseases are causing illnesses and the deaths of millions of people, nurses generally do not regard scholarship or action in this arena as part of their domain. It is predicted that the epidemics will get worse as the displacement of wild populations and their habitats caused by development activities continue. International multidisciplinary efforts are required to keep ecosystems intact, minimize habitat alterations, require planners to prepare for unanticipated consequences of development, and establish a reliable global surveillance system. Acting internationally in concert with other nurses, other disciplines, and other organizations, nurses could, if they had a global vision, bring their unique skills and perspectives to addressing this type of global environmental phenomenon.

Moving toward an ecocentric perspective will give nurses a common worldview, already held by a great proportion of the world's peoples, of oneness with a living planet, harmony, balance, interconnectedness, and transcendence. It will empower nurses to move beyond their present domain boundaries to align their efforts with other disciplines and organizations worldwide to address the devastating environmental problems affecting the earth and threatening all of existence.

REFERENCES

1. Brown LR, Flavin, French H. *State of the World 1995: A Worldwatch Institute Report on Progress Toward a Sustainable Society.* New York, NY: Norton; 1995.
2. Brown LR, Nicholas L, Kane H. *Vital Signs 1995: The Trends That Are Shaping Our Future.* New York, NY: Norton; 1995.
3. Chopoorian TJ. Reconceptualizing the environment. In: Moccia P, ed. *New Approaches to Theory Development.* New York, NY: National League for Nursing; 1986.
4. Kleffel D. Rethinking the environment as a domain of nursing knowledge. *ANS.* 1991; 14(1):40–51.
5. Schuster EA. Earth caring. *ANS.* 1990; 13(1):25–30.
6. Kuhn TS. *The Structure of Scientific Revolutions.* Chicago, Ill: University of Chicago; 1970.
7. Merchant C. Environmental ethics and political conflict: A view from California. *Environ Ethics.* 1990;12(1):45–68.
8. Miller AS. *Gaia Connections: An Introduction to Ecology, Ecoethics, and Economics.* Savage, Md: Rowman & Littlefield; 1991.
9. Roy C. Roy's adaptation model. In: Parse R, ed. *Nursing Science: Major Paradigms, Theories, and Critiques.* Philadelphia, Penn: W.B. Saunders; 1987.
10. Roy C. An explication of the philosophical assumptions of the Roy Adaptation Model. *Nurs Sci Q.* 1988;1(1):26–34.
11. Shortridge L, Valanis B. The epidemiological model applied in community health nursing. In: Stanhope M, Lancaster J. *Community Health Nursing: Process and Practice for Promoting Health.* 3rd ed. Chicago, Ill: Mosby/YearBook; 1992.
12. Sarter B. Philosophical sources of nursing theory. *Nurs Sci Q.* 1988;1(2):52–59.
13. Watson J. Nursing's caring–healing paradigm as exemplar for alternative medicine? *Altern Therapies.* 1995;1(3):64–69.
14. Schuster EA. Earth dwelling. *Holistic Nurs Pract.* 1992;6(4):1–9.
15. Kleffel D. *The Environment: Alive, Whole, Interacting, and Interconnected.* San Diego, Calif: University of California, San Diego; 1994. Dissertation.
16. Moccia P. *A Vision for Nursing Education.* New York, NY: National League for Nursing; 1993.
17. Callicott JB. Traditional American Indian and Western European attitudes toward nature: An overview. *Environ Ethics.* 1982;4(4):293–318.
18. Zaidi IH. On the ethics of man's interaction with the environment: An Islamic approach. *Environ Ethics.* 1981; 2(1):35–47.
19. Callicott JB. Toward a global environmental ethic. In: Tucker ME, Grim JA, eds. *Worldviews and Ecology: Religion, Philosophy, and the Environment.* Maryknoll, NY: Orbis Books; 1994.
20. Deutsch E. A metaphysical grounding for natural reverence: East-West. *Environ Ethics.* 1986;8(4):283–299.
21. Ames RT. Taoism and the nature of nature. *Environ Ethics.* 1986;8(4):317–350.
22. Wei-Ming T. The continuity of being: Chinese visions of nature. In Callicott JB, Ames RT, eds. *Nature in Asian Traditions of Thought: Essays in Environmental Philosophy.* New York, NY: State University of New York Press; 1989.
23. Cook FH. The jewel net of Indra. In: Callicott JB, Ames RT, eds. *Nature in Asian Traditions of Thought: Essays in Environmental Philosophy.* New York, NY: State University of New York Press; 1989.
24. Callicott JB. *Earth's Insights: A Survey of Ecological Ethics from the Mediterranean Basin to the Australian Outback.* Los Angeles, Calif: University of California Press; 1994.
25. Naess A. The shallow and the deep, long-range ecology movement: A summary. *Inquiry.* 1973;16:95–100.
26. Devall B, Sessions G. *Deep Ecology.* Salt Lake, Colo: Perigrine Smith; 1985.
27. Lovelock J. *Gaia: A New Look at Life on Earth.* New York, NY: Oxford University Press; 1979.
28. Lovelock J. *The Ages of Gaia: A Biography of Our Living Earth.* New York, NY: Norton; 1988.
29. Bohm D. *Wholeness and the Implicate Order.* London, England: Routledge & Kegan Paul; 1980.
30. Cheney J. Ecofeminism and deep ecology. *Environ Ethics.* 1987;9(2):115–144.
31. Warren KJ. Feminism and ecology: Making connections. *Environ Ethics.* 1987;9(1):3–20.
32. Warren KJ, Cheney J. Ecological feminism and ecosystem ecology. *Hypatia.* 1991;6(1):179–197.
33. Shaner H. Environmentally responsible clinical practice. In: Schuster EA, Brown CL, eds. *Exploring Our Environmental Connections.* New York, NY: National League for Nursing Press; 1994.
34. Todd B. An ecofeminist look at animal research. In: Schuster EA, Brown CL, eds. *Explor-

ing Our Environmental Connections. New York, NY: National League for Nursing Press; 1994.

35. Platt A. Breast and prostate cancer rising. In: *Vital Signs 1995: The Trends That Are Shaping Our Future.* New York, NY: Norton; 1995.

36. Women's Environment and Development Organization. Does the breast cancer epidemic have environmental links? *News & Views.* 1992;6(1):1,9.

37. Women's Environment and Development Organization. Women's coalitions battle breast cancer and other environmental health problems. *News & Views.* 1995;8(1–2):2.

38. Platt A. The resurgence of infectious diseases. *World Watch: Working for a Sustainable Future.* 1995;8(4):26–32.

Part IV

NURSING'S METAPARADIGM: CONCEPTUALIZATIONS OF HEALTH

Health has consistently been a major concept in nursing's metaparadigm, yet there is little agreement on the meaning of health among nurses and other health care professionals. Commonly accepted definitions of health include the absence of disease or symptoms of illness, the ability to perform one's roles satisfactorily, the ability to perform self-care activities, the ability to adapt to health problems, self-actualization, and exuberant well-being. Nurses' personal definition of health guides their goals for their clients and ultimately their nursing actions, or how they practice nursing. Within nursing, no two theorists define health in the same way. Several contemporary nurse theorists and scholars have expanded the meaning to include the client's own view of health. Four chapters are included that present various authors and theorist's unique perspective of health.

Toni Tripp-Reimer's chapter, "Reconceptualizing the construct of health: Integrating emic and etic perspectives," begins with three common views of health, citing several nurse theorists' views. She explains the differences between "emic" (culturally specific) and "etic"' (universally accepted) meanings of illness and disease. She provides an emic-etic health grid to help assist health care providers determine the meaning of health from both the client's culture and the provider's perspective.

The chapter "Perspectives on Health," by Mary Huch, is a dialogue among five renowned nurse theorists at a nurse theorist conference. Imogene King, Nola Pender, Betty Neuman, Martha Rogers, and Rosemarie Parse provide a fascinating and enlightening discussion on how their views of health are sometimes similar, yet more often divergent.

In her chapter, "Expressing Health through Lifestyle Patterns," Nola Pender describes the shift in nursing science toward a unitary view of humans, concommitant with a rejection of the health-illness continuum. Pender believes health is a primary life experience in which illness is superimposed. She compares her view with those of several other nurse scholars, and classifies and discusses five dimensions of health: affect, attitude, activity, aspirations, and accomplishments. She recommends that health should be defined in a positive, comprehensive, humanistic manner.

Afaf Meleis provides a critical analysis on the meaning of health in her chapter, "Being and Becoming Healthy: The Core of Nursing Knowledge." She begins with a discussion on the diverse definitions of health among nurses and health care providers, then suggests the need for a unifying definition. Examples of nurse theorists' definitions of health are provided. Meleis's major point is that health is more a social matter among poor people worldwide, because scarce community resources, limited access to care, and inadequate knowledge and ability to prevent disease have a far greater impact on their health and illness. For those well above poverty, health is often based on lifestyle choices and one's personal responsibility, a generalization that should not be applied to those constrained by societal conditions. Meleis challenges nurses to consider multiple societal contextual factors that influence health and move beyond the traditional view that health is the "client's responsibility."

16

Reconceptualizing the Construct of Health: Integrating Emic and Etic Perspectives

TONI TRIPP-REIMER, RN, PhD

Despite the importance of the health construct for nursing, there is not agreement on the nature of health. Various conceptualizations of health are reviewed, the emic-etic distinction between the concepts of disease and illness is delineated, and a new model of health is presented. This model is illustrated with examples from the folk and scientific domains of one cultural group, Greek Americans. Finally, implications for using this model in nursing practice are discussed and research directions are suggested.

Since Nightingale (1860) an association between the concepts of nursing and health has been identified. Recently, investigators analyzing major theories of nursing have proposed that the health construct is central to nursing (Fawcett, 1980; Flaskerud & Halloran, 1980; Stevens, 1979; Torres, 1980; Winstead-Fry, 1980). Fawcett (1980) contended that the phenomenon of interest in nursing science is encompassed by four essential concepts: person, environment, health, and nursing (p. 11). Similarly, Torres (1980) wrote "In nursing the most significant concepts that influence and determine its practice are man, society, health, and nursing . . . Without any of these concepts, nursing cannot evolve either as a science or as a professional practice field" (p. 2).

The concept of health also has evolved as a focal point in nursing curricula. In their review of 50 baccalaureate nursing programs, Yura and Torres (1975) found that the four concepts of man, society, health, and nursing,

were basic to most American nursing programs. It can be concluded, therefore, that health is a cardinal construct in nursing practice, research, and education.

In this chapter, various conceptualizations of health construct are reviewed, and a new model of health is presented. This model is illustrated by tracking the distinction between illness and disease in the folk and scientific domains of one cultural group, Greek Americans. Finally, implications for using this model in nursing practice are discussed.

CONCEPTUALIZATIONS OF HEALTH

Despite the importance of the health construct for nursing, there is not agreement on the nature of health. Winstead-Fry (1980) noted that "while health is a cherished goal in nursing care, there is a great deal of confusion about what it is and how to achieve it" (p. 1); she cited the conflicting definitions of health as a major reason for this confusion. Health has been variously defined as an absolute entity, a

Source: Tripp-Reimer, T. (1984). Reconceptualizing the construct of health: Integrating emic and etic perspectives. *Research in Nursing and Health,* 7 (2): 101-110. Reprinted with permission of and copyright © 1984 John Wiley & Sons, Inc.

state, a process, a goal, and an equilibrium. These varying definitions partly result from conceptualizing the health construct in three major ways: (1) a dichotomous variable, (2) a continuum, and (3) a more inclusive holistic state. Correspondingly, nursing theories can generally be categorized as approaching health according to one of these three conceptual modes.

Health as a Dichotomous Variable

The discipline of medicine generally defines health within a structural model. Primarily concerned with the appearance of conditions which interfere with biological functioning of the organism, medicine focuses on the identification and treatment of pathology. In this system, health becomes a residual category containing those individuals or states which manifest as normal. Health is considered present in the absence of pathological symptoms (Mercer, 1972). Taking this conceptualization to its extreme, health is sometimes viewed as "compensated illness" (Wilson, 1970, p. 4).

Weeks-Shaw (1905), an early nursing author, viewed health as a dichotomous variable. She wrote, "Health has been comprehensively defined as the 'perfect circulation of pure blood in a sound organism.' Any departure from either of these three conditions constitutes disease" (p. 1). Orem (1980), a more recent nursing theorist, also followed this dichotomous conceptualization, "Health and healthy are terms used to describe living things . . . when they are structurally and functionally whole or sound. Individual human beings are said to be healthy or unhealthy" (p. 118).

Health as a Continuum Variable

The second major conceptualization is that health is one end of a continuum. Although

the continuum may consist of a sequence of states ranging from health to illness (or sometimes death), it is essentially a bipolar construction. Absence of pathological symptoms constitutes one pole and abnormality (variously termed *disease, sickness, illness,* or *nonhealth*) constitutes the other. An individual may range along this continuum in various combinations of health/illness.

This linear view of health was best expressed by Roy (1976). Her health-illness continuum flows from peak wellness through high level wellness, good health, normal health, poor health, extreme poor health, and finally death. Rogers (1970) also can be characterized as viewing health and illness as linear categories. She wrote, "Health and illness are part of the same continuum. They are not dichotomous variables" (p. 125).

Health as a Utopian State

The third conceptualization has been termed the *eudaimonistic model* (Smith, 1981) comprised of "several views of human nature that extend the idea of health to general well-being and self-realization." Smith identified Maslow's hierarchy (1962) as this type in representing an ideal of human nature and personality. Another such scheme is Dunn's (1959) high-level wellness which promotes maximizing organic, psychological, and social functioning. The World Health Organization's definition of health as "a state of complete physical, mental, and social well-being and not merely the absence of disease and infirmity" is a third example of this model (Coe, 1970, p. 13).

In nursing, the eudaimonistic view of health can be identified in the writings of Peplau (1952): "Health . . . is a word symbol that implies forward movement of personality and other ongoing human processes in the direction of creative, constructive, productive, personal, and community living" (p. 12). King (1981) also can be characterized as following this holistic approach in her contention that "Health is defined as dynamic life experiences of human being, which implies continuous adjustment to stresses in the internal and external environment through optimum use of one's resources to achieve maximum potential for daily living" (p. 5).

Although these conceptualizations have roots in the basic sciences, they are not without criticism. Winstead-Fry (1980) pointed out that the health-illness continuum is based on the idea that health and illness are opposites. While the continuum model corrected the view that illness is a gross deviation of life processes, Winstead-Fry found that it is a "major obstacle to the proper view of health . . . because the continuum makes it difficult to formulate theoretical definitions of health" (p. 1-2).

In her chapter "Toward a Theory of Health," Newman (1979) also was critical of these three major conceptualizations. She pointed out that the dichotomous as well as the utopian (complete psychological and social well-being) are not useful models of health for nursing because "they are nonexistent in the complexity of our changing world" (p. 55). She contended that progress was made in understanding health when it was viewed linearly because "this conceptualization recognizes the dynamic, changing relationship portraying different degrees of health and illness" (p. 55-56). However, she clearly pointed out that this linearity maintains the dichotomy by polarizing health at one end of the continuum and illness at the other. To derive a more complete understanding, Newman (1979) called for a synthesis of the concepts of health and illness, based on Hegel's (1967) dialectical process of the fusion of opposites. Applying this process to health and illness, she took a condition specified as disease and its opposite, which she called non-disease. "The fusion of these two antithetical concepts brings forth a synthesis, which can be regarded as health" (p. 56).

However, even this new formulation is incomplete because it, as well as the other health conceptualizations, do not consider that health is perceived differently by the client than by health professionals. These perspectives can be reconciled by incorporating a division of the concepts of illness and disease. While formally beginning in sociology, the illness-disease distinction was elaborated in anthropology. This distinction has its theoretical foundation in the emic/etic approaches formulated by Pike in 1954 and elaborated by French (1963), Pike (1966), and Sturtevant (1964).

Emic-Etic Distinction

Following a distinction in linguistics between phonemic and phonetic, Pike (1954) coined the terms *emic* and *etic*. The study of phonemics involves examination of the sounds used in a particular language, while phonetics attempts to generalize from studies of individual languages to universals covering all languages. By analogy, emic categories are culturally specific while etic categories are culturally universal (Pike, 1954, 1966).

An emic analysis seeks to discover the significant distinctions made by the members of a particular culture. The main aim of emic study involves discovery of the native principles of classification and conceptualization so that the use of a priori definitions and models of cultural content can be avoided. An emic analysis is made from within each cultural system and therefore, culturally specific. Emic investigators attempt to penetrate a culture and see it as its own members do. The emic approach yields a description of a cultural system from the inside, from the viewpoint of the participant, not the observer. This is sometimes called "subjective culture" (Berry & Dasen, 1974; French, 1963; Segall, 1979; Sturtevant, 1964).

An etic analysis consists of observing behavior without learning the viewpoint of those studied. Using externally derived criteria, the etic investigator examines and compares several cultures (Barry & Dasen, 1974; French, 1963; Pike, 1954, 1966; Segall, 1979). Because etic categories can be applied across cultures, Pike (1954) called them culture-free features of the real world. The etic label also may be applied to features which are not truly universal but have been derived from the examination of several cultures (Sturtevant, 1964).

The categories of Western biomedicine can be viewed as an etic classification system according to which data from individual clients are analyzed. This etic approach imposes a measurement external to the phenomenon. However, these categories of explanation and definition, embedded in Western biomedicine, may not be appropriate when projected onto transcultural or lay explanatory systems (Kleinman, 1978). Price-Williams (1975) pointed out the difficulty in characterizing the health state of transcultural clients from only the etic perspective of Western biomedicine.

Opposed to this etic approach is the emic perspective which focuses on the culture of the client. The emic approach describes the phenomenon from the subjective perspective of the client. Emics show what categories a particular people use and how they classify their own health experience. An emic analysis defines the perceptions and classifications made by members of a particular community (including the choice of criteria for determining adaptive and maladaptive behavior). It is within nursing's domain to mediate between the biomedical (etic) model and the patient (emic) model; to understand, interpret, and intervene based on what both the physician and patient are perceiving. This can be accomplished by first synthesizing the concepts of disease and illness.

Disease

Disease may be viewed from the biomedical perspective as an etic category. Units of analysis from biomedicine can be applied universally. In the Western biomedical paradigm, disease is malfunctioning or maladaptation of biological and psychological processes in the individual. Disease is defined in terms that are objective, observable, and quantifiable (Coe, 1970; Eisenburg, 1977; Kleinman, Eisenberg, & Good, 1978; Suchman, 1963).

Disease is specifically related to changes in specific organs of the body caused by specific agents, which if allowed to affect the body would do so in predictable ways. Diseases are specific kinds of biological reactions to some kind of injury or change affecting the internal environment of the body. Diseases are indicated by certain abnormal signs and symptoms which can be observed, measured, recorded, classified, and analyzed according to clinical standards of abnormality (Idler, 1963). Such a physiologically based definition of disease, while obviously useful for biomedicine, is inadequate for the discipline of nursing.

Illness

On the other hand, illness is an emic category, which is only understood from the client's perspective. Illness is a subjective phenomenon in which individuals who perceive themselves as not feeling well modify their normal behavior. In contrast to disease (a concept of biology), illness is a personal phenomenon concerning an individual's altered perception of self. Illness refers to a social entity, a status defined in terms of social functioning in its broadest sense. It concerns the reactions of the individual and the social group toward the condition (Chrisman, 1977; Coe, 1970; Eisenburg, 1977; Idler, 1963).

Illness represents personal, interpersonal, and cultural reactions to disease or discomfort. Cultural factors govern the definition, perception, labeling, explanation, and evaluation of the illness experience. Illness, therefore, is a culturally constructed category. In addition, culture patterns the methods of coping with the illness experience (Kleinman et al., 1978; Maslow, 1962).

Illness and Disease

Illnesses are lay experiences of changes in states of personal being and in social function. Diseases, in the scientific paradigm of biomedicine, are abnormalities in the structure and function of body organs and systems (Eisenberg, 1977).

There is not automatic complementarity between these two perspectives. Physicians focus on disease problems (problems of biological malfunctioning) and offer appropriate disease interventions. Patients primarily are concerned with the nature and consequences of illness problems (ie, the way the sickness is perceived, experienced, and evaluated by the individual and his or her social network) (Fabrega, 1974, 1979; Kleinman et al., 1978).

There are many cases of illness which never come to the attention of health professionals. Zola (1972) estimated that 70 percent to 90 percent of all self-recognized episodes of illness are managed outside the health-care system. In most cases of illness, the popular and folk sectors (self-treatment, family care, self-help groups, religious and folk practitioners) provide a substantial portion of health care. In addition, it is possible for an individual to have a disease yet be unaware of it. It also is possible for an individual to feel ill without showing any objective evidence of pathology.

Kleinman et al. (1978) said that physicians diagnose and treat diseases whereas patients suffer illnesses. They noted that physicians often disregard illness problems because they look on the disease as the entire disorder. For patients, illness problems (difficulties in living) are usually viewed as constituting the entire disorder. In addition, Kleinman et al. (1978) contended that the professional training of physicians disregards illness and its treatment. Biomedicine increasingly has banished the illness experience as a legitimate object of clinical concern.

A NEW MODEL OF HEALTH

Clearly, each perspective (disease or illness) separately is insufficient. To facilitate a synthesis of the etic and emic perspectives, a health grid is useful. While the idea of using a grid to explicate the concept of health is not new (Dunn, 1959), changing the axes of the grid results in a different conceptualization. This new conceptualization of the health grid is useful for clinical practice because it assists the nurse to understand the situation from both perspectives, client and biomedicine. The concepts of disease and illness are synthesized in the health grid seen in Figure 16.1. The grid indicates that the health state inherently contains two dimensions: the etic (objective) and the emic (subjective). The horizontal axis consists of the disease to nondisease continuum. This etic axis represents the objective interpretation of the health state by a scientifically trained practitioner. The verticle emic axis ranges from illness at the bottom to wellness at the top. This illness-wellness axis represents the subjective perception and experiences of an individual and social group to the health state.

THE HEALTH QUADRANTS: A GREEK EXAMPLE

Because folk health systems are lay models which deviate from biomedicine, cross-cultural examples illustrate the distinction between the concepts of illness and disease. To

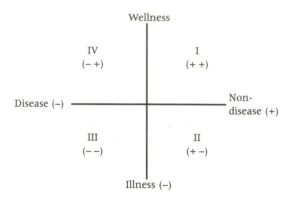

FIGURE 16.1. The emic-ethic health grid.
Quadrants specifying areas of congruence or incongruence resulting from the intersection of client and practitioner perspectives.

examine the quadrants formed by the bisecting axes, examples will be presented from one ethnic group, Greek immigrants (Tripp-Reimer, 1980, 1981).

The Greek immigrant population is a good illustration of the illness-disease distinction because, in addition to using orthodox Western medicine, the Greek community also retained traditional folk health practices which differ dramatically from the biomedical model. Members of the Greek population reported that the community had a history of seeking good medical care. Early in the century, a Greek immigrant from the area graduated from a university College of Medicine. Greek immigrants, unable to speak English, sought out this physician for formal medical care. Prior to his arrival, the community used the services of an Albanian doctor fluent in Greek. Thus, in seeking medical care, the population did not experience the significant language barriers of many immigrant groups. In addition, education and professional status are highly valued among the Greek people. As a result, fear of the professional was not as great as that reported by Clark (1970) for other immigrant groups. Finally, the rapid up-

ward mobility of the community members allowed them to afford formal medical care. However, folk medical beliefs and practices were maintained in conjunction with those of biomedicine.

Quadrant I

Quadrant I of the health grid represents the intersection of nonillness and nondisease. There is agreement between client and provider; the client subjectively feels fine and objective pathology is not detectable. Health behaviors in Quadrant I are wellness promoting and/or illness preventive. Normal developmental stages often have special wellness-promoting and illness-preventing prescriptions. For example, in many cultures childhood, infancy, and pregnancy are viewed as times in which the individual is particularly susceptible to various types of illness; special measures are prescribed or proscribed to ensure that wellness is maintained.

Although Greek immigrants seek orthodox Western prenatal care during pregnancy, folk beliefs and behaviors are followed concurrently. In Greek immigrant society, as well as in Greece, pregnancy is a time of great respect for women. Pregnant women are restricted from certain activities because these actions will "mark" the baby. Correspondingly, pregnant women are prohibited from attending funerals or viewing a corpse or other frightening sights. They pray to St. Simeon and refrain from sinful activity to prevent infant deformity (Tripp-Reimer, 1981).

However, the majority of pregnancy admonitions are related to diet. Pregnant women are encouraged to eat large quantities of food; foods high in iron and protein are thought to be particularly beneficial to both mother and child. Correspondingly, several folk tales surround the giving of food to pregnant women.

There are a number of folk practices which relax the woman during labor and delivery. After delivery, the mother is considered especially susceptible to illness for 40 days. Very traditional Greeks restrict the woman to her house during this time and the maternal grandmother runs the house. At the end of the 40-day period the mother and child attend church and receive the ritual blessing (Tripp-Reimer, 1981). In this example of Quadrant I, incongruence between biomedical and folk systems is minor. The emphasis of each is the same, to promote and maintain the wellness of mother and infant.

Quadrant III

In Quadrant III there also is congruence. The individual feels ill and there is objective pathology that can be identified by a scientifically trained practitioner. An example of congruence in Quadrant III can be seen with thalassemia major. Thalassemia (or Cooley's anemia) is a genetic disease manifested by a quantitative defect in the synthesis of hemoglobin A. In the homozygous state a serious anemia results, leading to early death in untreated cases. Thalassemia is found among populations throughout the Eastern Mediterranean, reaching frequencies of 20% in some Greek populations. Thalassemia also is found in the American immigrant populations. Research in the United States indicated that 5% of Italian Americans, 10% of Greek Americans, and .5% to 1% of Afro-Americans carry the gene for beta thalassemia (Garn, 1971).

Biomedical treatment (including supportive drug therapy and splenectomy) provide individuals with an average life expectancy of 15 to 20 years in the United States. Affected infants initially may gain weight normally but become progressively anemic. Pallor, diarrhea, recurrent bouts of fever, poor feeding, and progressive enlargement of the abdomen due to hepatosplenomegaly are common presenting features of homozygous beta thalassemia. Growth is slowed (after age 4) and skin discol-

oration (ranging from yellowish to gray-green hues) becomes apparent. The facial features are gradually distorted with boffing of the skull, hypertrophy of the maxilla, and prominence of the malar eminences at times so extreme as to obliterate the nasal passages. The skeletal features are distored especially in the skull and in the long bones and hands. The cause of death in thalassemia often is attributed to cardiac failure (Book, 1978; Harris, 1975; Kolata, 1980).

Not only do patients exhibit these obvious pathological changes, but they also consider themselves ill. In her study of thalassemia patients in Cyprus, Book (1978) reported "Some of the older patients who suffered from increasing complications as well as social ostracism openly expressed despair" (p. 16). She further pointed out from field observation and interview material that other social and situational factors assume importance in the adjustment of the patient and family to the illness. School problems, parents' attitudes about the disease, and reactions of relatives, teachers, and peers were areas of concern. In the case of thalassemia, therefore, scientifically trained observers can objectively identify pathology and the patients' subjective reports experiencing illness. They do not consider themselves well.

Summarizing evidence in Quadrants I and III, there is agreement between health professionals and clients. That is, in Quadrant I there is congruence because the client considers self well and the practitioner cannot identify disease pathology. In Quadrant III there also is congruence because the client considers self ill and the practitioner can objectively detect pathology.

Quadrant II

Quadrants II and IV are characterized by incongruence. That is, there is a mismatch between the way the provider and the client view the health state. In Quadrant II (nondisease/illness) there is no objective pathology that can be identified by a scientifically trained observer. However, the person considers self as ill. This quadrant includes categories that are often termed *folk illnesses*. Folk illnesses are generally attributed to nonscientific causes.

Individuals may identify conditions as folk illness and not seek professional health care because health professionals are not considered knowledgable about the treatment. In these instances assistance is sought from a folk practitioner.

The evil eye is an example of a pervasive folk illness known throughout the Mediterranean area. The evil eye generally is caused unintentionally and may result simply from envy or admiration. A common cause is for a woman to compliment another's child. Simply because the woman envies or admires the child she may unintentionally cause the "eye." The child may later feel lethargic, have a headache, or be irritable (Tripp-Reimer, 1981).

Among Greeks, the eye is known as *matiasma* or literally "bad eye." The most common method of detecting matiasma consists of placing olive oil in a glass of water; if the oil disperses then the eye has been cast. While some informants believed that matiasma would disappear after it had been detected, most felt that additional ritual acts were needed. These acts fall into two general categories. The first consists of physical acts such as taking three sips of the oil-and-water mixture, making three crosses over the glass, then washing the face with the water or making the sign of the cross over the affected part of the body. The second category consists of ritual prayers or sayings that have the power to remove the evil eye. A few informants believed that general prayers can be made for removal of the evil eye, but more believe that praying to the Virgin Mary was most effective. However, the majority held that there are special prayers to remove the evil eye. It was commonly believed that these prayers or "the words" are ef-

fective when said aloud. One saying was roughly translated as "Jesus Christ wins and sends away all of the bad things." This saying is repeated as the healer makes the sign of the cross (Tripp-Reimer, 1981).

Groups with belief in the evil eye also have methods for protecting against it. For example, Greek children may wear a phylacto, which is blessed wood or incense. Children also may wear gold crosses or blue beads, which are said to reflect the eye. Additionally, after complimenting a child the admirer may perform ritual acts to thwart any unintentional effects of envy.

Thus, Quadrant II is an illness category which does not correspond to a disease entity. In this example of matiasma, the illness has elaborate preventive, symptomatic, diagnostic, and treatment practices which surround it, and which are entirely outside the domain of biomedicine.

Quadrant IV

In Quadrant IV there may be obvious pathology which can be identified by a scientifically trained practitioner, but the patient does not consider self ill. Conditions which are readily identifiable by health professionals, but which are not considered illnesses may result from two major factors. The condition may be ignored, because the condition is considered normal among the reference group, or more commonly because it remains undetected. Many diseases (hypertension, diabetes, respiratory or kidney problems) do not have symptoms that are readily identifiable by lay people. These are hidden diseases detectable only by specialized equipment or laboratory tests.

Among Greeks, glucose-6-phosphate dehydrogenase (G-6-PD) deficiency is a relatively common pathological condition which is not considered an illness. In the erythrocyte, G-6-PD is the first enzyme of the pentose phosphate shunt. This pathway is essential to maintaining the integrity of the red blood cell. Some individuals are deficient in the enzyme G-6-PD or have a variant of this enzyme. Although there are well over 80 variant forms of G-6-PD deficiency, the GD-Mediterranean or Gd B- is the one most common in Greek Americans. The highest frequencies of this gene occur in individuals of Mediterranean descent where it reaches frequencies of 35 percent in parts of Greece (Garn, 1971; Harris, 1975).

Individuals with G-6-PD deficiency are asymptomatic unless they ingest an oxidizing agent and thereby precipitate acute hemolytic anemia. The Mediterranean type of G-6-PD deficiency is so threatening that the World Health Organization (1973) recommended that all hospitalized patients from populations at risk (including Greeks) should be screened for G-6-PD deficiency when hospitalized for any cause. In individuals with G-6-PD deficiency even such common medications as phenacetin and aspirin can induce hemolysis.

Because G-6-PD deficiency can be easily detected by electrophoresis and other laboratory tests, it is easily identified by a scientifically trained practitioner. However, unless the individual ingests an agent with oxidizing properties, the individual will not consider self ill because there are not any symptoms of the deficiency. Therefore, again, a mismatch exists between the health practitioner who can detect pathology and the client who may be wholly asymptomatic.

IMPLICATIONS FOR NURSING

In summary, two health grid quadrants manifest congruence: Quadrant I and Quadrant III. In Quadrant I there is agreement between both practitioner and client that the person is well and without pathology. In Quadrant III there also is congruence, the client feels ill and the health practitioner can detect objective pathology. However, in Quadrants II and IV there are mismatches between the client's and provider's perceptions of the client's health state. In Quadrant II where no disease pathology is evident, the client may consider self ill and have elaborate folk configuration surrounding the perceived condition. In Quadrant IV, although pathology is present, the client does not consider self ill because the condition is ignored or undetected. Health, then, can be visualized as the location on a grid where the subjective components of illness are combined with the objective components. Health in this conceptualization is not seen as a goal but as a state.

To locate the client's health state on the grid, the nurse uses two major assessments. The nurse derives the client's position on the etic (disease/nondisease) axis from the medical diagnosis. In addition to presence or absence of pathology, a number of other features surround this axis, including etiology, pathophysiology, prognosis, and treatment.

To determine the client's emic (wellness/illness) axis, the nurse may use the Explanatory Model (modified from Kleinman et al., 1978). This modified assessment tool includes the following questions:

1. Do you consider yourself well or ill? (If ill, continue; if well, stop).
2. What do you think caused this illness?
3. Why did this illness start when it did?
4. What does your illness do to you? How does it work?
5. How severe is this condition? Will it last a long or short time?
6. What have you [already] done for this problem?
7. What [else] do you plan to do in the future?
8. What kind of treatment do you think you should receive?
9. What are the most important results you hope to receive from this treatment?

10. What are the chief problems your illness has caused you?
11. What does your family think about this illness?
12. What do you fear most about your illness?

Locating the patient's position on the health grid is useful in understanding how the client perceives and interprets the health state, and in identifying areas of congruence or inconsistency between the client's perception of health and the biomedical one.

Where there is congruence (Quadrants I and III) there will be fewer misunderstandings in identifying a problem, even though there may be differences in the specific nature of the problem or what to do about it. But in Quadrants II and IV where incongruence exists, there will be greater misunderstandings between client and provider.

Ultimately this model may be used to prescribe nursing interventions. I suggest that:

1. *Quadrant I* (nondisease/wellness) nursing interventions consist of strategies for maintaining and promoting wellness.
2. *Quadrant III* (disease/illness) nursing interventions center on assisting the client with a pathological problem to cope with the condition; that is, gaining understanding of the pathological process, ministering to physical needs, and coping with life changes.
3. In *Quadrant II* (illness/nondisease) the clients may never seek health care. When they do, nursing interventions consist of fostering self-care activities, and referring to appropriate folk or traditional healers.
4. In *Quadrant IV* (wellness/disease) initial nursing interventions are to assist the patient to identify pathology and enter a treatment plan.

In all quadrants, the nurse may act as culture broker, translating the biomedical and client orientations. In Quadrant I, nurses assess the effectiveness of client activities promoting wellness. In Quadrants II and IV, nurses specify which model holds primacy: in Quadrant II, the client model will dominate; and in Quadrant IV intervention is directed toward assisting the client to see the validity of the biomedical model. In Quadrant III, intervention may be the mediation between the client's model of illness and the biomedical model of disease.

These are initial formulations which need investigation. Specifically, the following questions merit attention. What are the strategies and techniques used by nurses engaged in cultural brokerage? In what clinical situations are the biomedical and client orientations given differential importance? (In critical care situations, nursing interventions may be based on a biomedical framework; in long-term care situations, nursing intervention may focus more on the client model of illness.) In what clinical situations is cultural brokerage primarily unidirectional (focusing on one model); in what situations does brokerage consist of mediation between the two models?

CONCLUSION

By viewing the health state as a grid with the axes of disease/nondisease and illness/wellness, we have a tool to synthesize the health state from the perspectives of both the provider and the client. In thus doing, we have baseline interventions for each of the quadrants. In each of these quadrants, the baseline nursing interventions will be different.

Because folk health systems most clearly differentiate the client and provider perceptions, this health grid has been illustrated with examples from Greek-American culture. However, this emic-etic distinction obtains in all health-care situations. That is, the health state of each client can be located on this grid: a synthesis of the client's subjective perception (wellness/illness) and the objective perception of the scientifically trained health professional (disease/nondisease). While this grid is most clear when using a cross-cultural example, it has important implications for health-care delivery to all clients and to the understanding of the interaction between scientifically trained practitioners and lay patients.

REFERENCES

Berry, J., & Dasen, P. *Culture and cognition*. London: Methuen, 1974.

Book, P. Death at an early age: Thalassemia in Cyprus. *Medical Anthropology*, 1978, 2, 1-40.

Chrisman, N. The health seeking process: An approach to the natural history of illness. *Culture, Medicine, and Psychiatry*, 1977, 1, 351-377.

Clark, M. *Health in the Mexican-American culture*. Los Angeles: University of California Press, 1970.

Coe, R. *Medical sociology*. New York: McGraw-Hill, 1970.

Dunn, H. High-level wellness for man and society. *American Journal of Public Health and Nations' Health*, 1959, 49, 786-792.

Eisenberg, L. Disease and illness: Distinctions between professional and popular ideas of sickness. *Culture, Medicine and Psychiatry*, 1977, 1, 9-23.

Fabrega, H. *Disease and social behavior: An interdisciplinary perspective*. Cambridge, MIT Press, 1974.

————. The ethnography of illness. *Social Science and Medicine*, 1979, 13, 565-576.

Fawcett, J. A framework for analysis and evaluation of conceptual models of nursing. *Nurse Educator*, 1980, 5, 10-14.

Flaskerud, J., & Halloran, E. Areas of agreement in nursing theory development. *Advances in Nursing Science*, 1980, 3, 1-7.

French, D. The relationships of anthropology to studies in perception and cognition. In S. Kotch (Ed.), *Psychology: A study of science*. New York: McGraw-Hill, 1963.

Garn, S. *Human races*. Springfield: Thomas, 1971.

Harris, H. *Principles of human biochemical genetics*. Oxford, England: North-Holland, 1975.

Hegel, G. The phenomenology of mind. New York: Harper & Row, 1967. (Originally published, 1807.)

Idler, E. Definitions of health and illness and medical sociology. *Social Science and Medicine*, 1963, 13(a), 723-731.

King, I. *A theory for nursing: Systems, concepts, process*. New York: Wiley, 1981.

Kleinman, A. International health care planning from an ethnomedical perspective: Critique and recommendations for change. *Medical Anthropology*, 1978, 2, 71-96.

Kleinman, A., Eisenberg, L., & Good, B. Culture, illness and care: Clinical lessons from anthropologic and cross-cultural research. *Annals of Internal Medicine*, 1978, 99, 25-58.

Kolata, G. Thalassemias: Models of genetic diseases. *Science*, 1980, 210, 300-302.

Maslow, A. *Toward a psychology of being*. Princeton, NJ: Van Nostrand, 1962.

Mercer, J. Who is normal? In E. Jaco (Ed.), *Patients, physicians, and illness*. New York: Free Press, 1972.

Newman, M. Toward a theory of health. *Theory development in nursing*. Philadelphia: Davis, 1979.

Nightingale, F. *Notes on nursing: What it is and what it is not*. New York: Appleton, 1860. (Originally published 1859.)

Orem, D. *Nursing: Concepts of practice*. New York: McGraw-Hill, 1980.

Peplau, H. *Interpersonal relations in nursing: A conceptual frame of reference for psycho-dynamic nursing*. New York: Putnam, 1952.

Pike, K. *Language in relation to a unified theory of the structure of human behavior*. Glendale, CA: Summer Institute of Linguistics, 1954.

————. *Language in relation to a unified theory of the structure of human behavior*. The Hauge, The Netherlands: Mouton, 1966.

Price-Williams, D. *Explorations in cross-cultural psychology*. San Francisco: Chandler & Sharp, 1975.

Rogers, M. *An introduction to the theoretical basis of nursing*. Philadelphia: Davis, 1970.

Roy, Sr. C. *Introduction to nursing: An adaptation model*. Englewood Cliffs, NJ: Prentice-Hall, 1976.

Segall, M. *Human behavior in cross-cultural psychology: Global perspective*. Monterey, CA: Brooks/Cole, 1979.

Smith, J. The idea of health: A philosophical inquiry. *Advances in Nursing Science*, 1981, 3, 43-50.

Stevens, B. *Nursing theory: Analysis, application, evaluation*. Boston: Little, Brown & Company, 1979.

Sturtevant, W. Studies in ethnoscience. *American Anthropologist*, 1964, 66, 99-131.

Suchman, E. *Sociology in the field of public health*. New York: Russell Sage, 1963.

Torres, G. The place of concepts and theories within nursing. In J. George (Ed.), *Nursing theories: The base for professional nursing practice.* Englewood Cliffs, NJ: Prentice-Hall, 1980.

Tripp-Reimer, T. Genetic demography of an urban Greek immigrant community. *Human Biology,* 1980, 52, 255-267.

─────. Ethnomedical beliefs of Greek immigrants. *Transcultural Nursing Care,* 1981, 6, 126-140.

Weeks-Shaw, C. *A text-book of nursing: For the use of training schools, families and private students.* New York: Appleton, 1905.

Wilson, R. *The sociology of health: An introduction.* New York: Random House, 1970.

Winstead-Fry, P. The scientific method and its impact on holistic health. *Advances in Nursing Science,* 1980, 2, 1-7.

World Health Organization. *Pharmacogenetics technical report series* (524). Geneva: World Health Organization, 1973.

Yura, H., & Torres, G. Today's conceptual frameworks within baccalaureate nursing programs. *Faculty curriculum development III: conceptual framework—Its meaning and function.* New York: National League for Nursing, 1975. (NLN Pub. No. 15-1558)

Zola, I. Studying the decision to see a doctor. In Z. Lipowski (Ed.), *Advances in psychosomatic medicine.* Basel, Switzerland: Karger, 1972.

17

Perspectives on Health

MARY H. HUCH, RN, PhD

On May 12, 1989, in Pittsburgh, six nurse leaders participated in a panel discussion on health at Discovery International, Inc.'s Nurse Theorist Conference. The participants were Imogene King, Nola Pender, Betty Neuman, Martha E. Rogers, Afaf Meleis, and Rosemarie Rizzo Parse. The goal of the conference was to present views on the meaning of health from different perspectives. The panel discussion provided the nurse leaders an opportunity to engage in a dialogue about health. Five of the participants answered the questions posed and the conference keynote speaker Afaf Meleis responded. Four questions were posed to the panel relating to the meaning of health, the uniqueness of nursing, and nurse-person relationships. The dialogue of the panel discussions follows.

QUESTION: What is the meaning of health from your particular perspective?

Rosemarie Parse:
Health for me is a personal commitment. The individual in mutual interrelationship with the environment is coauthor of his or her own health. Each individual knows a personal way that is the incarnation of his or her values, and health unfolds as the person becomes more diverse. Health is recognized in one's own patterns of relating and is changed through interrelationship with the environment. Three ways in which a person changes health are creative imagining, affirming self, and glimpsing the paradoxical. Health is not a state of well-being. It is not something that human's strive for; it is the "who" that one is. The nurse in relationship with the person ac-

cepts the person's own description of health as the reality of health for that person. Health is not something related to societal norms.

Imogene King:
I think I'm going to change one word in my definition of health of eighteen years ago. Because I have the word *state* in it, and that's pretty static. So I would say that health is our dynamic life cycle. And several of the philosophers and theologians whose literature I reviewed recently gave me insight, too. You can hardly conceptualize health without conceptualizing human being. I went back to my 1971 book and would you believe that I have in my diagram that man's health is the overriding comprehensive concept? I'm so pleased to get all this confirmation from the recent review of literature. I've described my concept of health, and the characteristics of health. A characteristic to me describes the nature of something. And the characteristics are that health is genetic, it is perceptual, it's

Source: Huch, M. H. (1991). Perspectives on health. *Nursing Science Quarterly, 4* (1): 33-40. Reprinted with permission from Chestnut House Publications.

subjective, it's cultural, it's relative, it's functional; health is dynamic, and is influenced by environmental situations.

Nola Pender:
In looking at health, I take a multidimensional approach and consider it as patterning. So, I define health as a multidimensional approach of human beings as they actualize both inherent and acquired potentials, because I think both are possible. Individuals are born with certain potentials and then, as part of their experience, with the environment, they acquire others. Actualizing the potentials, being and becoming, is, indeed, health. The definition I used in my book has two primary modes of actualizing health, one is through competent personal care, and the other is through meaningful relationships with others. And those others can be individuals, aggregates, communities, and societies. I also differentiate health, or health promotion from illness prevention. Illness prevention is primarily a stabilizing phenomenon. Health and health promotion in particular are actualizing phemonena.

Betty Neuman:
I see health certainly as a dynamic concept. I like to view it as a process-based concept. I like to think of health as energy. From the perspective of the Neuman model of systems an excess of or a dearth of energy has to do with the wellness versus the illness state. I certainly see the environmental exchanges, internal and external, as influencing the health state in a major way. So health is energy used related to the newly developed concept, created environment. I hope you'll all ponder that, because I believe looking at causal factors will tell us more about health than perhaps we've known before. I know there's a lot of disagreement at present on whether health is on a continuum. But this is my view. It fits the view of the nursing

model that I have designed. Looking at it on a continuum reflects the degree of client wellness at any given time. I think it's easy to define. I know there are many factors that are at play when we talk about the health state. But if we can look at the Neuman model as being a health-oriented model then we're beginning from the viewpoint of health. So, it's a health orientation. The goal, then, in terms of health, is similar to what Imogene has said, optimal health for the client. And interestingly enough, the theory for the model has been defined as client-optimal system stability. So we're talking about stability, basically as being almost synonymous with the wellness state.

Martha Rogers:
I shall try to be independent. I feel health is a value term that we give to the human-environmental field integral process. Health is relative and it is infinite. In times of exploding acceleration, it changes in its meanings about as fast as we change our clothes, assuming we have some to change. The goal of nurses is to participate in the process of people achieving maximum health or well-being within the potential of each individual, family, and group. Potentials are not steady. Potentials are infinite, continuously changing; they are not just a scientific term in my book.

Afaf Meleis:
Well, we have healthy diversity in this group. Health is probably all these things. And I think the common theme here is that nurses participate in helping people through the process of health. I agree with that, but I think probably the other common theme that I would like to question and have us think about is that this is health in terms of an individual commitment and an individual situation. I would like to add another dimension. Health is a personal commitment, but it is also a social commitment. And it is a social

commitment within a group. We have had people whom we have interviewed who do not quite fit into that mode of thinking and reflecting about meanings in describing their situation. Health for them is being able to put food on the table. Health for them is being able to be connected to their own extended family. I really believe that we need to understand health, and bring in the environment perspective, and we need to bring in the cultural perspective. There is no way for us to understand the meaning of health from a personal point of view without understanding health within the culture or health within the society. It takes on a completely different meaning. So, I would like to ground our discussion and add to it that health is to manage, health is to negotiate, health is to achieve for a group, not to achieve for the self, because I heard it being described as achieved for the self. Health is to grow within a group, and have the group or the family grow, and health is to be part of that group. And health is to think about the environment and look at it, look at the entire environment to understand the person.

Rosemarie Parse:
I would like to just say that my definition of personal commitment does take into consideration your concern for culture and society and groups. I think that where we differ is in our definition of *personal*. When I talk about personal, I am talking about the nature of the human-environment interrelationship. And when I talk about a person's way of living health, that is coconstituted with others and the environment, which includes close family, and society. So I think in the definition of health as a personal commitment, an unfolding of values—the way I have identified it— does take into consideration the cultural and the societal aspects you speak about. I think it also applies to everyone. In a prior conversation that Afaf and I had, she mentioned that

it's like a middle-class view. And it's again because of our basic difference in the definition of personal. I think that health is inherent in being human. Our way of living is in patterns of relating and that is inherent in human existence. So, it's not a question of health as a personal commitment for a certain group of people; it's for the person in Biafra; it's for the person in the jungle with beri-beri; it's for all. The human way of being is participating in choosing health. It is health that one is living since it is inherent in being human, and the choices are inherent in being human. It's not only that we have different opportunities and options in the middle class, as she has suggested, but that the options are inherent in our being human. That is where we differ, in the definition of personal and what's entailed in being human.

Afaf Meleis:
I'm not talking about culture and environment as influencing health. I think that everybody at this table is talking about the relationship between person and environment and the effect of environment on the person. I'm not really talking about that. I am saying that the person's view of health is not a view that's a personal view of health. We cannot separate the person view of health from a group view of health, from an environment view of health, from a cultural view of health. These choices that we are speaking about here are the luxury that we see in some of the developed countries and even here, in a "so-called" developed country we see it more in the middle class. The idea being proposed is that the choices are there, and we make those choices and take advantage of them. Those choices are not there for many people. And it's not that they take advantage of them or not. They are not there, period. And, therefore, it is the structure that provides those choices. So, there is no way for us to understand personal commitment without

looking at the group commitment. "Person" is a Western phenomenon. Person is more a middle-class phenomenon, a Western phenomenon. It is "we" rather than "I". It's just a completely different perception of the whole thing. We come from "I" and the others come from "we."

Nola Pender:
I was just going to comment that as I look at the dimensions of health on the aspect of social contribution, what has been interesting to me is that we are now thinking about world community. I talked with some of the people at the American Cancer Society. They were talking about their programmatic thrust, and that they have really functioned on the idea of people helping people within their own neighborhoods. When one talks about social or societal contributions, we need to think in terms of a world community and not simply our own family, our own primary groups to which we relate, but in a much broader frame that will then allow changes to occur via shared energies that will make things different.

Imogene King:
I would like to again reintroduce you, in terms of Afaf's comments, to my conceptual framework: individual, personal systems, interpersonal systems, and social systems. Because it seems to me that health pervades and interacts with persons as individuals, with groups, and with the social system within a society, and the societies within a particular cultural orientation. And I think that has proven to be a structure to show these interactions.

Betty Neuman:
I have a brief comment to make and it has to do with our responsibility as nurse caregivers in helping those who do not realize they have an option for health to help to bring this to mind in some way or another. There are options in

health. I agree that we do have these options, but we don't always know what they are, and we may need to be shown. And, I don't know of any other body of caregivers who can do that except us. That is our charge as I see it.

QUESTION: How does the meaning of health from your particular perspective reflect the uniqueness of nursing and distinguish it from other disciplines?

Martha Rogers:
Well, let me say in the first place that the uniqueness of nursing is in the focus of the science of nursing which is unitary irreducible human beings and their respective environs. Now, one cannot generalize from parts to wholes and this is written up extensively in the literature. The use of the term *health* within this context refers to whatever we mean by the whole, by irreducible human-environment field process manifestations. So that whatever we're talking about, and I think this is where the uniqueness in terms of nursing would come, in reference to the whole. The criteria of healthy parts, or unhealthy parts, wouldn't matter—it tells you nothing about the health of the whole. And I think that is a lesson that we have to give great thought. We have not thought about it enough. One of the reasons being that there are those who still say the human is too complex, so you can't ever study the whole. Strangely enough, that isn't true and the other thing is that the wholes aren't going to go away. So, in that sense, whenever I use the term *health* I am referring only to unitary human beings and this is where our uniqueness is. Nobody else does or ever has studied unitary human beings as irreducible wholes. And, the only reason for our existence is that we have something that is different. If we're the same as everyone else, then they can get rid of us. I want to stay around a little while.

Betty Neuman:
Well, I said this in the literature, and I'll reiterate it here. The uniqueness of nursing, I find, is in looking at all variable areas of the client for analysis purposes only and considering how they fit into the whole in relation to their interaction with the environment. I always see this interplay taking place. However, we cannot deal with just a separate part, I would agree with Martha in this respect, that man is a whole, but to analyze the existing parts and the interplay with the environment is also important. And, then, we can put them back together again, so to speak, and integrate the parts of a whole. This is my belief in terms of my model's intent and purpose. That is not only in assessing, but also in nursing action. We may decide to deal with just one part. We have one priority or one variable of the client's condition. I believe that other disciplines are less holistic not only in their philosophies, but also in their functional approaches to client care. I doubt if any other health-care discipline is as concerned as we are with conceptualizing the domain of their function. I don't know for sure if that's true, but I suspect it is. If anyone can help to clarify that I would like to know myself.

Nola Pender:
In terms of the meaning of health from my perspective and its uniqueness to nursing, I think I commented on the fact that while we may and should develop a unique perspective, a secondary goal is to have that perspective adopted as a dominant worldview. But in terms of its uniqueness, I mentioned that I saw health as a dominant life experience. That is, illness experiences are secondary, superimposed on a primary health experience which is a part of living. Illness experiences are integrated into that primary experience. Also, I think a positive view of health is very different. We still struggle with, as Reynolds indi-

cated, where we are in terms of theory and concept development and where we are in describing and measuring health. So we have a gap between what we say we espouse in our current ability and in our current instruments. But, hopefully, that will change as we become more comfortable with a unitary view. Our instruments will reflect that orientation.

Imogene King:
I give credit to Martha for bringing this idea to our consciousness in a direct way. However, Martha, you know the history of nursing as well as I do, and health has been viewed as an integral concept and nurses have always been interested in maintaining people's health, helping them regain health and in health promotion. I think today the people are writing about it. But it's been my experience that nurses are unique as individuals and as a group because of what they know and how they use what they know. We are asked, and we expect it of ourselves, to conceptualize knowledge from every discipline in higher education, and put it together for ourselves. Now Martha's going to disagree with me. But knowledge is knowledge. It's available to everyone, no matter what the discipline. You put it together for yourself, and you use it, and you have to make decisions at a moment in time, no matter where your location is in terms of the position you hold. And I think it's our unique way of thinking about the world, about human beings, and about their health, that really sets us aside from any other health profession and any other discipline. I just think we should start to give ourselves credit for the kinds of things we've done.

Rosemarie Parse:
We're talking about the meaning of health from our perspective and how it reflects the uniqueness for nursing. It is not health that identifies our uniqueness, it is our knowledge

base. And for me the knowledge base that undergirds practice is lived experiences of unitary humans. And I think that's what distinguishes us from other disciplines. Many other disciplines do talk about health in every way that we have already spoken about it. I think that definitions of health will not identify or define us as particularly unique, but it is our unique focus on lived experiences of unitary humans.

Afaf Meleis:
I am reflecting on the concept of unique, because I think this is something that's probably a very predominant concept in nursing, more in the 1970s than in the 1980s, where we were trying to find a slice for ourselves, and find out what we are about. I think we are in a situation now where we have identified a perspective for nursing. So I think I'm sort of past that idea of trying to find out what's unique about nursing and what we do that is significant for humanity and makes a difference in the lives of the people we take care of. I do agree, however, that there are some unique aspects of our knowledge that sort of give us the perspective on what we look at as health. And the unique perspective is that we do look at the human being as a whole, and I think that everybody on this panel is talking about looking at the human being as a whole. We are also talking about looking at lots of variables. It's not like, perhaps, other disciplines, that we look at maybe the social variables or the cultural variables or the biological variables by themselves. I think nurses look at a number of variables and look at the human being in terms of the accumulation of those variables. When I say that, I think of Anita Mason who wrote a really excellent article in *Nursing Outlook* a few years ago. She was trying to differentiate between what she does with her clients and what her colleague, a physician, does with his clients. And they had both talked about it. And I think one par-

ticular comment is really pertinent here. She said she noticed that what she does is she casts a very wide net around the client and asks questions around what the client has come for. And she noticed that her colleague, and he agreed with her, does not cast a large net. He goes directly to the problem and sort of works outward with a checklist. I would add a couple of other things to what has been said. We look at health in terms of a pattern. And I think patterning is also a common theme here. But we probably also add to that look at health in terms of development, development of human beings and development in terms of social development. We look at it in terms of options. I think I'm seeing it at this panel. We look at it as a social obligation, and we look at it in terms of our options. I really want us all to think about what we do in our practice, because that's how I ground some of these ideas. When I see a client, and I think about energy, and I think about the personal commitment, and I think about obligations, I also think about what options does that person have. What are the perceptions of their options? What are the groups' perceptions of their options? Nobody else in the health-care system thinks about options, about development, about access, about pattern, as much as we do. So I think that is nursing's uniqueness.

Betty Neuman:
I'm in agreement with Afaf.

Rosemarie Parse:
Afaf talked about looking at a lot of variables, are these measurable variables? I talk about lived experiences and they are not measurable, they will not be measurable. If we are studying the lived experiences of the human being, and if the belief is that health is an unfolding process, then health will not be measured. Afaf, when you say unitary, and then go on to say that we do look at psychological

and sociological variables, it's inconsistent. It's the lens that you look through. There was a column in one of the issues of *Nursing Science Quarterly* that talked about lenses, and how we view humans. We put a lens on for the particulate and that lens shows us sociological, psychological, and physical variables. We cannot say that these are the same variables as when we look through the unitary lens. I see patterns there, and those patterns are not patterns of physiology or patterns of psychology. It is not a collection of what other disciplines study.

Afaf Meleis:
I'm in agreement with that. We do look at patterns. But there are, and I think I heard right here on this panel, that there are some variables that have an impact on the person in terms of their perceptions of health. I don't think it's an either/or kind of situation. There are some aspects in our environment that are reducible to variables. How much money are we making? How much food can we put on the table? I take all this into consideration when I'm looking at the life situation of human beings, which is a unitary analysis. I don't think that ethnography, qualitative approaches, or phenomenological approaches are the ways for us to get at some of the data related to lived experiences, to the exclusion of variables. Nursing will probably develop its unique methodological approaches to data collection and to understanding human health. And that uniqueness will come not from disregarding the present approaches to the development of knowledge, or adopting completely phenomenological and ethnographic approaches to the development of knowledge. It will probably come, and it is coming right now, from using all the perspectives together. I think the trick that we haven't mastered is how to do that. And the reason we haven't mastered that is that no other discipline has been able

to do that. It's up to us to do it. But it's not going to happen if we say that the lived experience will only be understood through phenomenological approaches and ethnographic approaches or that health is going to only be understood in terms of variables. It's not either/or.

Rosemarie Parse:
The worldviews underpinning the perspectives you talk about are different. If the worldviews can be combined at a conceptual level, then what you say would be possible. But when you approach persons to study health as a lived experience, you get the data from the descriptions of the people. And it's not a matter of checking the variables. It's important that the ontological base and the research methodology be consistent. I'm not saying that some particular frameworks will not be using quantitative methods. It's just that when you study lived experiences, you will use qualitative methods.

Nola Pender:
I was going to say something very much in line with what Afaf said, and that's that I have a real commitment to both approaches. And I think the excitement is what Phyllis Kritick has called the integrative tension that forces one to look at coming from two different perspectives for the richness in the blend, rather than from an either/or.

Betty Neuman:
Well, Nola. You just took the words out of my mouth, so to speak. I feel that we really need to integrate a lot of things in terms of our own ways of viewing health. And, perhaps, there is no one single way. The human is very complex. So is a small group, or a large group. So we need to integrate a lot of facts, which I happen to call variables. But that does not mean that I don't believe in the whole person, or Martha's concept, or Rose-

marie's. It's just that the integration factor, how we view it, and how we interpret the data is critically important.

Martha Rogers:
I think we get into a real problem here because the whole is different from the parts. And if we're going to talk about the whole, we're talking about a new worldview. And unless we recognize that these are two different worlds, it would be like saying I got up this morning on a flat earth, and right now I'm on a round one. I think if we're going to talk about people as wholes, we have to stick to what we're talking about. And, there's no point in our saying that the human is so complex. The human isn't complex. It's our perspective of it. If we ask questions that make humans complex and if we want to add up parts, of course, there are no answers. It's like these puzzles. Oh, I think you've probably seen the one with nine dots. And they say "with four lines connect all the dots and you can't cross anything." And everybody looks puzzled saying that it can't be done. It can be done if you go outside the dots. But sticking to the dots and going from one to the other, you can't do it. And I'm saying that the human being isn't the one that's complex. We are asking the wrong questions. And when we talk about these different fields and adding them up, I think of one psychologist who said that human psychology doesn't deal with people; it deals with a part of them. And these other fields do not deal with the whole field of people, either. It's confusing if you say we believe in irreducible human beings, then start talking about the parts. An irreducible human being is just that.

Imogene King:
In a book I read recently on "how to read," the author in one of the sections said we should continue to ask the questions that children ask their parents. Children ask the most piercing, inquiring questions about their world. But somehow, the day they go to school, something happens to them. The best questions are asked by children and we should continue to go back to ask the same questions.

Nola Pender:
One of the dilemmas that I certainly have struggled with and you may have, too, is our commitment to the whole versus the parts. Does that mean that when one starts thinking about the whole, there are dimensions? And, if there are, are they measurable? I have difficulty with the movement from part to whole, with the underlying assumption that once you get to the whole, nothing is measurable.

Rosemarie Parse:
You see, Nola, it's not going from the parts to the whole. If you look at the whole itself, it is different. It is a different look altogether. It is a different lens. It's not the same as a look at the parts. When you view the whole you cannot see the biological and the sociological parts and you cannot put these together to see it. As Martha said, it's the irreducible unitary human. And when you are studying it, you are studying a different phenomenon.

Nola Pender:
I agree with that totally. I'm still back to once you have the irreducible phenomenon, is it not in some way measurable? Are dimensions not measurable?

Martha Rogers:
Of course there are ways things can be measured. When one is viewing current holistic trends generally, one is having to learn to ask new questions. Tools that have been used to measure or evaluate or study psychological phenomena, or biological, or whatever you are talking about, are not valid for study in other fields. Tools developed in physics cannot

be taken and suddenly applied to psychological phenomena. They are not valid. Now, it doesn't mean that one can't take a tool and validate it. But, we're dealing with different kinds of things. This doesn't mean we throw out previous learnings. For example, the idea of a Q-sort can be used to develop a new tool. We do need new tools. We already have some. Many, I suspect, you're already familiar with, like Ference's human field motion tool and Elizabeth Barrett's power tool. But these are all tools developed by the individual that have been validated and tested. Questions that relate to parts are not valid questions if one's looking at the whole. And it is field-pattern that identifies the whole, not parts.

Imogene King:
I just want to say that in my review of literature, I mentioned the name, Nola Pender. She has been involved with three other nurses in developing instruments. They are among the few nurses who have really tried to design instruments to measure parameters of health. And I just wanted to call that to your attention, because she's sitting here now. The tools have reliability and validity.

Afaf Meleis:
I do have one more comment about worldviews. It is true that perhaps to some people the existing worldviews of the different approaches to developing knowledge may be incompatible. But we ought to be developing our own worldview.

QUESTION: Describe the nurse-person relationship in the context of your perspective of health.

Rosemarie Parse:
The nurse-person relationship from my view is a subject-to-subject engagement. It is the nurse in true presence with the person as the person unfolds in his or her own way. True presence is the nurse with the person illuminating meanings, synchronizing rhythms, and mobilizing transcendence. The person in the presence of the nurse explicates "what was," "is," and "will be," dwells with the rhythms of the situation, and moves beyond the moment. This presence with the person is the practice of nursing. Nursing practice in light of my view is different from the traditional view. The nurse's goal is not to restore health or prevent illness. But, rather, it is to "be with" the person as the person chooses ways of changing patterns of health in interrelationship with the environment. It's clearly different from other views of nurse-person relationships where the nurse is a conduit to pass information along from another discipline.

Imogene King:
My theory of goal attainment establishes the nursing process of nurse and client interaction. The nurse, by virtue of professional knowledge, gives that individual the knowledge that he or she thinks the person needs. The person gives knowledge about self. Between the two of them they mutually establish some goals for health promotion or regaining health for that individual and they agree about the means to achieve those goals. And both, then, exhibit behavior that will help that individual achieve a state of health which I say is a way to function in the usual roles of that individual.

Nola Pender:
I have identified the nurse-patient relationship in terms of certain verbs that I think describe a different kind of interrelationship with patients or clients than we traditionally think of in nursing. And that is the role of working together for informing about options, enabling creation of options, what I call empowering, supporting, advocating, and

"caring about" rather than in the traditional sense of "caring for." And these verbs would sum up what I view as a different essence of the nurse-client relationship, than "caring for" or "doing for" within the parameters, particularly of health promotion.

Betty Neuman:

My response to this question is that the nature of the nurse-client relationship within the context of the Neuman Systems Model is reciprocal in terms of clarifying perceptual differences, negotiating mutually acceptable and relevant goals, and focusing on increasingly existing strengths toward the best use of energy to retain, attain, and maintain an ultimate client system stability which is synonymous with wellness, whatever that wellness state.

Martha Rogers:

It's awful. There "ain't" no such thing as a nurse-person relationship. The process of change is through human and environmental field process and the relationship is a human field-environmental field relationship. If you want a relationship, you know, like me and you, it's impossible. I can't take you out of your environment. You can't take me out of my environmental field. The field process and the pattern changes are just that. One might also have a group field in which all of the same principles would apply, but a group does not respond like the individuals within a group. If you're going to study a family, you study the family. Studying the members *as a* family does not tell you about *the* family. And there are plenty of illustrations I could use to clarify that, but there is no nurse-person or nurse-client process. Rather, in this human-environmental field process we are participants in making possible change directed toward whatever we hope is going to be maximum health. So, I think this represents a whole new way of thinking.

Afaf Meleis:

You know, I'm thinking that this is really exciting listening to these perspectives because I believe we are coming to some sense of agreement about what it is, not that we are searching for agreement. But that there is really a perspective about nursing, and what the nurse-person relationship is like. What I heard was that nurses have to be really present, with their whole being in a relationship. That's what a relationship is about. And I think Rosemarie Parse is saying something about that presence and the significance of that presence. I heard also that nurses give knowledge and give information and we certainly all give knowledge and information at certain points. It's not the whole goal, but it is one of the goals for a particular situation. I also heard that it's working together. It's giving options. It's an empowering. It's caring. It's dealing with these parameters that will enhance health. We can't empower unless we have some knowledge to give. And we can't empower and become an advocate unless there is some access to something that we want our clients to get into. We can't increase strength unless we empower, and we empower by giving knowledge and being present. So, what I'm hearing here, and I hope the you are hearing the same thing, too, is that this nurse-client interaction or environment-environment interaction is important because it is the environment of the person. It's the nurses, who they are and what they are about, that interact with client, the group, and who they are and what they are about, that is the interaction. Components of it are being present, providing knowledge, exchanging and working together.

And I don't see real differences. I see that each one of these wonderful nurse theorists sitting at this table is looking at a part of what nursing is all about. And all together they are providing us with what nursing is about. When we ground that in terms of what we do clinically or what we do in terms of research, it's not possible for us to see only one of these perspectives. It's not possible for us to actually work with only one of these perspectives. We cannot be imparting knowledge at all times, we cannot be empowering at all times. But we can be doing part of that in every encounter.

Rosemarie Parse:
Afaf, please elaborate on empowerment.

Afaf Meleis:
Actually, that's a constant I'm working with. But, Nola also mentioned it, so maybe we should ask Nola to say what she thinks first.

Nola Pender:
In terms of empowerment, as I see it, it's essentially creating options, helping people not only to recognize existing options, but actually creating options that may not exist at one time and yet can exist in the future.

Afaf Meleis:
Thank you, Nola. Part of empowerment is raising consciousness. Helping the group of people to see the situation from a different perspective. Seeing the different options, the potential of access, the potential for some changes. And then allowing the person, not really allowing, because the person is allowed that, or the group is allowed that, but allowing ourselves to allow others to then take charge and go from there.

Rosemarie Parse:
It's what I thought you were going to say. Empowerment has to do with the nurse giving to or telling the person what's right, in terms of health. Is that where you are?

Afaf Meleis:
It's working together. It's the negotiating. It's opening up. It's consciousness raising. A good

example is being with some colleagues and talking about feminist perspectives. Now, I'm not making anybody do anything. But, I'm dialoguing. It's dialoguing, it's providing a perspective. A new whole comes out of this dialogue. It's not, "I am doing this or you could do this," it's rather, as we dialogue, something comes up that we probably both are able to do.

Rosemarie Parse:
Yes, but that is not the definition of empowerment.

QUESTION: Pose a research question related to your perspective that you believe is significant.

Martha Rogers:
Oh, I have to always put in a lot of words. We need two kinds of research: basic research in the science of nursing, and applied research. Applied research does not create knowledge, rather it tests knowledge already available. And new knowledge comes about through basic research. By this I mean in the science of unitary human beings. Now we need extensive basic research. Applied research can never really go beyond basic research. I'm talking now about things that were well known to scientists in other fields. I didn't dream these up myself. I just happen to agree with them. But we do need new questions in terms of holistic trends. We need the development of tools for evaluation. We need particularly basic research in the whole construct of patterning. When I use the term *pattern* I am referring only to field pattern, human field pattern, and environmental field pattern. These refer to wave frequencies if you like. They are patterns, abstractions. We cannot see them, but they show up in the manifestations. We need research of that sort. Research that will get us into wave frequencies and their significance in terms of develop-

ment. In the area of applied research we need a great deal on the effectiveness of noninvasive modalities in relation to human health. So, you just take your pick. It's wide open, and it is fun!

Betty Neuman:
In relation to my own perspective of health, we need to explore the relationship of the Neuman concept of the created environment. It's very new and we need to look at that in terms of health, how does it relate to health and what meaning does it have? And we need to look at health as a process on a continuum again. And I know that this is very debatable, but this is my personal view.

Nola Pender:
One of the fascinating questions for me relates to human development, particularly adult developmental processes. The data from 2,000 people that I have studied have raised the question, Do patterns of health differ across the life span? And I think that's an interesting question when one considers patterns, and health patterns, and what kind of configurations we see. Can we identify some commonalities of configurations, that may then show an interesting transition throughout the life span?

Imogene King:
I would like to see nurses and graduate students engage in some philosophical inquiry which is a little different from the usual traditional scientific mode, and the first question I would pose would be, How do you describe your health? And I would collect data on as many people as I could find in whatever environment I could find. If I were going to test hypotheses in terms of my own theory, I would test one something like this. "Mutual goal setting will increase functional abilities in human beings." I do have a reliable valid instrument called a *criterion reference measure*

of goal attainment that was recently published and could be used to gather data to test this hypothesis.

Rosemarie Parse:
I think the next move in nursing is to develop unique research methodologies congruent with the frameworks and theories. The Parse Research Methodology has evolved from the theory, has been published, and is being tested. It seeks to uncover the structure of lived experiences. Some questions might be, What is the structure of the lived experience of suffering? and What is the structure of the lived experience of laughter? It would be the lived experience that the researcher was interested in studying using the new methodology. Knowledge about the structure of lived experiences expands the theory, the expanded theory then guides practice and further research.

Afaf Meleis:
I am looking at patterns of health and patterns of coping for women from different cultures, who have no or low income, and I'm looking at that with some colleagues from different countries and also in San Francisco. We are including the immigrant population. We are looking at those in and within the context of their lived experiences that include the multiple roles that they play. So we're looking at women not as reproductive beings, but rather as productive beings.

SUMMARY

In the dialogue the panelists specified their perspectives on the meaning of health. Through the lively discussion, similarities and differences in views were explored and new ideas surfaced. When nursing leaders come together to share divergent views, issues are clarified and in the process nursing science is enhanced.

18

Expressing Health through Lifestyle Patterns

NOLA J. PENDER, RN, PhD, FAAN

Few concepts have received more attention from health professionals and the public during the last decade than health. This is largely due to the emergence of disease prevention and health promotion as global priorities. Unfortunately, the nature of health as a positive life process is poorly understood. Theoretical formulations of health often lack specificity and existing measures almost without exception reflect a narrow clinical perspective of health as the absence of disease. The purpose of this chapter is to propose a system for classifying expressions of health of persons in their entirety and to suggest related indicators of high-level health.

During the last decade nursing, as well as other health disciplines, has recognized the limitations of medical and technological approaches for improving the quality of life and health of the world's population. Major changes in social, political, and environmental conditions of living and the life ways of large segments of society are necessary, if significant improvements in health are to occur during the next century. Thus, disease prevention and health promotion have become global agendas with the potential for achieving health goals unattainable previously through curative interventions. The escalating commitment to health promotion among nations raises important questions concerning the nature of health. What is the *critical essence* of that which is to be promoted? A review of relevant scientific literature confirms that health as a human life span process is poorly understood.

Historically, illness, not health, has been the primary concern of the health professions and mortality and morbidity the indicators of "health" used most frequently (Smith, 1981). Therefore, it is not surprising that in reviewing studies of health, Terris (1975) identified the following illness-related approaches to health assessment: measurement of impairment, assessment of physiological systems in relation to established norms, and measurement of performance in the context of potential decrements. The concept of health has not fared much better in nursing. Although health along with person, environment, and nursing constitute the commonly accepted metaparadigm of the discipline (Fawcett, 1984), the concept of health seems to elude clear theoretical descriptions and, to an even greater extent, useful empirical specifications. Reynolds (1988), in reviewing the measures of health used in reports of nursing research, found that, despite articulation of a holistic concept of health in dominant theoretical views within

Source: Pender, N. J. (1990). Expressing health through lifestyle patterns. *Nurse Science Quarterly, 3* (3): 115-122. Reprinted with permission from Chestnut House Publications.

the discipline, nurse scientists tended to use indicators derived from a clinical model as the absence of disease.

Is health such a complex human process that it cannot be studied qualitatively or quantitatively? Is high-level health a utopian state, a mirage to be fantasized but never achieved (Dubos, 1965)? On the other hand, if health can be the object of systematic investigation, can it *only* be defined by negation, that is as the absence of disease? Unwilling to settle for such a narrow definition, various health disciplines have attempted to define health from fragmented perspectives placing primary emphasis on psychological, sociological, cultural, or spiritual dimensions. Some attempts have been made to synthesize these perspectives to achieve a complete view of health. Parse (1987) refers to this approach as the totality paradigm, in which persons are considered as biopsychosocial spiritual beings responding and adapting to their environment. A major question about this additive approach is whether the whole is equal to or greater than the sum of the parts.

PERSON AND HEALTH: NEW VIEWS OF OLD CONCEPTS

Within the past two decades in nursing, there has been a significant conceptual shift toward viewing persons as unified wholes possessing integrity and manifesting characteristics that are more than and different from the sum of the parts. According to Rogers (1970),

> The unity of man is a reality. Man interacts with his environment in his totality. Only as man's wholeness is perceived does the study of man begin to yield meaningful concepts and theories. Only as man's oneness is apprehended is it possible to identify man's distinctive attributes. (p. 44)

This shift in nursing toward a unitary view of human beings has resulted in increasing reliance on the tenets of human science in addition to the reductionistic paradigm of traditional science for understanding health. How do individuals *experience* health and what *meanings* do they give these experiences have emerged as central questions within the discipline. Tripp-Reimer (1984) suggested that within nursing, health be reconceptualized to incorporate both etic and emic perspectives. In the etic perspective, objective observations without input from those observed are used to determine health. In the emic perspective, the meaning of health to individuals within their particular culture is ascertained. Concerns relevant in the latter perspective include, How is health expressed? Is the expression of health universal or culture specific? Are expressions of health qualitatively different at various developmental phases throughout the life span?

In contrast to the totality paradigm based primarily on the etic perspective, the simultaneity paradigm (Parse, Coyne, & Smith, 1985) captures the emic perspective. Within the latter paradigm each person is viewed as a synergistic being in open, mutual, and simultaneous interchange with the environment. In this context health is a wholistic unfolding of humans in interaction with the environment in which all the elements or dimensions of health are experienced as a unitary phenomenon. Based on Rogers's theory of unitary human beings, Newman (1979) defined health as the totality of the life process evolving toward expanded consciousness. Parse (Parse et al., 1985), also in the Rogerian tradition, described health as a "process of becoming uniquely lived by each individual . . . a nonlinear entity that cannot be qualified by terms such as *good, bad, more,* or *less.* Unitary man's health is a synthesis of values, a way of living . . . a continuously changing process that man cocreates" (pp. 9-10). Definitions with similar themes have been offered by Pender (1982), who described health as the actualization of inherent and acquired human potential and Watson (1988) who defined health as harmony with self and environment. A new approach for combining objective (etic) and subjective (emic) health perspectives is needed to avoid a conception of health in which observable physical and behavioral aspects are viewed as separate or in oppositional relationship to experiential aspects. It is the author's belief that both perspectives are valuable and can coexist within the discipline of nursing.

Along with acceptance of a unitary view of health, there is an increasing tendency in nursing to reject the health-illness continuum which Newman (1979) criticized on the grounds that it maintains a false dichotomy by polarizing health at one end of the continuum and illness at the other end. If nursing is to facilitate a client's movement toward health on the health-illness continuum, this must *always* be away from illness. An "either-or" dichotomy precludes the existence of high levels of health in the presence of a disability or chronic illness. This belief, if carried to its logical conclusion, would imply that health promotion efforts are futile for millions of Americans young and old who have a chronic disease incurable by existing medical means. Health promotion would only be considered appropriate for the favored few without any evidence of disease, thus disenfranchising the poor, the old, and the disabled of services directed toward optimizing their health. To address this dilemma, Newman (1979) suggested a synthesis of the concepts of diseases and nondisease into an integrative concept of health.

Taking another theoretical approach to the problem posed by the health-illness continuum, Pender (1987) described health as the primary life experience with illness superimposed on health. Health can exist without illness, but illness never exists without health as its context. When illness occurs, it is synthesized as part of the ongoing health experience modifying it in varying ways—changing the quality of the experience, and *decreasing* or *increasing* overall feelings and perceptions of health. Unlike Parse (1981), who rejects the idea of health as existing to varying degrees, Smith (1981) views health as a comparative term. It has long been recognized that all persons free of disease are not equally healthy. It is the degree to which health is present from both objective and subjective points of view that should be mutually assessed by nurse and client. It is only on the basis of both perspectives that effective efforts can be directed toward appropriate health enhancement activities.

The dominant definition of health espoused by a society has profound political and economic implications because the dimensions of that definition and their associated measures often become major social concerns. Frequently, programs of national and international scope are established to bring about positive changes in the identified indicators of health (McDowell & Newell, 1987). Thus, the discipline of nursing faces one of its biggest challenges in decades—how to best articulate the dimensions of health of persons in their entirety and develop valid and reliable indicators of health as a unitary phenomenon. Such indicators must be articulated with a level of conceptual clarity that permits communication of this perspective to other health disciplines and the public. The clinical view of health as the absence of disease has been the dominant definition in the United States for decades. It is time for a paradigmatic shift to a unitary conception of health that will enable society to deal capably with the multiplicity of factors now known to have an impact on health status.

As nursing moves forward in developing a unitary concept of health, strongly influenced by the tenets of human science, the discipline should not lose sight of empiricism as a viable approach to health-related research. Some questions asked about health are best addressed within a traditional science paradigm. For example, health processes outside of conscious awareness may be observable using highly sophisticated methods and techniques (Norbeck, 1987). Nursing can provide leadership to the health disciplines in blending the approaches of traditional and human sciences. Differences between the two paradigms should not be interpreted as conflict but as integrative tension that promotes creativity in scientific endeavors (Kritek, 1989).

HEALTH AS PATTERN

Rogers (1970) identified the energy field as the fundamental unit of the universe for the science of nursing. The human and environmental fields are coextensive and in an intimate relationship. Pattern is the distinguishing characteristic of an energy field, which becomes more complex throughout the life span. Persons shape their own health experiences to a considerable extent as they make choices from the options available to them (Parse, 1981). Innate to energy fields are generative powers that can facilitate positive patterning and repatterning, resulting in progressively healthier conditions of being, as objectively measured and subjectively reported.

There is no single, universal health pattern that all human beings share. Health when viewed as a lived experience, that is, within the emic perspective, represents many alternative realities. Only individuals can reveal the hidden meanings that they create for health. Although health has many different shades of meaning, there are recurring themes or commonalities that persons report as expressions of health when queried as to what health means to them. The critical question is, What are the varying human patterns most indicative of health?

DIMENSIONS OF THE HEALTH EXPERIENCE

In 1981, Smith proposed a model of health with four dimensions reflective of existing lit-

erature: the clinical dimension defining health as the absence of disease, the role performance dimension describing health as competent performance of socially defined roles, the adaptive dimension characterizing health as flexible adjustment to changing life situations, and the eudaimonistic dimension viewing health as exuberant well-being. Laffrey (1986) operationalized Smith's model in a scale intended to determine the extent to which individuals viewed health along each of these dimensions. In further research Woods and colleagues (1988) supported the health conception model of Smith in a study of 528 women who were asked, "What do you mean when you say you are in good health?" Their work contributed to the further elaboration of the eudaimonistic view of health identifying nine images consistent with this dimension: actualizing self, practicing healthy life ways, positive self-concept, positive body image, social involvement, fitness, effective cognitive function, positive mood, and harmony.

Parse (Parse et al., 1985) conducted a phenomenological study of 400 men and women who were asked to write descriptions of a personal situation in which a feeling of health was experienced. Recurring themes were identified for persons of differing ages. As an example, the recurring themes for persons between 20 and 45 years of age as expressed within the theoretical framework of man-living-health were: spirited intensity, fulfilling inventiveness, and symphonic integrity.

CLASSIFYING EXPRESSIONS OF HEALTH

In this section, a system for classifying human expressions of health is proposed. Five dimensions of human health expression are organized further into 15 subcategories as shown in Table 18.1. This framework for studying health has emerged as a result of discussions with colleagues, review of the literature, and

TABLE 18.1. Classification System for Expressions of Health

Affect			
Serenity	*Harmony*	*Vitality*	*Sensitivity*
Calm	Close to God	Energetic	Aware
Relaxed	Contemplative	Vigorous	Connected
Peaceful	At one with the universe	Zestful	Intimate
Content		Alert	Loving
Comfortable		Fit	
Glowing		Buoyant	
Happy		Exhilarated	
Joyous		Powerful	
Pleasant		Courageous	
Satisfied			

Attitudes		
Optimism	*Relevancy*	*Competency*
Hopeful	Useful	Purposive
Enthusiastic	Contributing	Initiating
Open	Valued	Self-motivating
Reverent	Caring	Self-affirming
Trustful	Committed	Innovative
	Involved	Masterful
		Challenged

Activity		
Positive Life Patterns	*Meaningful Work*	*Invigorating Play*
Eating a healthy diet	Setting realistic goals	Having meaningful hobbies
Exercising regularly	Varying activities	Engaging in satisfying leisure
Managing stress	Undertaking challenging tasks	activities
Obtaining adequate rest	Assuming responsibility for self	Planning energizing diversions
Avoiding harmful substances	Collaborating with coworkers	
Building positive relationships	Receiving intrinsic or extrinsic	
Seeking and using health information	rewards	
Monitoring health		
Coping constructively		
Maintaining a health-strengthening environment		

Aspirations	
Self-Actualization	*Social Contribution*
Growth or emergence	Enhancement of global harmony and interdependence
Personal effectiveness	Preservation of the environment
Organismic efficiency	

Accomplishments		
Enjoyment	*Creativity*	*Transcendence*
Pleasure from daily living	Maximum use of capacities	Freedom
Sense of achievement	Innovative contribution	Expansion of consciousness
		Optimized harmony between man and environment

reflection on 5 years of quantitative and qualitative research conducted by a health promotion research team (S. N. Walker, K. R. Sechrist, M. F. Stromborg, & N. J. Pender.) in which the health and health practices of approximately 2,000 adults were studied. The following assumptions undergird the proposed classification:

1. Integration of the views of clients as well as health professionals is essential to derive a useful definition of health.
2. Health is a manifestation of person/environment interactional patterns that become increasingly complex throughout the life span.
3. Some human health patterns can be directly observed, others must be self-reported.

The five dimensions within the classification are expressed in common language and the alliteration, although originally unintended, may be useful. Each of the five dimensions of health expression—affect, attitudes, activity, aspirations, and accomplishments—should be assessed in terms of daily fluctuations as well as evolving patterns over time. The five dimensions are proposed as culture-free whereas some of the 15 subcategories and potential indicators may be culture-specific. Tools already exist to measure some of the suggested indicators; for others, approaches to description and/or measurement remain undeveloped. Consistent with a unitary view of human beings, a comprehensive assessment tool could be constructed to assess all of the dimensions simultaneously.

AFFECT

Sensation and emotion are fundamental attributes of humanness that are expressions of wholeness or unity (Rogers, 1970). *Affect* as used here is intended to denote emotions and feelings as subjectively experienced. Affect can be assessed best through personal report, but facial expressions, body positions, or gestures, as well as an increasing array of technologic measures (biofeedback, electromagnetic resonance imaging), can provide some indication of internal emotional states. The link between emotions and illness has been suspected for centuries, but little has been known about feelings as an expression of health. Recent research in psychoneuroimmunology indicates that person/environment interactions and accompanying emotional responses may moderate immune function (Kiecolt-Glaser & Glaser, 1987). Certain emotional patterns such as serenity and harmony may enhance immune competence; their polar opposites may impair immune capabilities. There is also considerable evidence that physiological changes related to activity have an impact on emotions. For example, production of endogenous opiates or internal tranquilizers can contribute to emotional experiences of comfort and calm (Watkins & Mayer, 1982).

Feelings and emotions have a direct effect on the quality of the lived experience of health. The emotions identified in Table 18.1 are those frequently reported as expressions of high-level health. *Serenity* is a sense of tranquility, a peaceful inner state, amid life's ebb and flow. *Harmony* emanates from feelings of relatedness to God and/or the universe and is sometimes described as a feeling of being at peace with nature and fellow humans. *Vitality* is a sense of energy and power. *Sensitivity* is intense knowing of self and others. Feelings of serenity, harmony, vitality, and sensitivity at any moment reflect much more than the current life situation. Human beings have the unique ability to evoke emotions in response to remembered events from the past or anticipated events in the future. This capacity provides persons with the power to transcend current situations; to be unbound by time and space. Persons may be calm, content, or even joyous in the face of difficult situations because of their vision of a greater good to be attained in the future.

Exploration of emotions as important expressions of health presents many exciting challenges to the research community. Current research on the connections between emotions and illness need to be recast in a positive perspective. Research questions from this viewpoint might be, What person/environment interaction patterns encourage positive emotions? Which emotional patterns or fluctuations in patterns are healthful, which are unhealthful, and are these effects general or person-specific? Are different emotional profiles expressive of health at different points in the life span? What interventions on the part of health professionals assist clients in achieving positive emotional patterns? What self-care strategies can increase the frequency of positive emotions? Do emotions perceived as negative detract from or at times promote health?

Emotions can be a positive integrative force (Rogers, 1970). It is the richness of emotional experience that is uniquely human. Research approaches must be used that capture this richness as well as rhythms and fluctuations in emotional patterns. Recent scientific breakthroughs in understanding emotions will fuel increased interest and expanded research efforts in this area in the next decades.

ATTITUDES

Language, thought, and the ability to form attitudes and beliefs characterize unitary human beings and result from innate capacities to abstract and image features or person/environment interaction. Humans not only think in concepts and relationships but give meanings to such abstractions. According to Rogers (1970) persons seek to organize the world of experience and make sense of it and can do so because of the capacity for rational thought. Attitudes structure the way persons see their world and, like emotions, express persons' values and priorities.

Attitudes can be developed in relation to specific situations, events, or actions. Life in its entirety can be viewed as an event. As such, persons develop attitudes or beliefs about their own personal lived situation as well as the life process as a shared experience with others. It is these general attitudes or beliefs that are proposed to profoundly influence health.

Attitudes expressive of high-level health are presented in Table 18.1. These are recurring cognitive themes in the literature and in more than 75 in-depth interviews conducted by the author and her colleagues with persons considered to have stellar health behaviors. Three subcategories of attitudes have been proposed: optimism, relevancy, and competency.

Attitudes toward life, its value, meaning, and ultimate worth are reflected in the subcategory of *optimism*. Beliefs that all will end well despite life's changing circumstances and that there are possibilities for personal growth even in difficult situations is expressed through an optimistic outlook. Optimism is enhanced by reverence for life and trust in God or the orderliness of the universe. Optimism expands openness to creative possibilities in life patterns.

Relevancy is grasping one's place in the world with an appreciation for unique, personal contributions. Relevancy is expressed through self-respect and a feeling of acceptance by others as a useful and contributing member of society. Persons experiencing a sense of relevance are caring, committed, and involved in life. Relevancy also has an eternal time frame by which persons come to appreciate the importance of their personal existence within infinite time and space.

Competency is expressed in personal clarity about actual and potential capabilities and belief in the power to channel capabilities into meaningful patterns of work and play. Competent persons actively initiate challenging life situations. They are interactive rather than passive, challenged rather than threatened, and self-affirming rather than self-debasing. Perceptions of personal competency are transferred to fellow humans with resultant appreciation of their unique patterns and emergent potential.

Positive attitudes and beliefs express high-level wellness. They are an integral part of health as a lived experience.

ACTIVITY

Movement is an alternative to language for communicating thought (Engle, 1984). Activity reflects patterns of energy distribution as well as person/environment rhythmicity. Movement is a means whereby space and time become experienced reality (Newman, 1979). Movement augments awareness of human and environmental fields. According to Newman, the total pattern of movement reflects the organization or disorganization of the thought and feeling processes of the individual. Activity expressive of health facilitates the fuller emergence of personal potential. Three dimensions of activity considered expressive of health are positive life patterns, meaningful work, and invigorating play (see Table 18.1).

Positive life patterns go beyond isolated health practices to action patterns that are an integral part of life ways. Thoughtful patterning and repatterning of daily routines and rhythms through informed decision making based on an awareness of options enhance human capacity for optimal well-being. Clusters of behaviors with empirical support for their health-enhancing properties are the backbone of positive life patterns. Eating well,

exercising regularly, obtaining adequate rest, and managing stress represent behavioral clusters comprising positive life patterns. Such patterns must be sustained over time to optimize health. Exercise as one behavioral cluster expressive of health is a good example of unitary characteristics. If exercise is to be maintained, it must be of appropriate rhythmicity, periodicity, complexity, and intensity for a given human field. Human and environmental fields must have compatible activity rhythms and patterns to optimize health.

Health is also expressed through *meaningful work*. More energy is expended on work than on any other human activity. Work that is health-promoting has been characterized as challenging, varied, well-directed, interpersonally satisfying, and both intrinsically and extrinsically rewarding. In recent years attempts have been made to achieve greater harmony between human fields and work patterns. Child care, flexible time, job sharing, and use of home as a satellite work site are only a few of the examples of greater awareness of the need for compatibility between person/environment patterning and work.

The rhythm between work and *invigorating play* changes throughout life. For most children, play constitutes the major activity in which they engage. In fact, meaningful work as an expression of health may not be relevant until the preschool or school years when confronted by the "tasks" of learning. The harmonious integration of work and play often becomes disrupted in young, middle-aged, and older adult years. Young and middle-aged adults, in striving to be successful, to achieve adequate pay, and to contribute meaningfully to society, may neglect play. Some compensate for this imbalance by focusing on enjoyable aspects of work and reinterpreting work as play. Older adults often have considerable discretionary time for play but lament lack of resources for recreational pursuits or the absence of meaningful work. It is predicted that leisure time will expand for many persons in the United States in the future as efforts are made to maximize the employment rate in a large and diverse population (Bezold, Carlson, & Peck, 1986). For both younger adults on shortened work weeks and the aging population in part-time employment, meaningful hobbies, satisfying leisure activities, and energizing diversions will be increasingly important as expressions of personal health.

ASPIRATIONS

Human beings are inherently purposeful. Life is not a random series of events, but an organized unfolding of each individual in light of personal aspirations and choices. Persons choose the directions in which they evolve in light of the range of options within awareness. Unfortunately, for persons in disadvantaged groups such as the poor and some ethnic/racial minorities, the range of choices is often constricted, limiting options for self-realization. Unnecessary limitations on self-expression is dehumanizing as well as detrimental to the continuing viability and vitality of a society.

The capacity of human beings to bring about changes in human and environmental fields is important for achievement of aspirations and goals. By modifying the nature of person/environment interactions, individuals can maximize available choices. Although persons usually have considerable freedom of choice concerning the goals they will pursue, the goals selected must be compatible with those of society. Social and cultural values as well as the needs of significant others provide a context for setting goals. Inherent in humanness is the moral responsibility for the ethical selection of goals and the means used to accomplish them.

Aspirations within a society often reflect normative patterns—the usual rather than the unusual, the average rather than the exception. Fitting in to societal norms rather than exceeding them is often condoned and encouraged to the detriment of creative change. Individuals possess unique capabilities for self-transcendence (Sarter, 1988). It is only as society encourages people to achieve their uniqueness unconstrained by normative expectations that we will have instances of maximized human health potential for systematic study.

Self-actualization and social contribution are proposed as two subcategories of aspirations needing further clarification and study in relation to human health patterns. Self-actualization is not a new term. Maslow (1970) popularized the concept in his writings as a high-level need for human organisms. *Self-actualization* is predicated on fulfilling a more basic need for self-preservation. Suggested empirical indicators for self-actualization are growth or self-emergence, personal effectiveness, and organismic efficiency. Self-actualization is an orientation toward being all one can be and fulfilling one's personal potential.

Social contribution enhances global harmony, creates health interdependence, and promotes an ecologically balanced environment for present and future generations. The community in which we live is a world community in which annihilation is an ever present threat. Social contribution as an expression of health is a sensitivity to the needs and potentials of all people, which results in responsible social actions within a particular life situation. It is through shared aspirations of aggregates that social changes supportive of health are realized.

ACCOMPLISHMENTS

Accomplishments as expressions of health can be identified as the payoffs for a life well lived. They are unencumbered by time and space and may be viewed as daily achievements, life attainments, or states to be experienced only after death. Regardless of the time frame, persons need bench marks to measure their progress, their emergence as unique human beings. Accomplishments confirm a person's selfhood as well as his or her oneness with the evolving universe.

In modern society, accomplishments are often viewed as measures of worth rather than as expressions of health. Too frequently, being and becoming are sacrificed to doing, thus destroying the balance among affect, attitudes, activity, aspirations, and accomplishments. When kept in proper perspective, accomplishments contribute to the richness of human experience. Creative achievements of human beings throughout history have markedly enhanced the quality of life for others.

Enjoyment, creativity, and transcendence are accomplishments proposed as expressive of health (see Table 18.1). *Enjoyment* is a condition in which there is heightened aesthetic awareness of the multiple dimensions of human and environmental fields. Positive emotions and thoughts predominate. Daily experiences are sources of joy. Human unfolding, its challenges and exigencies as well as successive stages of development provide continuing sources of pleasure.

The capacity for *creativity* is inherent in all human beings. It is expressed through envisioning new configurations within human and environmental fields and restructuring reality or abstractions consistent with these envisioned patterns. Creativity is experienced as performing at one's optimum, maximizing human capabilities, and accelerating diversity and complexity.

Transcendence is stretching beyond the realm of human experience toward new options and possibilities (Parse, 1981). It is experienced as freedom from constraint and expansion of human consciousness to encompass infinite time and space. It is the experience of optimum mutuality and harmony between person and environment.

Accomplishments are the expression of life purpose and thus the expression of health. Their pursuit directs human patterning and evolutionary emergence.

CONCLUDING COMMENTS

Health is a life span process, a largely subjective and private experience, only partially observable by traditional scientific methods. Although defining health only in terms of negation, that is, as the absence of disease, has been common practice for more than a century, this approach will no longer suffice in an era of increasing concern about the promotion of health and the quality of life for human populations. Health as an experience is not fragmented, it only becomes fragmented in the minds of health professionals with differing perspectives. A new view of health is needed that is positive, comprehensive, unifying, and humanistic. This article represents one attempt to move toward that goal. It is imperative that an increasing number of nurse scientists direct their efforts toward expanding our understanding of human health processes and the personal, social, political, and environmental factors affecting the health of differing populations if significant progress is to be made in optimizing health for a larger segment of the world population in the years ahead.

REFERENCES

Bezold, C., Carlson, R., & Peck, J. (1986). *The future of work and health*. Dover, MA: Auburn House.

Dubos, R. (1965). *Man adapting*. New Haven, CT: Yale University Press.

Engle, V. F. (1984). Newman's conceptual framework and the measurement of older adults' health. *Advances in Nursing Science, 7*(1), 24-36.

Fawcett, J. (1984). *Analysis and evaluation of conceptual models of nursing*. Philadelphia: Davis.

Kiecolt-Glaser, J., & Glaser, R. (1987). Psychosocial moderators of immune function. *Annals of Behavioral Medicine, 9*, 16-20.

Kritek, P. (1989, April). *Nursing research enterprise in clinical practice: An agenda for the future*. Paper presented at Northern Illinois University Annual Research Conference, DeKalb, IL.

Laffrey, S. C. (1986). Development of a health conception scale. *Research in Nursing and Health, 9*, 107-113.

McDowell, I., & Newell, C. (1987). *Measuring health: A guide to rating scales and questionnaires*. New York: Oxford.

Maslow, A. H. (1970). *Motivation and personality* (2d ed.). New York: Harper & Row.

Newman, M. (1979). *Theory development in nursing*. Philadelphia: Davis.

Norbeck, J. S. (1987). Empiricism and health promotion research. In M. E. Duffy & N. J. Pender (Eds.), *Conceptual Issues in Health Promotion: Report of Proceedings of a Wingspread Conference* (pp. 110-120). Indianapolis, IN: Sigma Theta Tau International.

Parse, R. R. (1981). *Man-living-health: A theory of nursing*. New York: Wiley.

————. (1987). *Nursing science: Major paradigms, theories, and critiques*. Philadelphia: Saunders.

Parse, R. R., Coyne, A. B., & Smith, M. J. (1985). *Nursing research: Qualitative methods*. Bowie, MD: Brady.

Pender, N. J. (1982). *Health promotion in nursing practice*. Norwalk, CT: Appleton-Century-Crofts.

Pender, N. J. (1987). *Health promotion in nursing practice* (2nd ed.). Norwalk, CT: Appleton & Lange.

Reynolds, C. L. (1988). The measurement of health in nursing research. *Advances in Nursing Science, 10*(4), 23-31.

Rogers, M. E. (1970). *An introduction to the theoretical basis of nursing*. Philadelphia: Davis.

Sarter, B. (1988). *The stream of becoming: A study of Martha Roger's theory*. New York: National League for Nursing.

Smith, J. A. (1981). The idea of health: A philosophic inquiry. *Advances in Nursing Science, 3*(3), 43-50.

Terris, M. (1975). Approaches to an epidemiology of health. *American Journal of Public Health, 65*, 1037-1045.

Tripp-Reimer, R. (1984). Reconceptualizing the construct of health: Integrating emic and etic perspectives. *Research in Nursing and Health, 7*, 101-109.

Watkins, L. R., & Mayer, D. J. (1982). Organization of endogenous opiate and monopiate pain control systems. *Science, 216*, 1185-1192.

Watson, J. (1988). *Nursing, human science, and human care*. New York: National League for Nursing.

Woods, N. F., Laffrey, S., Duffy, M., Lentz, N. J., Mitchell, E. S., Taylor, D., & Cowan, K. A. (1988). Being healthy: Women's images. *Advances in Nursing Science, 11*(1), 36-46.

19

Being and Becoming Healthy: The Core of Nursing Knowledge

AFAF IBRAHIM MELEIS, RN, PhD, FAAN

Health has been described as a central concept and the goal of nursing. The incongruence between that centrality in nursing and in other disciplines and the public's view is discussed. Other issues and views of health also are considered, including diversity and unity in conceptualizing health, the social nature and societal obligations toward the health of the individual, the lack of congruency between conceptual and empirical views of health, and health as viewed in nursing and in the international arena. Several conditions to be included in nurses' attempts in the theoretical development of health are articulated. The need for focusing on an understanding of the health-care needs of underserved populations, the potential advantage in using a feminist framework, and the integration between a static conception of being healthy and a process/dynamic/becoming conception of health are some of the strategies that can be used to develop a contextual conception of health.

Becoming healthier is a popular goal in the United States, and in the media, health has been dramatized, glamorized, fictionalized, and popularized. If one can only lose weight, exercise regularly, eat oat bran, refrain from high-fat diets and decrease cholesterol, caffeine, and alcohol intake, one will be healthy. If one can just be more beautiful, more autonomous, take a bit more control over one's life, one can be healthy. Indeed, this nation has become preoccupied with ways by which health is maintained and promoted.

Two general observations can be made about this avalanche of information on health. First, the preoccupation and focus on healthy lifestyles appear to be more a popular media endeavor than an actual reflection of social and health policies. The second interesting point is that nursing, itself, is demonstrating an equally persistent fascination with health, both as a cause and a consequence. Health phenomena figure dominantly in the writings of nurse theorists and in the research that is done by nurses. Such a focus on health is not new to nursing. In the nineteenth century, Florence Nightingale conceptualized nursing in terms of a healthy environment and focused on the nurse's ability to assist the personal healing potential of clients. This interest in health has evolved to current conceptualization and inquiry.

The purpose of this chapter is to challenge the reader to think critically about the current state of knowledge surrounding health in nursing. To facilitate this critical analysis, some

Source: Meleis, A (1990). Being and becoming healthy: The core of nursing knowledge. *Nursing Science Quarterly, 3* (3): 107-114. Reprinted with permission from Chestnut House Publications.

issues, questions, and challenges that need to be considered and confronted by nurses as professionals and as citizens of the world are delineated. The *first* is that, when health is considered in the United States, it is rarely associated with nurses. The public tends not to think of nurses or nursing when it considers health and well-being. In other countries, including Egypt, Saudi Arabia, Brazil, Colombia, India, and People's Republic of China, health is associated with medicine, physicians, or local healers, or more recently, with community and primary health-care workers—but not necessarily with nurses. Why is it that nurses claim health to be the focus and goal of nursing? Why do they fail to receive the recognition and acknowledgment that nursing makes a difference in the health of a nation? The *second* aspect of health that should be questioned is the ethnocentric framework for health that has emerged and is gaining support in the scientific and popular literature in the United States.

HEALTH IN NURSING

There are several ideas about health that represent the status of the concept of health in nursing today: Each of these is shared here with related questions.

Centrality of Health in Nursing

That health is central to nursing is demonstrated in discussions by theorists, curriculum developers, and metatheorists. Indeed, some metatheorists suggest that theories in nursing must be inclusive of a definition of health as both a process and an outcome (Payne, 1983). A number of disciplines may be interested in the same phenomenon, for example, how women juggle their multiple roles of mother, worker, and spouse, while maintaining an in-

tegrative self-identity. A nursing perspective necessitates the consideration of ways by which this integration is manifested in healthful patterns of living and how these patterns can be developed, maintained, or promoted.

Health also is central to medicine, public health, and the lay person who comes from a certain background, namely the lay person who has the luxury of thinking of health as a central point of life. In what way is this centrality similar to or different from the centrality of health that is claimed by nursing? What does it mean when health is said to be a basic or central concept in nursing? Does it mean that any time a research project about a significant question in nursing is developed, health must be included as an outcome? Is a theory in nursing differentiated from theories in other disciplines by its focus on health? Does health have to be defined in all works or analyses of any other concept in nursing? *The question of centrality needs to be carefully considered, particularly in view of the fact that such centrality of health in nursing is not recognized by the public or by other disciplines.*

Diversity and Unity

Another comment about health is the diversity of definitions of health in nursing. Health has been conceptualized as a state, a process of development, an actualization, an outcome, and a style of life. A number of researchers and theorists have raised questions about this diversity and the need for agreement.

The way the question is raised presupposes that there is the potential for unity of thought in the way nurses view health and that there is value in that unity. The question of diversity versus unity of thought is important and is reflected in the many debates in nursing about one theory, one philosophy, one conceptual framework. The question is not whether there should be unity or diversity of definition but what aspects of health can be agreed upon and what aspects demand diversity. Understanding of the whole experience of health would be much better served if the tension and the syntheses between unity and diversity were considered.

Recently, diversity in conceptualization has been more supported in nursing and the medical literature. There are several reasons for this support. Nursing is predominantly a female profession. Therefore, ways of knowing in nursing may be different than in other disciplines and the knowers in nursing may follow a different approach to knowledge development (Belenky, Clinchy, Goldberger, & Tarule, 1986; Schultz & Meleis, 1988).

The second point in favor of diversity of conceptualization is that types of knowledge may be different because of the nature of nursing and the diversity of nursing clients. Nursing is practiced in so many different clinical areas in so many parts of the world that a multitude of definitions for health are requisite. A definition of health that fits in a modern coronary care unit where patients recover from acute myocardial infarctions is quite different from a definition of health for patients recovering from kwashiorkor in a rural area of Zimbabwe. Recovery in the United States may involve health in terms of mobility and sleep, whereas recovery in Zimbabwe may require the ability to find food, water, and adequate nutrition.

Likewise, there are multiple levels of meaning of the wellness/illness experience in the medical literature. In presenting these meanings, Pietroni (1987) has supported the idea that clinicians should be able to understand and speak clearly about each one and apply the appropriate level of meaning to a particular practice situation. Among these levels of meaning is the *classical scientific view* of health, that is, the medical, material, and molecular indications of the presence or absence of illness. In this view the task is to repress symptoms, remove the cause, or replace the diseased part or function of the part. There also

is the *psychological/psychosomatic/psychoanalytical* view in which health and illness are considered an expression of deeper meanings. In this mode, personality structures are related to health and illness; and behavioral approaches of stress reduction, relaxation, biofeedback, and other direct interventions are used. The *preventive/promotional or anticipatory view* of health speaks the language of health risk assessment, seeking meaning through individual choices, self-care, yoga classes, fitness clubs, and control of health by clients. The *cultural/social/political view*, on the other hand, addresses the role of environment in both the disease and health processes. It dictates interventions within the context of societies, cultures, and political systems. A fifth view, or level, is the *archetypal, metaphorical,* and *symbolic*. Meanings of health are found in intuition and symbolism. Interventions within this mode are relaxation, exercise, visual imagery, psychodrama, group care, and connecting with the universe.

A final level within which health and illness can be understood is *space/time/energy and the "rhythm of spheres."* This view represents some of the writers who are well known to nurse metatheorists, such as Dossey (1982), Capra (1983), and Bohm (1980). In this mode the person is conceptualized as a "bioenergetic organism" who is governed by energy, bound by the illustration of time, but universally connected to all others. Healing is, therefore, a universal and collective concern; and health is defined in terms of the meaning given to it, to time, to space, and to the balance in the collective field forces. All of these meanings of health are interactive, and a holistic approach involves all of them.

Pietroni's (1987) view supports the need to accept diversity in definitions of health. There are appropriate times for the use of each of these modes. Health-care providers tend to have one prominent way of thinking about health; yet, the health-care needs of the client preclude the possibility of focusing only on one level of meaning. Pietroni's conceptualization also is an example of academic discussions about health in which no reference is made to nursing scholarship or practice related to health. One must ask whether nursing has no interdisciplinary influence, and if not, how can that be changed?

The quest for a single definition of health is not appropriate, possible, or useful. Keller (1981) is correct when she wrote, "Has it now become a game to create a definition of health? Or is it safer and easier to continually talk and write about health than to do something about it?" (pp. 43-44).

Although diversity should be accepted and reinforced, there is a need for unity in perspective that represents the territory of investigation, the territory for theoretical development. Human responses to health and illness situations, self-care behaviors in health and illness, client-nurse interactions, client-environment interactions, the subjective world of ill or healthy clients, coping styles, therapeutic actions that enhance recovery, and a sense of well-being are all part of that perspective, part of what provides nursing its territory. In addition, there are conditions that are essential to understanding this territory, such as patterns, trends, context, responses, and perceptions. It is not possible to study, analyze, or conceptualize health from a nursing perspective without considering these conditions.

If health is so considered and it is discovered that there are different definitions that emerge, then there is no rationale to continue the search for one definition and one approach to health. It is more useful to dialogue about the nature and degree of unity, as well as the nature of and degrees of diversity. As long as certain basic conditions that emanate from a nursing perspective are met, it is important to understand health from different philosophical approaches.

In reviewing nursing theories, research reports that focus on health, analyses of research on health, and clinical narratives, seven current models of health emerge that are being used in nursing practice, research, and theory. One way nurses have traditionally conceptualized health is as an absence of disease, a model that relies on medical knowledge (Smith, 1982). A second involves internal homeostasis, as represented by Johnson (1980). Another is the adaptation model of health, which takes Johnson's ideas one step further from internal regulatory mechanisms to adaptation with external regulatory mechanisms (Roy, 1984; Smith, 1982). A fourth is the role functioning/self-care model, which is predicated on being able to perform those role functions that society expects from a person (Orem, 1980; Smith, 1982). A fifth is the existential meanings model, which focuses on symbolism and the place of the self in an intricate web of relations among objects, subjects, nature, and in the relations that include objects, subjects, nature, and the supernatural (Patterson & Zderad, 1976; Travelbee, 1971). Another model is that which relies on space/time/energy and consciousness expansion; health is viewed in terms of awareness, personal control, personal empowerment, and mastery over body (Newman, 1986; Rogers, 1970). A final model that guides an understanding of health is the crucial/social/political model, which has been discussed by cross-cultural and critical theorists (Allen, 1986; Tripp-Reimer, 1984). An effective approach to the theoretical development of health is to address the nature of unity and diversity in these models.

Health as a Social Matter

One predominant unifying theme in these models is the role of the individual in maintaining and enhancing health. What most of these models demonstrate is that health is increasingly defined as a personal matter, one in which the individual has an obligation. The underlying assumption is that individuals are responsible for their health; families, communities, and societies are not as accountable. This perception of health is reflected in such definitions as "reaching one's optimum," "ability to take care of self," "exercising," "watching one's diet," "feeling in control," "ability to adjust to the environment," "eating a diet to prevent cancer and heart diseases," "avoiding stress," "modifying type 'A' personality." But is health really a personal matter? Can one feel and become healthy in isolation from structural constraints in the environment? Is it possible that individuals can achieve total control over their environment? Are there some groups of individuals who cannot master and control their bodies' well-being because their environments are oppressive or because they have no choices, or because they have never had the opportunity to think of their optimum capacity? Could nursing not be conceptualized in terms of the environment and interactions with the environment and, at the same time, health be considered a personal matter?

Health may be a personal matter for those individuals who are privileged and come from a white, middle-class background. For others in the United States and the rest of the world, health is a social matter. Certainly, for poor people, health is social. Pill and Scott (1982) interviewed a sample of 41 working-class women in the United Kingdom and found that half of them held fatalistic views about health and illness. This view, the authors maintain, is bound to have influenced readiness for health education, consultation behaviors, and expectations about what they want from the health-care system. What are the structural conditions that have created these fatalistic views of health? When health is viewed as a personal matter, those people in the world who are constrained by societal conditions and who represent the majority of nursing clients are assessed as abnormal. They do not fit the mold of personal perse-

verance and personal control over one's health. A framework of individualizing strategies for health curtails any plan of action to develop societal mechanisms for enhancement of health.

In addition to the danger of conceptualizing health as a personal matter, there is a tendency to reduce the conceptualization of health to one's bodily function or system. Health for women or women's health, for instance, has become synonymous with reproductive and maternal capacities.

> In a society that values a woman primarily for her capacity to perpetuate the species, "women's health" exists as a euphemism for obstetrics and gynecology. This view of women has existed historically in most Western cultures and helps to explain the myth that all women's problems can be attributed to wandering wombs or raging hormones. (Webster & Lipetz, 1986, p. 87)

Although this view has been changing within the last two decades, as evidenced by the increasing research in nursing about other aspects of women's health, such as violence against women, women's work, and women's aging, there still is a predominant view of women's health as reproductive health.

Broadening the conception of health of women beyond one system is not enough to capture the totality of their health. A conceptualization of health that does not encompass the views of women reduces a discussion of health to a cliche. In some current research that the author is doing in collaboration with a number of international colleagues, women have said that one of the most stressful aspects of their multiple roles is worry. They spend a great deal of their energy worrying. They worry about the economic situation, about whether they are going to be paid on time, whether their children are going to take drugs, whether their landlord is going to evict them, and whether they will have a job the next day. Well-being for these women is in relief from their worrying. Worrying for them is not a personal matter; it is a public and social matter. Health for them incorporates family, community, work, and society. It is not mastery of their body; it is strategizing with the constraints and resources of their environment to achieve a sense of well-being. Nursing can understand the health of individuals if the perspective of group, family, community, and society orientation is considered. For many individuals health cannot be separated from that of their parents, children, extended family, neighbors, and friends. Individualism is not the norm for these people and, consequently, their isolated experiences are not meaningful nor are they representative of the core of health for them.

Access to health care is another aspect of health that needs consideration. Health professionals cannot afford to address health as a concept without also addressing access to it. Definitions of health are bound by access to health care and how options for health care are perceived, and a conceptualization of health that does not include access is limited at best and erroneous at worst.

When health is seen as a community and as a social and societal obligation rather than only a personal objective, it increases the potential for structural changes. Health is relief from worry. Health is relief from fear of rape, of violations to one's self, to one's body, and to one's integrity. Health is not being robbed of defenses. Health is access and options for health care. To include innovative definitions of health is to take an activist role in helping people realize health from the perspective of social obligation. Nurses need to consider whether they have taken a proactive role theoretically, empirically, clinically, and politically in issues related to the social obligations of health.

Conceptual and Empirical Views

The incongruity between a conceptual view of health and an empirical approach to studying health in nursing has been delineated and discussed by Reynolds (1988), who views health conceptually as encompassing the whole person and incorporating the relationship between the person and the environment. Reynolds' informative review of nursing research has shown that there are very few operationalizations of health that encompass these conceptual ideas. Research about health depends on the clinical manifestations of health, that is, the number of physical and psychological symptoms. When health is considered as an outcome variable, there is a tendency to separate clinical manifestations from the experience of being healthy. Nurse scientists have not yet demonstrated a way to measure or to understand the total experience of health in a way that goes beyond the mere absence of symptoms and individual perceptions of wellness, to incorporate more than role performance or functioning. The questions to be asked here are, What do nursing's operational definitions represent? and How is health conceptualized?

In the absence of more comprehensive measures of health that are congruent with a nursing perspective, Meleis, Norbeck, and Laffrey (1989) have employed two measures of health in their research about roles of women and health. One is an objective measure that focuses on clinical manifestations of illness, and the other is a subjective measure that encompasses subjective aspects of health as perceived by the person. The Cantril ladder was used for a rating of self-health. The importance of the self-rating measure has been demonstrated by Mossey and Shapiro (1982), who found that the way people view their health is highly correlated with subsequent health outcomes. As others have repeatedly indicated, there are no measures that encompass a holistic view of health (Pender, 1987; Reynolds, 1988). Should health measures be developed to correspond with each of the different conceptualizations of health in nursing? Or should a set of conditions be developed that can be incorporated into whatever measure is used? Should the development of one holistic measure of health be abandoned in exchange for a more realistic approach that measures several dimensions of health?

Webster and Lipetz (1986), among others, have claimed that the clients' experiences of wellness and illness only can be understood in the context of their everyday lives and with information about their usual health practices and health beliefs. Clients' descriptions of their health concerns in their own words are essential in assessment, planning health care, implementing interventions, and evaluating their effectiveness. Given these criteria, what are the most effective methodologies for describing health empirically, and what are the most appropriate strategies for theory development?

Health and Primary Health Care

International colleagues are considering health from the perspective of the Alma Ata Declaration of 1978 (World Health Organization, 1978). If the potential of maintaining, regaining, or developing health and well-being are discussed without careful consideration of primary health care as a strategy to attain it, then nursing in the United States will be increasingly isolated from international nursing. Concepts that are central to primary health care are community participation, consciousness raising, appropriate local resources, access, options, and empowerment. Primary health care provides a strong community orientation. Questions to be considered include, Are any of these primary health care concepts manifestations of health? Are conceptualiza-

tions of health in nursing congruent with this view of health? Should they be?

CONDITIONS FOR THE DEVELOPMENT OF THEORY

Conceptual development must take into consideration the diversity of nursing philosophies, as well as the diverse populations served by nurses. One approach to the diversification of philosophies would be to use feminist epistemological principles as an approach to theoretical formulations related to health. Feminist researchers have identified several important epistemological principles that are congruent with the goals of nursing and that have been used as guidelines in nursing practice, although not so readily in nursing theory-building and research. These principles, as outlined by Cook and Fonow (1986), suggest that nursing (a) attend to the significance of gender and lack of gender sensitivity as a basic feature of all social life, (b) consider consciousness raising as a central and specific methodological tool in research and clinical practice, and (c) include advocacy in defining the role of the theorist, the researcher, and the clinician. Feminist theory also challenges the norms of objectivity, which assume that the subject and object of research could or should be separated, and that lack of subjective involvement is the basis for human science. One should be sensitive to the potential for exploitation of research participants, the biased participation of particular groups over others, and to ethical issues inherent in research.

Nursing could empower clients and research participants by providing them information from research and clinical expertise that assists them in changing the structural constraints that impede their well-being. These feminist principles are congruent with the nursing mission, a predominantly female constituency, the caring work of nursing, and its humanitarian values.

To consider gender as a focal theoretical category is as important as considering class and ethnicity. Careful attention to all of these concepts should sensitize nursing to the extent to which it may have built knowledge related to health based on white, male, middle-class values.

Yet, to define and describe health in ways that are not culturally, ethnically, and socially biased is a difficult task. In discussing the relationship between health and environment Allen (1981) has said,

> We may look at nursing for healthy living as providing an environment in which individuals, families, or groups can learn. This means that nursing shapes the structure for learning (through) access to knowledge and information; situations in which to discuss, share, and work with others engaged in similar pursuits; opportunity to examine, analyze, plan, and test out aspects of health behaviors with health professionals; opportunities for the community to participate in educational programs for health and to evaluate its own health status and that of its families. (p. 153)

To discuss health as a personal matter constrains the potential of understanding health as a social/environmental/societal/political one.

Conceptually, there is a need to articulate conditions that are essential to understanding health, regardless of what theory is used. These conditions, such as pattern, human rights, societal obligation, and development, can form a framework for theory development and research. Health as development implies

> progressive improvements in the living conditions and quality of life enjoyed by

society and shared by its members. It is a continuing process that takes place in all societies; few would claim that their development is complete. (WHO, 1978, p. 44)

Finally, there is a need to develop and implement nursing therapeutics that create, maintain, and promote healthy social/environmental/political contexts that emanate from lack of access and options. There is also the need for the development of frameworks to enhance health in hospitals, at home, or in administration, schools, or families.

Strategies for the Development of a Contextual Conception of Health

Several strategies could be used for the development and refinement of a conceptualization of health that is more congruent with societal needs and the mission of nursing. The *first* is to focus on investigations and theories about populations who have not been particularly central to the discipline of nursing before but are in need of nursing services; these are the underserved, the stigmatized, and the disenfranchised.

It is easier to recruit white middle-class subjects in our research studies. However, if predominantly white, middle-class heterosexual women are being selected for research, one must ask whether health is being conceptualized as having the same values as them. If we disagree, then one must ask whether there are strategies to improve the participation of other groups in research. A discipline that purports to care for the homeless and the ethnically and socially diverse should not engage in scholarship that tends to exclude women of color, working-class women, immigrants, lesbians, or any other disenfranchised group. Nursing can discuss their views only if they are included in nursing studies and theoretical work.

One of the *most important agenda items for the development of a meaningful conceptualization of health and well-being is to develop some means by which representative research participants can be recruited.* Theorizing about and investigating populations who are disenfranchised or stigmatized takes a tremendous amount of time, effort, and energy. Utilizing these populations is not cost effective. From an economic perspective, many are not likely to understand the pencil-and-paper instruments nor to respond meaningfully to structured interview questions.

There are approaches to increase participation of diverse groups in research. Cannon, Higginbotham, and Leung (1988) have demonstrated that white women who were raised in middle-class families and whose occupations were male dominated tended to volunteer and respond to request letters and media solicitations for research subjects more than other women who represented other ethnic, class, and occupational backgrounds. To get underrepresented women to participate in research, researchers have had to use what Cannon et al. (1988) termed *labor-intensive recruitment strategies,* including verbal contact, face-to-face approaches, more extensive interviews, and the conviction that the research was worthwhile. Sixty percent of the black working-class women in their sample, for instance, were recruited through such interview strategies versus 30 percent of the white working-class women. Reasons for difficulty in recruiting nonwhites included less leisure time, more skepticism about research and its motives, a fear of stereotyping, and less control over time. These constraints have to be carefully addressed and removed to enhance recruitment of diverse populations.

There are other approaches to increase diversity in research participants. Lipson and Meleis (1989) found that developing trust, modifying interviewing styles and consent procedures, providing structure for reciprocity with subjects, and nontermination of relationships were important strategies in getting first-generation immigrant subjects to participate. In another research project the provision of a modest reimbursement for time to complete the interview may have increased the diversity of the sample to more than 50 percent nonwhite participants (Meleis et al., 1989). Such an increase in participants enhances the theoretical development of health and, in turn, allows further diversity in the definition of health. International work also could help in the development of conceptualizations that represent diverse populations.

It is not enough to work in disciplinary isolation in developing a contextual conceptualization of health. It is imperative to receive recognition from members of other disciplines, as well as the public, for the roles of nurses in the health and well-being of societies. Such acknowledgment can enhance that role in influencing policies related to health. Focusing on significant questions related to health also will enhance nurses' potential in being involved in health policies.

Although there is a body of literature that either defines health, or claims it to be a central concept, or uses health as a correlate variable (eg, Shaver, 1985; Smith, 1981), it has not adequately informed clinical practice or the public. The questions to be asked are, Is the information disseminated to the public? Is the message compelling and valuable? What would be more compelling? Some questions are those that address the processes of becoming healthy and nurses' activities in bringing health to people. The "being healthy" focus in definitions of health and the "becoming healthy" questions in the face of illness, lack of access, lack of resources and within such constraints as stigma, bias, and handicap are those to which the public needs answers. These are significant questions and are more urgent and germane in terms of potential impact on social and health policy. Nurses cannot afford to spend time only on definitions. The need to develop more definitions can be supplemented with engagement in creating substantial changes for people whose health is compromised in some form or another. Some of the philosophical, theoretical, and definitional questions need to be grounded in socially significant health issues.

One can do so by asking such questions as, Is the public or legislators aware that the central focus of nursing is health? What platform is congruent with the mission of nursing as it has been defined? What platform is significant for the public, for legislators? What will make nursing visible so that it can make a statement that will be heard? One way to do so is to challenge each other to come up with questions that are not only significant but are at the cutting edge of the discipline and profession of nursing.

Instead of defining health from different perspectives, maybe it should be described and explained in terms of how people are kept healthy in spite of positive HIV or a diagnosis of AIDS, or by the strategies by which Alzheimer's patients and their caregivers become more healthy than they were before confronting the disease. How can nursing make them more healthy than they were before? How can nursing make a difference in helping overburdened single working mothers maintain their own and their children's health, or the health of the single homebound elderly? Questions such as these should be the business of nursing. Health should be considered in terms of the consumer who needs specific answers and demands specific actions.

If the view of health is broadened beyond a personal focus to include social, political, and cultural contexts, other significant questions will emerge. The development of measures that focus on clinical manifestations, subjective and objective perceptions of health, meanings associated with health, priorities, relations with the environment, and individual health as part of group health are all essential strategies in developing health as a central focus in nursing. Answers to significant questions through the development of measures that represent a nursing perspective will help provide the necessary substance for the development of middle-range theories to describe, explain, and predict health.

Being healthy, as viewed empirically, provides a static view of health that can be measured by existing measures, such as the general well-being scale, omnibus personality inventory, Cornell medical index, or the Cantril ladder. These measures represent a limited view of health that may not address what the public may consider significant. Being healthy can be reconceptualized in ways that nursing constituents and clients can relate to and understand.

Being healthy need not provide a static view of health. When considered from the perspective of clients, it is a way of life, an attitude, an outlook, a history, a context with sociocultural norms, a belief, and a tradition. Being healthy is managing, negotiating, achieving, growing, becoming, and helping others grow and become. Being and becoming healthy may be parts of a whole perception of health. Becoming healthy is hopefulness, transcending worries, realizing options, advocating, and accessing resources. Being and becoming healthy incorporate awareness, resources, opportunity, development, access, enabling, empowerment, and advocacy.

REFERENCES

Allen, D. G. (1986). Using philosophical and historical methodologies to understand the concept of health. In P. L. Chinn (Ed.), *Nursing research methodology: Issues and implementation* (pp. 157-168). Rockville, MD: Aspen.

Allen, M. (1981). The health dimension in nursing practice: Notes on nursing in primary health care. *Journal of Advanced Nursing, 6*, 153-154.

Belenky, M. F., Clinchy, B. M., Goldberger, N. R., & Tarule, J. M. (1986). *Women's ways of knowing: The development of self, voice, and mind*. New York: Basic Books.

Bohm, D. (1980). *Wholeness and the implicate order*. Boston: Routledge.

Cannon, L. W., Higginbotham, E., & Leung, M. L. A. (1988). Race and class bias in qualitative research on women. *Gender and Society, 2*, 449-454.

Capra, F. (1983). *The turning point: Science, society, and the rising culture*. New York: Bantam.

Cook, J. A., & Fonow, M. M. (1986). Knowledge and women's interests: Issues of epistemology and methodology in feminist sociological research. *Sociological Inquiry, 56*(1), 1-19.

Dossey, L. (1982). Space, time, and medicine. New York: Random House.

Johnson, D. E. (1980). The behavioral system model for nursing. In J. P. Riehl & C. Roy (Eds.), *Conceptual modes for nursing practice* (2nd ed.). New York: Appleton-Century-Crofts.

Keller, M. J. (1981). Toward a definition of health. *Advances in Nursing Science, 4*(1), 43-52.

Lipson, J. G., & Meleis, A. I. (1989). Methodological issues in research with immigrants. *Medical Anthropology, 12*(1), 103-115.

Meleis, A. I., Norbeck, J. S., & Laffrey, S. C. (1989). Role integration and health among female clerical workers. *Research in Nursing and Health, 12*.

Mossey, J. M., & Shapiro, E. (1982). Self-rated health: A predictor of mortality among the elderly. *American Journal of Public Health, 72*, 800-808.

Newman, M. A. (1986). *Health as expanding consciousness*. St. Louis: Mosby.

Orem, D. E. (1980). *Nursing: Concepts of practice* (2nd ed.). New York: McGraw-Hill.

Patterson, J. G., & Zderad, L. T. (1976). *Humanistic nursing*. New York: Wiley.

Payne, L. (1983). Health: A basic concept in nursing theory. *Journal of Advanced Nursing, 8*, 393-395.

Pender, N. J. (1987). *Promotion in nursing practice* (2nd ed.). Norwalk, CT: Appleton-Century-Crofts.

Pietroni, P. C. (1987). The meaning of illness-holism dissected: Discussion paper. *Journal of the Royal Society of Medicine, 80*, 357-360.

Pill, R., & Stott, N. C. H. (1982). Concepts of illness causation and responsibility: Some preliminary data from a sample of working class mothers. *Social Sciences & Medicine, 16*, 43-52.

Reynolds, C. (1988). The measurement of health in nursing research. *Advances in Nursing Science, 10*(4), 23-31.

Rogers, M. (1970). An introduction to the theoretical basis of nursing. Philadelphia: Davis.

Roy, C. (1984). *Introduction to nursing: An adaptation model* (2nd ed.). Englewood Cliffs, NJ: Prentice-Hall.

Schultz, P., & Meleis, A. I. (1988). Nursing epistemology: Traditions, insights, questions. *Image: Journal of Nursing Scholarship, 20*, 217-221.

Shaver, J. F. (1985). A biopsychological view of human health. *Nursing Outlook, 33*, 186-191.

Smith, J. (1981). The idea of health: A philosophical inquiry. *Advances in Nursing Science, 3*(3), 43-50.

———. (1982). Letters to the editor. *Advances in Nursing Science, 4*(3), xi.

Travelbee, J. (1971). *Interpersonal aspects of nursing* (2nd ed.). Philadelphia: Davis.

Tripp-Reimer, T. (1984). Reconceptualizing the construct of health: Integrating emic and etic perspectives. *Research in Nursing and Health, 7*, 101-109.

Webster, D., & Lipetz, M. (1986). Changing definitions: Changing times. *Nursing Clinics of North America, 21*(1), 87-97.

World Health Organization. (1978). *Primary health care: Report of the International Conference on Primary Health Care*, Alma Ata, USSR. 6-12, September 1978, Geneva.

Part V

NURSING'S METAPARADIGM: CONCEPTUALIZATIONS OF NURSING

Nursing is usually described as both a science and an art, however within these boundaries, theorists' and scholars' definitions of nursing are very diverse. Joy Johnson critically examines and analyzes relevant literature on the art of nursing in her chapter, "A Dialectical Examination of Nursing Art." Her five conceptualizations of the art of nursing include the nurse's ability to (1) grasp meaning in patient encounters, (2) establish a meaningful connection with patients, (3) skillfully perform nursing activities, (4) rationally determine an appropriate course of nursing action, and (5) morally conduct nursing practice. Each conceptualization is discussed with supporting examples from nurse theorists' and others' models or work.

Based on expanding Carper's "esthetic ways of knowing" the art of nursing, Anne Boykin, Marilyn Parker, and Savina Schoenhofer describe how nurses utilize aesthetic knowing in practice. In their chapter, "Aesthetic Knowing Grounded in an Explicit Conception of Nursing," these authors critique Carper's work and criticize her failure to explain the patterns and structures nurses use in performing the art of nursing. They conceptualize aesthetic nursing as a knowledgeable, professional service whose goal is to "nurture persons [in] living, caring, and growing in caring," and explain both the meaning of their definition and how to practice aesthetic nursing in a case example. These authors believe that knowledge of the aesthetic pathway is essential for synthesis of all four ways of knowing, and that since aesthetic nursing is both unique to the individual and universal to other nursing situations, the outcome cannot be predicted. Thus, aesthetic knowing includes application and synthesis of multiple ways of knowing, and is both the process and product or outcome of nursing practice.

Several nurse theorists and scholars view nursing as synonymous with caring, but there is much controversy about this issue. Kristen Swenson conducted three phenomenological studies of caring in perinatal contexts. Her theory of caring, derived from these studies, is described in her chapter, "Empirical Development of a Middle Range Theory of Caring." She presents a brief review of caring definitions from the literature, then explains how she developed and tested her theory of caring. Swenson identified five essential processes that women clients viewed as helpful, which she classified as "caring behaviors": knowing, being with, doing for, enabling, and maintaining belief. She illustrates each process with examples from her studies, and includes references to other research studies.

In 1993, five nurse theorists participated in a panel discussion on several topics related to nursing: (1) caring as an essence of nursing, (2) the value of developing nursing theory, (3) what constitutes nursing research, and (4) the role of advanced practice nurses. Mary Huch's chapter, "Nursing and the Next Millennium," provides a transcript of the theorists'—Imogene King, Madeleine Leininger, Rosemarie Parse, Hildegard Peplau, and Martha Rogers—responses to these relevant issues in nursing. The divergent viewpoints on nursing by these renowned theorists may challenge and stimulate one's own perspective about the future of advanced practice nursing.

20

A Dialectical Examination of Nursing Art

JOY L. JOHNSON, RN, PhD

Literature relevant to the art of nursing is immensely diverse and fragmented. This state is problematic in that progress in understanding nursing art cannot be made until the subject of nursing art is clearly delineated. In light of the need for conceptual clarity regarding nursing art, a dialectical study was undertaken to identify the distinct conceptions of nursing art that are represented in the nursing literature. The examined discourse was that contained in the works of 41 nursing scholars published between 1860 and 1992. The analysis revealed five distinct conceptualizations that can be identified as the art of (1) grasping meaning in patient encounters, (2) establishing a meaningful connection with the patient, (3) skillfully performing nursing activities, (4) rationally determining an appropriate course of nursing action, and (5) morally conducting one's nursing practice.

It is often said that nursing is an art and a science. Unfortunately, what is meant by the term *nursing art* is not well delineated or understood. In examining the theoretical issues nurses have concerned themselves with, it is clear that the majority of time and effort has been spent considering the nature of nursing science. Although numerous descriptions and definitions of nursing art have been suggested, little effort has been expended to analyze those definitions or to enter into a dialogue regarding the nature of nursing art.

Science alone will not solve all of the problems of nursing. Nursing is, after all, a practice discipline. Guidance regarding the use or application of scientific findings does not emanate from nursing science itself. As Ellis indicated, nursing is much more than the application of scientific findings. The practitioner cannot just "select from a rack of ready-to-wear theories."[1(p1434)] It is therefore essential that the manner in which knowledge, judgment, and skill are used in the clinical setting be carefully considered. These phenomena fall generally under the rubric of the art of nursing. Ultimately, an understanding of nursing art will further an understanding of how excellence can best be pursued and achieved in nursing practice.

The characterization of nursing as an art is not a recent development, and the literature relevant to the art of nursing is immensely diverse. It includes works such as Nightingale's[2] *Notes on Nursing* and Benner's[3] *From Novice to Expert*. Despite the abundance of writings on the topic of the art of nursing,

Source: Johnson, J. L. (1994). A dialectical examination of nursing art, *ANS, 17* (1): 1-14. Reprinted with permission from and copyright © 1994 Aspen Publishers, Inc.

there have been few instances in which nursing scholars have addressed one another's positions. This failure is due in part to the fact that nursing scholars have tended to pursue their conceptions of nursing art in isolation and have not considered other conceptions. Nursing scholars have not confronted one another in light of their differences, resulting in the current situation in which a plethora of diverse views concerning the art of nursing are relatively unquestioned and unexplored.

Schlotfeldt[4] pointed out that the future of the nursing profession depends on the ability of its members to identify and resolve issues. Yet nurses will be unable to resolve issues related to the art of nursing unless the subject at issue is clearly set forth. Walker identified the need for such an analysis when she argued that the controversy regarding the art of nursing "has been difficult to resolve for the point of contention has not been clearly set forth."[5(p118)] The tremendous diversity of ideas regarding the art of nursing expressed in the nursing literature will remain a source of confusion unless the diversities are put in order and rendered intelligible. When differences of opinion remain implicit, or even concealed, as in the nursing discourse relevant to the art of nursing, they cannot serve as the basis for the collective effort required to further thought.

In light of the state of fragmentation that characterizes the nursing literature relevant to the subject of nursing art, a philosophic study was undertaken to discover the common ground that underlies the differences of opinion regarding the art of nursing and to transmute the current diversity into rational and intelligible controversy. This study sought to render the existing diversity more intelligible so that a rational debate of fundamental issues can proceed and a better understanding of nursing art can be attained.

METHOD

The approach that was taken for this study was a critical examination and systematic analysis of the nursing discourse concerning the art of nursing. The method is one developed by Adler[6] and his colleagues at the Institute for Philosophical Research in Chicago to examine the controversies that surround such philosophic ideas as freedom, love, and equality. The aim of this method, which Adler[6] referred to as a *dialectical approach*, is to outline and clarify the structure of a controversy, and it involves a process of constructive interpretation. The goal of this philosophic method is to explicitly formulate patterns of agreement and disagreement. The challenge of the dialectical method is to achieve a nonpartisan treatment of positions or views. The dialectical task, therefore, involves rendering an objective, impartial, and neutral report of a many-sided discussion. Using this approach, the dialectician examines and clarifies what is implicit in the discourse. By way of constructive interpretation, the researcher attempts to find similarities and dissimilarities among the various conceptions.

Although the works examined in this study are historical in the sense that they date to a specific time and place, the intent of this study was to examine the ideas contained in them apart from their historical context. The study was in no way historical in its aim or its method. Therefore, for the purpose of this study, it was assumed that the authors concerned with the art of nursing are engaged in a continuing dialogue, even though they belong to different historical periods.

The point of departure for this study was the manifold and often confusing diversity that exists on the subject of nursing art. The general subject of nursing art includes a broad field of discourse and covers a variety of themes. Rather than seeking to include the work of every nursing author who has written on the subject of nursing art, a sample of works was required that was representative of the existing diversity of views regarding the art of nursing. Literature that was broadly related to the topic of nursing art was included in the study. In total the works of 41 authors composed the examined discourse. The findings reported here are part of a larger study[7] that examined the issues and controversies that exist regarding nursing art.

DISTINCT CONCEPTUALIZATIONS OF NURSING ART

Based on an examination of the nursing literature related to the art of nursing, it was concluded that there are diverse answers to the question, What is the art of nursing? The use of the term *art of nursing* in no way ensures that those involved in the discourse refer to the same subject. Part of the dialectical task involved determining whether there are distinct conceptions of the subject within the examined discourse. The questions that guided this determination included, Is *art* being used in the same sense? and, Does the discussion involve one subject or several distinct subjects? To identify the distinct conceptualizations of nursing art, each work was carefully read, and relevant passages believed to be germane to the topic were noted. Ties of relevance that connected the various authors were sought, and points of agreement were established. These points of agreement served to delineate each distinct conceptualization.

In examining the discourse, it was found that there were five separate senses of "nursing art." They can be described as

1. The nurse's ability to grasp meaning in patient encounters,
2. The nurse's ability to establish a meaningful connection with the patient,
3. The nurse's ability to skillfully perform nursing activities,
4. The nurse's ability to rationally determine an appropriate course of nursing action, and
5. The nurse's ability to morally conduct his or her nursing practice.

It should be pointed out that although the authors who have written about nursing art provide evidence for the construction of these conceptions, the identification of these conceptions is not theirs per se. It should also be noted that although these subjects are mutually exclusive, most authors have conceptualized nursing art as consisting of more than one ability; therefore, these authors are viewed as addressing more than one conception of nursing art. Finally, it cannot be concluded that an author's apparent silence on a particular conceptualization of nursing art indicates a denial of that conceptualization. The descriptions that follow focus primarily on the similarities of thought regarding each conception, rather than the issues, or points of disagreement, that exist regarding these conceptions.

Ability to Grasp Meaning in Patient Encounters

The situations that confront nurses are often characterized by uncertainty, ambiguity, and indeterminacy.[8] This is due in part to the fact that nursing practice situations are complex. The complexity of a patient's situation can be further compounded when patients are unable to articulate their needs, either because they are unaware of the needs or because they are incapacitated.[9] Consequently, the nurse must grasp the meaning of each particular patient situation and determine what in the situation is relevant. For select authors,[3,8-33] nursing art involves the ability to grasp meaning in patient encounters. According to these authors, the artful nurse, as compared to the nurse who lacks art, can grasp what is significant in a particular patient situation. The term *grasping meaning* is used here to describe the process of attaching significance to those things that can be felt, observed, heard, touched, tasted, smelled, or imagined, including emotions, objects, gestures, and sounds.

Although marked variation can be found among the descriptions of the authors who have been construed to conceptualize nursing art as the grasping of meaning, several points of agreement can be found. First, nursing art is seen as based in an immediate perceptual capacity and is not affected by the intellect. This capacity to grasp meaning is often referred to as intuition. Rather than being based in reflection, or reasoning, the art of nursing according to this view is based in an immediate perceptual capacity that is more integrated than simple sensation and more concrete than intellection; it is based in a capacity that involves the external senses as well as the imagination.

Using this capacity, the artful nurse attributes meaning to things that are felt, observed, or imagined. It is the artful nurse who can *sense* the meaning or significance of a situation, such as when a patient is distraught; *perceive* patterns, such as the set of signs and symptoms that indicate when a patient is going into cardiogenic shock; have a *feel* for what he or she is doing; or *sense* what should be done, such as *knowing* when to use humor to help relieve the tension of a situation. Thus, Chinn and Kramer stated, "Esthetic knowing is what makes possible knowing what to do with the moment, instantly, without conscious deliberation."[14(p10)] Nursing art is thought to involve the direct apprehension of what is to be done, or what is the case, and is unmediated by concepts. The immediacy of the art of grasping meaning was emphasized by Benner and Wrubel, who argued that "the person does not assign meanings to the situation once it is apprehended because the very act of apprehension is based on taken-for-

granted meanings embedded in skills, practices, and language."[9(p42)]

A second point of agreement is that the art of grasping meaning results in a form of understanding that defies accurate or complete description. The insights gained by this perceptual ability are thought to be tacit, non-propositional, personal, and as such incommunicable. Carper, for example, argued that esthetic knowing is gained by "subjective acquaintance, the direct feeling of an experience"[13(p149)] and that this knowing defies discursive formulation. The meanings that the artful nurse grasps are concrete and individual, pertaining to a particular patient situation (e.g., this particular patient that I am nursing and can observe in front of me who happens to have had an appendectomy), rather than abstract, pertaining to patients in general (eg, appendectomy patients). Orlando emphasized this distinction when she stated that the nurse must distinguish between general principles and "the meanings which she must discover in the immediate nursing situation in order to help the patient."[25(p1)]

A third point of agreement to be found is that the art of grasping meaning is a perceptual ability that can be honed and developed over time. Rew,[31] for example, argued that the nurse can learn to become sensitive to the signals and feelings that he or she experiences and, over time, can learn to understand their significance. Similarly, Newman[21] argued that nurses can learn to attend to and trust their inner experiences. Benner[3] contended that perceptual abilities are formed by previous experiences and by immersion in the present perceptual environment. Consequently, the information taken in by the senses is endowed with meaning. According to Benner,[3] it is through experience that the nurse learns to immediately focus on what is relevant in a patient situation and to grasp its meaning. Using past experiences, or foreknowledge, the artful nurse has the ability to recognize patterns and can therefore make sense of ambiguous, unstructured situations. According to Benner, "Past concrete experience . . . guides the expert's perceptions and actions and allows for a rapid perceptual grasp of the situation."[3(pp8-9)]

Finally, according to those who affirm this first conception of nursing art, the art of nursing is a holistic capacity. The nurse's perceptual ability allows him or her to immediately grasp the meaning of a situation, instead of piecing together an understanding of what is happening. In contrast, the nurse who is not artful must assess every minute detail, breaking down a situation into its component parts to discover what is of significance. Benner and Wrubel described the artful capacity as " a perceptual awareness that singles out relevant information from irrelevant, grasps a situation as a whole rather than as a series of tasks, and accomplishes this rapidly and without incremental deliberative analysis of isolated facts or bits of information."[10(p13)]

Ability to Establish a Meaningful Connection with the Patient

The connection between the nurse and the patient is considered by many authors* to be of particular importance, particularly in the current era of increasing technology. Many emphasize that it is the artful nurse's interactions that can bridge the gap introduced by technology and that such interactions can promote "wholeness and integrity in the personal encounter, the achievement of engagement rather than detachment, and . . . [denial of] the manipulative impersonal orientation."[13(156)] *Connection*, as it is used here, refers to an attachment, or union, that occurs between patients and their nurses. The term *connection* is used because, unlike the term *relationship*, it

encompasses short-term or fleeting encounters as well as long-term associations. According to these authors, a meaningful connection between the nurse and the patient is central to the provision of nursing care, since it is through this connection that services such as physical and emotional support are offered and accepted. Kim,[39] for example, pointed out that the core of nursing resides in human-to-human actions. Similarly, Gadow suggested that the central question in nursing is not, How can we help them [patients] to recover? but, instead, How can we recover them [and] overcome the distance between us?[16(p12)]

The second conception of nursing art is distinguished by four major points. First, it is contended that nursing art is nondiscursive; that is, it is expressed in the nurse's actions or behaviors. According to those who hold this second conception of nursing art, the art of nursing is "unmediated by conceptual categories."[13(p154)] It cannot be expressed through words; instead, it is expressed in the concrete actions and gestures of the artful nurse in response to a particular patient. Paterson and Zderad argued that "nursing is an experience lived between human beings"[28(p3)] and that nursing art is evident in the synchronicity between the nurse and the patient.

Second, it is contended that its expressive nature constitutes an essential characteristic of nursing art. Chinn and Kramer maintained that this expression takes the form of "human actions—words, behaviors, and other symbols—that give communicable form to what we know."[14(p6)] Although it is agreed that nursing art is expressive, there is little agreement regarding what exactly is expressed in nursing art. For some authors, emotions play an important role in the origin of art. For example, Watson[41] argued that through their art, nurses express emotions or feelings. The work of Peplau[29] suggested that the expression of nursing art is appropriately limited to the expression of sentiments such as concern, compassion, and

---

caring. Paterson and Zderad,[28] on the other hand, suggested that nursing art involves the expression of the nurse's state of being.

Third, it is argued that the art of nursing occurs in relation to another human being. The ideas of philosopher Martin Buber[44] are echoed frequently in the works of authors who have conceptualized nursing art as the ability to establish a meaningful connection. Buber[44] posited that relationships are of two kinds. The first is a subject-to-subject, or "I-Thou," relationship, which is a relationship of connectedness and affirmation of another person's being. The second type of relationship is subject to object, or "I-It," which arises out of a stance of separation and detachment, in which the individual is differentiated over and against a world of objects. Authors who hold that nursing art is establishing a meaningful connection with the patient contend that nursing art can only occur when the nurse stands in a subject-to-subject relationship with the patient. For example, Paterson and Zderad stated, "If she enters into genuine relation with the patient (I-Thou) her effective power (caring, nursing skills, hope) brings forth form (well-being, more-being, comfort, growth)."[28(p92)]

Finally, the authors who support the view that nursing art is the ability to establish a meaningful connection are in agreement regarding the necessity of authenticity on the part of the nurse. Bishop and Scudder argued that "the inauthentic nurse merely plays the role of nurse rather than really *being* a nurse."[34(p102)] It is held that the artful nurse must be genuine; any attempt to mask or hide feelings will serve only to distance the nurse from the patient, thereby threatening the relationship between the nurse and the patient. Parse[26] referred to this authenticity as genuine or true presence. Similarly, Watson asserted that "the degree of transpersonal caring (in this sense of unity of feeling) is increased by the degree of genuineness and sincerity of the nurse."[41(p69)]

Ability to Skillfully Perform Nursing Activities

The conceptualization of nursing art as the skillful performance of nursing activities is one of the earliest conceptions of nursing art found in the nursing discourse.[2,3,5,9-12,45-59] It is from this view that we see in early nursing curricula the attainment of nursing skills being referred to generally as the "nursing arts." Price contended that nursing art involves the ability to "recognize the nursing needs of the patient and to develop skill, through practice, in various procedures designed to answer those needs."[54(p19)] According to the authors who hold the view that nursing art is the ability to skillfully perform nursing activities, the artful nurse is one who has a demonstrable capacity to effectively carry out nursing procedures and techniques. *Skill*, as it is used here, refers to a developed proficiency or dexterity. *Nursing activities* are all those tasks, procedures, and techniques that a nurse carries out in his or her practice.

The focus of these authors' conceptualizations of nursing art is an array of activities both manual and verbal in nature. For example, we see in the work of Nightingale[50] a list of behaviors that the good nurse must demonstrate. These behaviors include such things as moving silently through the sickroom, keeping constant watch over the sick, and airing out the sickroom on a regular basis. Nightingale[50] expected the artful nurse to do more than understand these edicts. She expected these behaviors to be instantiated in the nurse's practice; the artful nurse knows more than what is to be done, she knows "how to do it."[50(p1)] Wiedenbach[58] numbered among the skills the nurse must possess the ability to perform back rubs, to take a pulse, and to help a patient walk as well as the ability to handle necessary equipment, such as a cardiac pacemaker and the circular-electric bed: "These skills involve manipulations and techniques—

executed with finesse to achieve desired results."[58(p28)]

Those who hold this third conception of nursing art were found to be in agreement regarding three central points. First, according to the authors, the art of nursing is primarily a behavioral ability; that is, it involves observable actions and focuses on the process of doing, rather than the process of knowing. As such, it is concerned with the nurse's demonstrable ability, not his or her knowledge per se. Heidgerken made this distinction clear when she stated, "The principles, procedures, and technics, or science, of nursing are learned in the classroom. The art, or skill, of nursing is learned on the ward."[48(p9)] Although there is agreement among the authors who hold this third conception that nursing art is ultimately a behavioral ability, there is no consensus regarding the role that one's intellectual capacity plays in the art of nursing. Some theorists argue that the activities must be intelligently performed. Montag,[49] for example, contended that skill without understanding is mere imitation. Similarly, Heidgerken[48] contended that the memorization and demonstration of step-by-step procedures will not produce an artful nurse. Tracy, on the other hand, contended that "the nurse should have so mastered her procedures that the minimum of thought is needed for their use."[57(p29)] Similarly, Benner and Wrubel[9] argued that nurse's everyday actions are effective not because they think about them, or base them on theory, but because they have a sophisticated repertoire of reactions.

Second, those who conceptualize nursing art as skillful performance of nursing activities are in agreement about the claim that nursing art can be learned. Key to learning the art of nursing are persistent practice and repetition. Goodrich maintained that practical experience for student nurses should be "sufficiently long to allow of a constant repetition of procedures."[47(p42)] Heidgerken, however, warned that practice alone is not enough and that "the atti-

tude of the learner, the will to improve, and eradication of mistakes are all equally as important as practice."[48(p54)]

Finally, there is also evidence of agreement regarding the fact that certain criteria can be used to judge the art of nursing. When discussing the art of nursing, these theorists inevitably use descriptors such as fluidity of movement, adroitness, coordination, and efficiency. Stewart indicated that nursing art involves "manual dexterity, lightness, steadiness, quickness of movement, strength, endurance, and that complete coordination of head and muscle which cannot be acquired except by long, directed training."[55(pp324-325)] Similarly, Heidgerken[48] argued that the artful nurse's activities must have the appropriate form; elimination of excess movements, appropriate timing, force, and coordination are among the qualities that characterize the activities of the artful nurse.

Ability to Rationally Determine an Appropriate Course of Nursing Action

For those* who support the fourth conception of nursing art, intellectual activity is essential to the performance of nursing care. According to this fourth conception, nursing art refers to the nurse's ability to rationally determine an appropriate course of nursing action. The term *rational ability*, as it is used here, refers to the intellectual ability to effectively draw valid conclusions from existing knowledge.

This fourth conception of nursing art is characterized by five points of agreement. First, it is argued that nursing art is practical in nature. According to these authors, the aim of this ability is the determination of an appropriate course of action. Nursing art, it is argued, is action oriented and not simply aimed at understanding. Beckstrand,[60] for example, contended

---

*References 2, 4, 5, 25, 39, 40, 45, 46, 48-53, 55, 56, 58-78.

that the aim of nursing art is the control of practice. Dickoff and James[62] concluded that nursing art is concerned ultimately with producing nursing situations. Similarly, Orlando contended that nursing art is a rational capacity that is aimed at "helping the patient."[25(p70)]

Second, it is contended that there is an underlying discipline on which nursing art rests. All of the authors who contend that nursing art is a rational ability emphasize the importance of knowledge, specifically scientific knowledge, to nursing art. Orem stated, "The art of nursing is the nurse's quality or habit of reasoning and judging correctly about the design and production of the kind and amount of nursing needed according to the principles or laws of nursing itself. Science and technique are 'the first necessary conditions for honest art.' The point of view of nursing as art therefore encompasses the point of view of *nursing as knowledge*."[52(p24)]

Arguments about the importance of knowledge for nursing art are often tied to the claim that nursing is a profession. Abdellah and her colleagues, for example, argued, "Professionalization of nursing requires that nurses identify those nursing problems that depend for their solution upon the nurse's use of her capacities to conceptualize events and make judgments about them. Nurses need to become skilled in recognizing both overt and covert nursing problems, in analyzing them in terms of relevant principles and in working out courses of action by applying nursing principles."[45(p11)] It was assumed by Abdellah et al.,[45] as it was by all of the authors who support this fourth conceptualization of nursing art, that the nursing profession possesses a distinct body of knowledge and that this body of knowledge provides the foundation for nursing practice.

Leininger[73] also contended that nursing art is based on scientific knowledge. She believed that nurses must, if they are to be effective, "scientifically care" for their patients. *Scientific caring*, according to Leininger, "refers to those judgments and acts of helping others based upon tested or verified knowledge."[73(p46)] The importance of knowledge to artful practice is echoed by all of the authors. Kim stated, "Knowledge is antecedent to action."[39(p146)] And Diers contended that "nursing practice is done consciously, if not always with a formal plan, that it is not done mindlessly."[65(p31)] Finally, Rogers claimed that "the art of nursing develops only as it incorporates more and more of science unto itself. The nature of its art lies in the core of scientific knowledge it embodies."[75(p32)]

The third point of agreement regarding the art of rationally determining an appropriate course of nursing action is that it presupposes that nurses possess a thorough understanding of what is before them and the actions they should take. According to this perspective, the artful nurse solves problems by selecting the intervention that is best suited to the intended end. This process of instrumental problem solving involves a thorough consideration of the facts of a situation and is made rigorous by the application of scientific theory. For example, Johnson[70] argued that an artful nurse thinks "logically, soundly, and searchingly" about the causes and effects in a given nursing situation. The key point is that the artful nurse's actions are not "automatic" or "blind" but instead are grounded in an intellectual activity, in which knowledge or information of certain kinds is considered to determine which actions will result in the best possible patient outcome.

Fourth, it is contended that the art of rationally determining an appropriate course of nursing action involves a process of logical reasoning in which scientific principles and theories are applied to problems identified in practice. According to this view, the artful nurse uses evidence to reason through the best course of action to be followed. Beckstrand described this process in the following manner:

Once the conditions requiring changes in the client's situation are determined, a practitioner examines the situation to identify the possibility of making the changes desired. First, a practitioner uses scientific knowledge of necessary and sufficient conditions to determine if desired changes are realizable. Next, a practitioner examines the situation to determine whether conditions for achieving the desired changes exist. . . . As a result, the set of realizable outcomes in practice is determined by what is scientifically possible within the exigencies of the practice situation.[61(p177)]

The steps of the nursing process (assessment, planning, implementation, and evaluation) are seen as the steps that an artful nurse takes to ensure quality patient care. The emphasis of this approach is on deliberate, systematic, and scientifically based care.

Finally, it is contended by those who hold the fourth conception of nursing art that the art of nursing can be judged according to certain standards. They agree that the appropriateness of a nursing action can be judged on the basis of whether the identified course of action enabled the practitioner to attain his or her identified goals or standards. For example, Henderson[37] contended that a nurse's art can be evaluated according to the degree to which the patient has reestablished independence. Some authors have suggested additional criteria for evaluation. Dickoff, James, and Wiedenbach,[63] for example, suggested that nursing art can be evaluated using the criteria of coherency, palatability, and feasibility.

Ability to Morally Conduct One's Nursing Practice

For a final group of authors,* nursing art involves the ability of the nurse to practice

morally: The nurse is obligated to practice in such a way that seeks to avoid harm and to benefit the patient. The term *moral*, as it is used here, refers to that which is good, or desirable, for human beings. These authors are in agreement regarding four central points. First, it is held that good or excellent nursing practice is, by necessity, moral in that it is directed toward the good of the patient. As Goodrich stated, "So much is nursing of the essence of ethics that it is consistent to assert that the terms good and ethical as applied to nursing practice are synonymous."[47(p5)] Conversely, the view that nursing art can under any circumstances be amoral or immoral is antithetical to this position. Indeed, for these authors, the moral aspect of nursing cannot be separated from the notion of excellence in nursing, either existentially or analytically. This is the case, it is argued, because unlike the fine arts, nursing is an art that deals directly with human beings. Artful nursing, Curtin[79] asserted, is inextricably entwined with human life and the achievement of particular human ends.

According to those who hold that nursing is a moral art, a nurse may be technically competent and knowledgeable, yet if he or she does not make moral choices in the performance of patient care, he or she is not artful. Lanara[81] argued that values and ideals must guide the nurse's care. In a similar fashion, Gadow[17] posited that good nursing is more than a cluster of techniques in that it involves a commitment to a moral end and is directed and judged by that end. This position is also supported by Bishop and Scudder, who argued that the artful nurse's ability consists in more than the ability to efficiently complete tasks: "[The] technician uses techniques which are evaluated by efficiency; whereas, the professional makes decisions which are evaluated by the good."[34(p69)]

Second, it is held that the possession of skill and knowledge are necessary, but not sufficient, conditions for the moral conduct of nursing practice. Indeed, it is presupposed by

---

*References 2, 3, 9, 11, 15-18, 34-38, 47, 48, 50-53, 60, 61, 67, 68, 79-81.

many of these authors that the artful nurse must be competent in his or her practice. As Curtin[80] pointed out, the license to practice nursing does not include permission to practice poorly. In stating that one is a professional, one is claiming a certain level of competence.

Third, it is argued by those who hold that nursing art is the ability to morally conduct one's practice that nursing art involves a commitment to care competently for patients. Curtin stated that "although knowledge and skill are integral to the practice of a profession, the foundation consists of the performative declarations professed by its practitioners and the fidelity of the practitioner to these promises."[80(pp101-102)] The moral responsibility to nurse well involves a commitment not only to nurse a patient competently, but to "sustain excellent practice in the face of unreasonable demands and lack of appreciation on the part of patients."[35(p37)] The artful nurse not only must be competent, but must also consistently demonstrate competence in his or her practice, no matter how arduous the circumstances.

Finally, the notion that the artful nurse must possess moral virtues is reiterated in various forms by all of the authors who ascribe to the notion that the art of nursing is of a moral nature. Expressed in all of their works is the belief that the artful nurse must be properly motivated in his or her action. Rather than being motivated by self-aggrandizement or expediency, the artful nurse is motivated by care and concern for others. Benner and Wrubel suggested that the same act done in a caring and uncaring way may have different effects and that only a nurse who cares about his or her patients will notice small differences in their behaviors and create unique solutions to patient problems: "Caring makes the nurse notice which interventions help, and this concern guides subsequent caregiving. Caring causes the nurse to notice subtle signs of improvement or deterioration in the patient. In fact, caring . . . is required for expert human practice."[9(p4)]

Accordingly, the nurse who does not care about his or her patient cannot nurse well. Lanara[81] argued that the ability to care about patients rests on the nurse's capacity to love others and that nurses, inspired by the ideal of love, will care not only for, but about, their patients. It is love, according to Lanara,[81] that allows the nurse to transcend obstacles and become heroic in his or her nursing practice.

CONCLUSION

Through the identification of these five conceptions of nursing art, nurses can begin to understand the structure of the discourse regarding nursing art. Once one goes beyond the description of the five conceptions identified, differences of opinion can be found among the authors who affirm a particular conception of nursing art. Indeed, each of the five conceptions is a subject of controversy in that each comprises numerous conceptual, existential, and normative issues.

It is evident that although nursing scholars have written about the subject of nursing art, few have acknowledged one another's conceptions. Indeed, to date there has been little recognition that different conceptions of nursing art exist. When one examines the discourse regarding the art of nursing, it is clear that not all of the authors agree about the nature of nursing art. This state of affairs is consistent with the state of the nursing discourse in general. Kikuchi and Simmons accurately characterized this state of affairs when they stated,

Although nursing scholars are prone to speak or write on the same topic, use the same words, or express a common interest in knowledge development, there is very little in their productions to indicate that they share to any great degree a common understanding, a coming-to-terms, that would allow for the minimal topical agreement required before questions can be commonly interpreted, controversies identified, issues debated, and answers commonly agreed upon.[82(p3)]

It is hoped that the identification of distinct conceptions of nursing art will facilitate productive debate and analysis among nursing's scholars.

The method employed in this research is limited in that it does not answer the question, What is nursing art? The next step must be taken: to examine each of these conceptualizations in detail to determine which conceptualization or group of conceptualizations is sound. The findings of this study provide the groundwork for future philosophic analyses, thereby bringing nursing one step closer toward a sound conception of nursing art. It is only when a sound conception of nursing art is developed that nursing will be able to answer questions regarding how nursing art should be pursued and developed. It is hoped that nursing scholars in the future will dispute the nature of nursing art more explicitly and extensively.

REFERENCES

1. Ellis R. The practitioner as theorist. *Am J Nurs.* 1969;69:1434-1438.
2. Nightingale F. *Notes on Nursing: What It Is, and What It Is Not.* New York, NY: Dover; 1969.
3. Benner P. *From Novice to Expert: Excellence and Power in Clinical Nursing Practice.* Menlo Park, Calif: Addison-Wesley; 1984.
4. Schlotfeldt RM. Resolution of issues: An imperative for creating nursing's future. *J Prof Nurs.* 1987;3:136-142.
5. Walker LO. *Nursing as a Discipline.* Bloomington, Ind: Indiana University; 1971. Dissertation.
6. Adler MJ. *The Idea of Freedom, I: A Dialectical Examination of the Conceptions of Freedom.* Garden City, NY: Doubleday; 1958.
7. Johnson JL. *Toward a Clearer Understanding of the Art of Nursing.* Edmonton, Alberta, Canada: University of Alberta; 1993. Dissertation.
8. Tanner C. Curriculum revolution: the practice mandate. In: *Curriculum Revolution: Mandate for Change.* New York, NY: National League for Nursing; 1988:201-216.
9. Benner P, Wrubel J. *The Primacy of Caring: Stress and Coping in Health and Illness.* Menlo Park, Calif: Addison-Wesley; 1989.
10. ———. Skilled clinical knowledge: The value of perceptual awareness. *Nurs Educ.* 1982; 7(3):11-17.
11. Benner P. The role of experience, narrative, and community in skilled ethical comportment. *ANS.* 1991;14(2):1-21.
12. Benner P, Tanner C, Chesla C. From beginner to expert: Gaining a differentiated clinical world in critical care nursing. *ANS.* 1992;14(3):13-28.
13. Carper BA. *Fundamental Patterns of Knowing in Nursing.* New York, NY: Teachers College, Columbia University; 1975.
14. Chinn PL, Kramer MK. *Theory and Nursing: A Systematic Approach.* 3rd ed. St. Louis, Mo: Mosby–Yearbook; 1991.
15. Gadow S. Clinical subjectivity: Advocacy with silent patients. *Nurs Clin North Am.* 1989; 24:535-541.
16. ———. Beyond dualism: The dialectic of caring and knowing. Presented at the conference "The Care-Justice Puzzle: Education for Ethical Nursing Practice" at the University of Minnesota; October 13, 1990; Minneapolis, Minn.
17. ———. Nurse and patient: The caring relationship. In: Bishop AH, Scudder JR, eds. *Caring, Curing, Coping: Nurse, Physician, Patient Relationships.* Tuscaloosa, Ala: University of Alabama Press; 1985:31-43.
18. ———. Body and self: A dialectic. *J Med Philos.* 1980;5:172-185.
19. Moccia PA. A critique of compromise: Beyond the methods debate. *ANS.* 1988;10(4):1-9.
20. ———. *A Study of the Theory-Practice Dialectic: Towards a Critique of the Science of Man.* New York, NY: New York University; 1980. Dissertation.
21. Newman MA. The spirit of nursing. *Holistic Nurs Pract.* 1989;3(3):1-6.
22. ———. *Health as Expanding Consciousness.* St. Louis, Mo: Mosby; 1986.
23. ———. Newman's theory of health as praxis. *Nurs Sci Q.* 1990;3:37-41.
24. ———. Sime AM, Corcoran-Perry SA. The focus of the discipline of nursing. *ANS.* 1991; 14(1):1-6.
25. Orlando IJ. *The Dynamic Nurse-Patient Relationship: Function, Process and Principles.* New York: G.P. Putnam's Sons; 1961.

26. Parse RR. Human becoming: Parse's theory of nursing. *Nurs Sci Q.* 1992;5:35-42.

27. ———. *Man-Living-Health: A Theory of Nursing.* New York, NY: Wiley; 1981.

28. Paterson JG, Zderad LT. *Humanistic Nursing.* New York, NY: National League for Nursing; 1988.

29. Peplau HE. The art and science of nursing: Similarities, differences, and relations. *Nurs Sci Q.* 1988;1:8-15.

30. ———. *Interpersonal Relations in Nursing: A Conceptual Frame of Reference for Psychodynamic Nursing.* New York, NY: G.P. Putnam's Sons; 1952.

31. Rew L. Nurses' intuition. *Appl Nurs Res.* 1988;1:27-31.

32. ———. Intuition in decision-making. *Image J Nurs Schol.* 1988;20:150-153.

33. Tanner CA. The nursing care plan as an instructional method: Ritual or reason? *Nurs Educ.* 1968;11(4):8-10.

34. Bishop AH, Scudder JR. *The Practical, Moral, and Personal Sense of Nursing: A Phenomenological Philosophy of Practice.* Albany, NY: State University of New York Press; 1990.

35. ———. Nursing ethics in an age of controversy. *ANS.* 1987;9(3):34-43.

36. ———. *Nursing: The Practice of Caring.* New York, NY: National League for Nursing Press; 1991.

37. Henderson V. The nature of nursing. *Am J Nurs.* 1964;64(8):62-28.

38. ———. Excellence in nursing. *Am J Nurs.* 1969;69:2133-2137.

39. Kim HS. *The Nature of Theoretical Thinking in Nursing.* Norwalk, Conn: Appleton-Century-Crofts; 1983.

40. ———. Structuring the nursing knowledge system: A typology of four domains. *Schol Inq Nurs Pract.* 1987;1:99-114.

41. Watson J. *Nursing: Human Science and Human Care: A Theory of Nursing.* New York, NY: National League for Nursing; 1988.

42. ———. The lost art of nursing. *Nurs Forum.* 1981;20:244-249.

43. ———. Caring knowledge and informed moral passion. *ANS.* 1990;13(1):15-24.

44. Buber M; Smith RG, trans. *I and Thou.* 2nd ed. New York, NY: Charles Scribner's Sons; 1958.

45. Abdellah FG, Martin A, Beland IL, Matheney RV. *Patient-Centered Approaches to Nursing.* New York, NY: Macmillan, 1960.

46. Abdellah FG, Levine E. *Better Patient Care Through Nursing Research.* New York, NY: Macmillan; 1965.

47. Goodrich AW. *The Social and Ethical Significance of Nursing: A Series of Addresses.* New York, NY: Macmillan; 1932.

48. Heidgerken LE. *Teaching in Schools of Nursing: Principles and Methods.* Philadelphia: Pa: Lippincott; 1946.

49. Montag MI. *The Education of Nursing Technicians.* New York, NY: G.P. Putnam's Sons; 1951.

50. Nightingale F. *Training of Nurses and Nursing the Sick* [Microfiche, Adelaide Nutting Historical Nursing Collection]. London, England: Spottiswoode; 1899.

51. ———. *Suggestions for Thought to the Searchers After Truth Among the Artizans of England* [Microfiche, Adelaide Nutting Historical Nursing Collection]. London, England: George E. Eyre & William Spottiswoode; 1860.

52. Orem DE. *Nursing: Concepts of Practice.* 4th ed. St. Louis, Mo: Mosby-Yearbook; 1991.

53. ———. The form of nursing science. *Nurs Sci Q.* 1988;1:75-79.

54. Price AL. *The Art, Science and Spirit of Nursing.* 2nd ed. Philadelphia, Pa: W.B. Saunders; 1960.

55. Stewart IM. The aims of the training school for nurses. *Am J Nurs.* 1916;16:319-327.

56. ———. Practical objectives in nursing education. *Am J Nurs.* 1924;24:557-564.

57. Tracy MA. *Nursing: An Art and a Science.* St. Louis, Mo: Mosby; 1938.

58. Wiedenbach E. *Clinical Nursing: A Helping Art.* New York, NY: Springer; 1964.

59. ———. The helping art of nursing. *Am J Nurs.* 1963;63:54-57.

60. Beckstrand J. The notion of a practice theory and the relationship of scientific and ethical knowledge to practice. *Res Nurs Health.* 1978;1:131-136.

61. ———. The need for a practice theory as indicated by the knowledge used in the conduct of practice. *Res Nurs Health.* 1978;1:175-179.

62. Dickoff J, James P. A theory of theories: A position paper. *Nurs Res.* 1968;17:197-203.

63. Dickoff J, James P, Wiedenbach E. Theory in a practice discipline: Part II. Practice oriented research. *Nurs Res.* 1968;17:545-554.

64. Dickoff J, James P. Taking concepts as guides to action: Exploring kinds of know-how. In: Nicoll LH, ed. *Perspectives on Nursing Theory.* 2nd ed. Philadelphia, Pa: Lippincott; 1992:576-580.

65. Diers D. *Research in Nursing Practice.* Philadelphia, Pa: Lippincott; 1979.

66. ———. Learning the art and craft of nursing. *Am J Nurs.* 1990;90:65-66.

67. Dock LL. *Short Papers on Nursing Subjects*. New York, NY: M. Louise Longeway; 1900.

68. Dock LL, Steward IM. *A Short History of Nursing: From the Earliest Times to the Present Day*. 3rd ed., rev. New York, NY: G.P. Putnam's Sons; 1937.

69. Donaldson SK, Crowley DM. The discipline of nursing. *Nurs Outlook*. 1978;26:113-120.

70. Johnson DE. A philosophy of nursing. *Nurs Outlook*. 1959;7:198-200.

71. ———. The nature of a science of nursing. *Nurs Outlook*. 1959;7:291-294.

72. ———. Theory in nursing: Borrowed and unique. *Nurs Res*. 1968;17:206-209.

73. Leininger M. Caring: A central focus of nursing and health care services. In: Leininger MM, ed. *Care: The Essence of Nursing and Health*. Thorofare, NJ: Slack; 1984:45-59.

74. ———. *Care, Discovery and Uses in Clinical and Community Nursing*. Detroit, Mich: Wayne State University Press; 1988.

75. Rogers ME. *Reveille in Nursing*. Philadelphia, Pa: F.A. Davis; 1964.

76. ———. *An Introduction to the Theoretical Basis of Nursing*. Philadelphia, Pa: F.A. Davis; 1970.

77. ———. Nursing science and art: A prospective. *Nurs Sci Q*. 1988;1:99-102.

78. Schlotfeldt RM. Structuring nursing knowledge: A priority for creating nursing's future. *Nurs Sci Q*. 1988;1:35-38.

79. Curtin LL. The nurse as advocate: A philosophical foundation for nursing. *ANS*. 1979;1(3):1-10.

80. Curtin L. The commitment of nursing. In: Curtin LL, Flaherty MJ, eds. *Nursing Ethics: Theories and Pragmatics*. Bowie, Md: Robert J. Brady; 1982:97-102.

81. Lanara, VA. *Heroism as a Nursing Value: A Philosophical Perspective*. Athens, Greece: Sisterhood Evniki; 1981.

82. Kikuchi JF, Simmons H. Prologue: An invitation to philosophize. In Kikuchi JF, Simmons H, eds. *Philosophic Inquiry in Nursing*. Newbury Park, Calif: Sage; 1992:1-4.

21

Aesthetic Knowing Grounded in an Explicit Conception of Nursing

ANNE BOYKIN, RN, PhD

MARILYN E. PARKER, RN, PhD

SAVINA O. SCHOENHOFER, RN, PhD

This article presents an expanded perspective of aesthetic knowing in nursing grounded in the theory of nursing as caring. The authors highlight Carper's contributions to nursing, applauding the value of her work. However, a major limitation of Carper's work on aesthetic knowing is the failure to provide an explicit conception of nursing to guide the search for patterns and structure of nursing knowledge, thus the limited development of the aesthetic pattern of knowing in nursing. The authors propose that aesthetic knowing in nursing is the creating experience in the nursing situation, expression of the experience, and appreciation of it through encounter. [Keywords: Aesthetic knowing, Caring, Nursing theory]

Most current literature which addresses epistemological issues in nursing references Carper's (1975; 1978) philosophical analysis of the fundamental patterns of knowing. Using Phenix's (1964) model of "distinguishing types of meaning" (Carper, 1975, p. 142), Carper's analysis of nursing literature yielded four patterns of knowing: "(1) empirics, the science of nursing; (2) esthetics, the art of nursing; (3) the component of a personal knowledge in nursing; and (4) ethics, the component of moral knowledge" (1978, p. 14). The purpose of this article is to propose a new understanding of aesthetic knowing in nursing, based on a critique of Carper's work and grounded in an explicit conception of nursing.

Many nursing scholars recall the experience of first reading Carper's work about the fundamental patterns of knowing in nursing. The work was revolutionary, stimulating visions and motivating actions. It was published during the time when the call for naming and developing nursing as a unique discipline of knowledge had been issued and increasing numbers of nursing scholars were responding by offering conceptions and structures for organizing the knowledge and practice of the field. Many were discouraged with structures borrowed from other disciplines and weary from demands for clarity in a field which lacked a consensus of identity. Carper's "Fundamental Patterns of Knowing in Nursing" (1978) appeared at that point in the evolution of the discipline. The initial work, presented in her dissertation (1975) and later in *Advances in Nursing Science* (1978), recognized the stress of

Source: Boykin, A., Parker, M. E., Schoenhofer, S. O. (1994) Aesthetic Knowing Grounded in an Explicit Conception of Nursing. *Nursing Science Quarterly* 7(4):158–161. Reprinted with permission by from Chestnut House Publications.

the times for educators, practitioners, and learners in nursing. She noted that the development of a body of knowledge for use in nursing practice and education was both a concern and controversy in nursing, often leading to conflict and confusion.

The thesis of her work on the fundamental patterns of knowing in nursing is that the knowledge used in nursing practice and education has patterns and structure which provide the discipline with particular perspectives (Carper, 1975; 1978). From this thesis, Carper's study proceeded. The significance of this work to nursing, according to Carper (1975), is threefold: (1) teaching and learning require reference to the context of the structure of knowledge; (2) each of the fundamental patterns of knowing represents a way to approach the discipline; (3) all knowledge is subject to revision. Her work offered hope for defining and structuring nursing knowledge in ways which would truly belong to nursing.

BEYOND CARPER: POINTS OF DEPARTURE

The authors' development of aesthetic knowing in nursing, while initially stimulated by an appreciation for Carper's contribution, is based on several interrelated points of criticism: first, her failure to articulate an explicit conception of nursing; second, lack of clarity in discussing knowing vs. knowledge; and third, her interpretation of the role of the aesthetic pattern of knowing.

Carper (1975) theorized that "the body of knowledge that serves as the rationale for nursing practice has patterns . . . that serve as organizing principles" (p. 3). The authors reject the thesis that patterns of knowing structure that which is known in nursing. On the contrary, the conception of nursing, explicit or implicit, provides that structure. Major criticisms of Carper's work are her failure to provide an explicit conception of nursing to guide the search for patterns and structure and the limited development of the aesthetic pattern. Carper (1978) acknowledges that "it is the general conception of any field of inquiry that ultimately determines the kind of knowledge the field aims to develop as well as the manner in which that knowledge is to be organized, tested, and applied" (p. 13). Although these key assertions were made, her investigation was conducted without an articulated general conception of the field to guide her inquiry. The degree to which Carper (1975) was able to develop and demonstrate aesthetic knowing as an essential pattern of knowing in nursing was limited by her conclusion that "each of the fundamental patterns of knowing represent one way of approaching the problems and questions in the discipline and are less than the whole of the subject matter" (p. 165).

Carper (1978) fails to distinguish between knowing and knowledge, for example, when she labels one pattern of knowing "personal knowledge" (p. 18). This lack of clarity may lead to a criticism of her work as fragmenting the integrity of nursing knowledge, implying that pathways of knowing lead to particular types of nursing knowledge. The authors' understanding focuses on patterns of knowing as ways of knowing, rather than on specific types of knowledge known or constructed. The unity of nursing is an enduring essence, the nursing situation is the ground of nursing knowledge, and the aesthetic pathway of knowing enables direct access to that essence.

Although multiple lenses are used to view and know the content of nursing, the authors assert that the essence of nursing is whole and unchanging. From any given lens, it is the explicit conception of nursing that specifies the patterned content and structure. Indeed, it is the explicit conception of nursing that guides review and study of related disciplines of knowledge as well. In order to understand the nature of knowing in the discipline, it is necessary to identify the domain of nursing. The essential point is that a conception of nursing is necessary in order to appreciate fully the patterns of knowing in nursing, and particularly in this case, the aesthetic pattern of knowing in nursing. Further development of the meaning of aesthetic knowing in nursing can be facilitated by using various conceptions of nursing such as those previously offered by Henderson (1964), Orem (1991), Parse (1992), Rogers (1992), or Watson (1985), as well as the conception the authors propose.

Carper asserted that aesthetics is the art of nursing (1978, p. 14). Her understanding of aesthetics was based on works from writers in philosophy (Dewey, 1958; Langer, 1957; Rader, 1960). It was primarily from these writers and from Phenix (1964) that Carper's conceptualization of the aesthetic pattern of knowing was developed. Carper (1978) acknowledged that art in nursing has had a restricted meaning (p. 16). Her treatment of aesthetic knowing in nursing suggests, indeed, a limited range of meaning of nursing as art. These authors agree with Carper's (1978) assertion that art in nursing has had a restricted meaning but do not concur with her implication that the aesthetic pattern of knowing is synonymous with the art of nursing (pp. 14, 16). The meaning conveyed in Carper's work is more in the realm of nursing arts and the use of art in nursing, rather than as a creative artistic expression of the appreciation of the unity that is nursing. Classic authors have informed our understanding of art and aesthetics. All art unites; it is a means of communication and moves humanity toward increased well-being (Tolstoy, 1930). Beardsley (1969) argued for the validity of the aesthetic experience as a personal encounter with the object of the art. Tomas (1968) wrote that "to create is to originate. And it follows from this that prior to creation the creator does not foresee what

will result from it" (p. 4). Richards (1962) and Berensohn (1972) suggest that the processes of creating art are primary; the artist has essential interest in acts of creation rather than in the created. The authors believe that aesthetic knowing is the creating experience, the expression of the experience, and the appreciation of it through encounter. Each experience of creating and appreciating is unique and cannot be predicted; it is the experience of aesthetic knowing that is primary in nursing, rather than either the process of creating or the product. The authors intend to offer a fuller description of aesthetic knowing as essential to understanding and doing nursing, approached from our general conception of nursing.

AN EXPLICIT CONCEPTION OF NURSING

The conception of nursing which has facilitated the authors' development of the meaning of aesthetic knowing is offered here. Specifically, nursing is viewed as a discipline of knowledge and a professional service which has as its goal nurturing persons living caring and growing in caring (Boykin & Schoenhofer, 1993, p. 21). This view, grounded in the assumption that persons are caring by virtue of their humanness, respects and acknowledges each person as a caring person. Further, the authors hold that all nursing takes place within nursing situations, "shared lived experiences in which the caring between the persons of nurse and nursed enhances the process of living and growing in caring" (Boykin & Schoenhofer, 1993, p. 3). This perspective is congruent with Watson (1985). It recognizes that the process is enhanced through nurturing relationships with the caring other (Boykin & Schoenhofer, 1993, p. 21). Caring in nursing is viewed as "the intentional and authentic presence of the nurse with another who is recognized as a person living caring and growing in caring" (p. 25). All nursing and nursing-related knowledge and activities are grounded in nursing situations. It is through understanding, appreciating, and being open to the aesthetic pathway that the fullness of the nursing situation is known.

The articulation of an explicit conception of nursing frames a human situation as nursing, assuring its coherence and integrity. Any explicit conception is generated from using the aesthetic pathway of knowing and engenders fuller appreciation of the nursing situation. Aesthetic knowing is a more central pathway of knowing in certain conceptions of nursing. In an effort to explore and communicate the centrality of aesthetic knowing as an integrated nursing way of knowing, a reflection of a particular nursing situation is offered.

FOUR WOMEN

There were three women, and a call from each. Nana was dying; Laura, her granddaughter had peace to make and love of family to share; Ruth, Nana's daughter and Laura's mother, had anger and fear and frustration and anger and fear and loneliness. Nana was dying but this didn't keep her from living—the drama, the pleasure, the red/gray hair to style and the blue nightgown (saved for 26 years) to wear for the ride to Hospice.

Nana saw bats and bugs, all black in a strange place with no sunshine and no fresh air. Sleep was fear; awake was fear. Then there was the possibility of warm sun on her shoulders as she walked high on the bluff above the Pacific. She could see blue and white—the sky and ocean. The birds soared and floated and were at peace in their world. She smiled, her eyes closed, and the skin over her eyes smoothed. Maybe she could choose this vision. Maybe she could join the birds.

Ruth asked for listening, accepting, understanding. Ruth asked for protection. From her daughter? her mother? her self? from years of living apart? from fear to join? Ruth went away. Yet, Ruth was there at the end, with her daughter, to send her mother, Nana, on her way. Ruth was grateful for listening without judgment, for unconditional love, for being there.

Laura asked for loving, supporting, for advising, for affirming, for information. Laura needed to care for Nana as Nana had cared for her. Nana was in Laura's bed; Laura slept near on the floor. The house was full of babies and children, of friends bringing food and reading Psalms, of Ruth and her other grown children. It was Christmas, and New Year's, and a few days of a new decade. Laura was left with no one to help and with no milk, and with no sleep, and with only sobs of hurt. Laura needed love to give love, and there was so much of all there can ever be.

And there was another woman, and another call. To trust and learn to be, to listen for more than the sounds, to know that knowing doesn't matter, to speak more than the words. To wonder at the chaos and harmony in the same place and what to do, how to be. Gifts.

Nursing is the offering and choosing of a holding of each and all together as birthing continues, the mysteries unfold; its strength and power is enough; its possibilities a gel (Parker, 1990).

In this reflective description of a nursing situation, the fourth woman, the nurse, enters into the shared world of three women in a family. She comes to know each of them as persons living caring and growing in caring: "I am nurse. I am with the inner person to respond to calls for help, to be what she can be and for assistance to become what she can become" (Parker, 1992). Each is known as caring person, as person expressing caring and moving toward fuller expressions of caring. This situation, using the above described conception of nursing, will be used to suggest the richness of nursing experienced through aesthetic knowing.

The nurse knows Nana as caring person—dying while living, living while dying. The nurse and Nana join in a rhythm that is spontaneous, mutual, and natural. Nana's dying is to be her fully expressed self, fully engaged in the moment, red/gray hair, blue nightgown and all. The nurse hears Nana's call for caring, for someone to be fully engaged with her in the alternating rhythm of living and dying. Through this rhythmicity the nurse is attuned to calls for caring and responds with caring. By offering vision of warm sun, walking above the blue ocean and joining the soaring birds, the nurse helps Nana create her own way of living dying. The nurse, recognizing Nana's courageous struggle to transcend limits and live her own dying, transcends her own helplessness and fear and participates fully in responding to Nana's call for caring. For each of the four women, there is movement, letting go, and reconnectedness.

A NEW SENSE OF AESTHETIC KNOWING IN NURSING

Each moment in a nursing situation is both unique and universal. If the moment were only new, the value would be minimal as there would be no connectedness. A reflected experience of nursing allows one to know, all-at-once, the uniqueness and the universality of the nursing situation. The nurse artist val-

ues unique individual experiences (Parker, 1992) and also values knowing the fullness of nursing. Expressing nursing as art requires understanding of the art of nursing. A communicated expression of nursing as art, such as the one offered above, encourages further appreciation by self and others.

Thus, the nursing situation reflected and communicated continues to be experienced as each nurse who shares the illustration enters into the world of the nursing situation and becomes participant. It is the aesthetic pathway that fosters full realization of the interconnection of persons and objects. It is in the appreciation that the nursing situation lives anew. Knowledge of the aesthetic pathway is essential for bringing empirical, ethical, and personal knowing to the nursing situation. The nurse may bring science and empirics to the nursing situation, yet can never actually predict the outcomes. Indeed, understanding of the aesthetic pattern of knowing reveals that the result of the nursing cannot be foreseen. The practice of nursing is not linear; the focus is on the continuing and dynamic process, the unfolding, rather than on the product. The nurse follows the call of the client and responds in concert, with mutuality, consonance, and harmony of action.

This article offers an expanded view of aesthetic knowing grounded in an explicit conception of nursing. It is nursing art that is reflected in the aesthetic experience of the nursing situation. It is the aesthetic experience which is then shared in descriptions of nursing situations, opening the pathway of aesthetic knowing to others. The nursing artistry expressed and given to others helps them to know the experience of nursing. In the sharing, the nursing situation is lived anew and the nursing art is known in new and unique ways. Because the nursing has now been expressed, in whatever form, it is not over.

The fuller understanding of aesthetic

knowing requires that one not view art in terms of process and product. The experience of participating with the art creates moments anew, and the work lives for each person in a unique and special way. Art is not in component parts. Nursing art, like a painting on the wall, is never a finished product. It is not a description of the process of sequential nursing actions. The art of nursing cannot be objectified. It must be appreciated, known, and studied using the aesthetic way of knowing. Nursing as a phenomenon is characterized by unity and connectedness, by uniqueness and universality all-at-once. Nursing therefore can be known in its fullness only from within the nursing situation; this requires use of the aesthetic pattern of knowing.

REFERENCES

Beardsley, M. (1969). Aesthetic experience regained. *Journal of Aesthetic and Art Criticism, 28,* 3–11.

Berensohn, P. (1972). *Finding one's way with clay.* New York: Simon & Schuster.

Boykin, A., & Schoenhofer, S. (1993). *Nursing as caring: A model for transforming practice.* New York: National League for Nursing.

Carper, B. (1975). Fundamental patterns of knowing in nursing. Unpublished doctoral dissertation, Teachers College, Columbia University, New York.

Carper, B. (1978). Fundamental patterns of knowing in nursing. *Advances in Nursing Science,* 1, 13–23.

Dewey, J. (1958). *Art as experience.* New York: Capricorn Books.

Henderson, V. (1964). The nature of nursing. *American Journal of Nursing,* 64, 62–68.

Langer, S. (1957). *Problems of art.* New York: Charles Scribner's Sons.

Orem, D. (1991). *Nursing: Concepts of practice* (4th ed.). St. Louis: Mosby-Year Book.

Parker, M. (1990). Four women. *Nightingale songs.* P. O. Box 811535, Boca Raton, FL 33481-1535.

Parker, M. (1992). Exploring the aesthetic meaning of presence in nursing practice. In D. Gaut (Ed.), *The presence of caring in nursing* (pp. 25–38). New York: National League for Nursing.

Parse, R. R. (1992). Human becoming: Parse's theory of nursing. *Nursing Science Quarterly,* 5, 35–42.

Phenix, P. (1964). *Realms of meaning.* New York: McGraw-Hill.

Rader, M. (Ed.). (1960). *A modern book of esthetics* (3rd ed.). New York: Holt, Rinehart & Winston.

Richards, M. (1962). *Centering: In pottery, poetry, and the person.* Middletown, CT: Wesleyan University Press.

Rogers, M. (1992). Nursing science and the space age. *Nursing Science Quarterly,* 5, 27–34.

Tolstoy, L. (1930). *What is art? and Essays on art.* London: Oxford University Press.

Tomas, V. (1968). Creativity in art. *The Philosophical Review,* 67, 1–15.

Watson, J. (1985). *Nursing: The philosophy and science of caring.* Boulder, CO: Colorado Associated University Press.

22

Empirical Development of a Middle-range Theory of Caring

KRISTEN M. SWANSON, RN, PhD

A middle-range theory of caring was inductively derived and validated through phenomenological investigations in three separate perinatal contexts. Caring was described in Study I by 20 women who had recently miscarried, in Study II by 19 careproviders in the newborn intensive care unit, and in Study III by 8 young mothers who had been the recipients of a long-term public health nursing intervention. The empirical development and refinement of the theory is discussed. The five caring processes and an overall definition of caring are presented. Finally, study findings are compared and contrasted with Cobb's (1976) definition of social support, Watson's (1979, 1985) "carative" factors, and Benner's (1984) description of the helping role of the nurse.

As evidenced by our history, practice, and scholarship, caring has long been recognized as central to nursing. Nursing's service to humanity is to care for the client experiencing actual or potential health deviations until such time as the client (individual or aggregate) is able to independently care for the self. Whether caring is self or other directed, the meaning of caring and the essential components of caring remain unclear.

Noddings (1984) analyzed caring from a philosophical standpoint and noted that the one caring is motivated to resolve or ameliorate the discomfort of the other as a result of having let the self become engrossed in the other's plight. Noddings' use of the term *engrossment* incorporates being able and willing

to perceive the other's reality in an "as if" fashion, as if the other's reality were one's own. Benner and Wrubel (1989), like Nodding, propose that caring is central to assessing and intervening on behalf of another. They claim that the focus of a nurse's caring actually defines the areas in which attention is paid to a client's stress and coping needs.

Gilligan (1982) and Ray (1987) place caring in an ethical framework. Gilligan (1982), in her examination of women's development, noted that caring and connectedness are central to a woman's sense of morality and ethics. Ray (1987), in a phenomenological investigation of eight critical care nurses' expressions of caring, identified five caring themes: maturation, technical competence, transpersonal caring, communication, and judgment/ethics. The pervasiveness of an ethic of caring led Ray (1987) to conclude that "the ability of these critical care nurses to apply ethics and morality in distinguishing right from wrong in the attitudes and behaviors associated with the uses of technology was the common denominator of their experiences as a whole" (pp. 167-168).

Several nurse investigators have focused on identifying caring acts. Leininger's (1988) ethnoscientific studies in 52 different cultures led her to conclude that "cultural care has more diverse than similar meanings, and the patterns of care expression have major implications for building an extensive body of nursing knowledge" (pp. 158-159). Brown (1986), Riemen (1986), and Larson (1987) have examined nurse caring behaviors and descriptions from the perspective of those cared for. Clients perceive as caring those nursing ministrations that are person-centered, protective, anticipatory, physically comforting, and that go beyond routine care. Larson (1984) noted a difference between nurses' and clients' perceptions of which caring behaviors were the most important. Whereas clients tended to value physical nursing ministrations, nurses believed they were most valued for their psychosocial supportive interventions.

Watson (1988), who views caring as a moral ideal, suggested that both nursing and medicine are moving out of an era in which cure is dominant into one in which care takes precedence. She noted, however, that more is known about treatment and cure than about healing and caring processes. Watson (1985) claims that nurses practicing, researching, and educating from a stance of caring will ultimately lead to "the promise of human preservation in society" (p. 29).

A universal definition or conceptualization of caring does not exist. Controversy exists within and outside of nursing as to the role of caring in personal and professional relationships. Is caring a process observable only in the context of two or more persons relating? Is it an intent embedded in the behavior of a caregiver? Or is it a perception identifiable only through the eyes of a care recipient? Can caring be taught? Is it a moral ideal? Or is it a way of being in the world? Caring has been discussed and described from each of these perspectives; yet little inquiry exists from a phenomenological inductive stance whereby caregivers, care receivers, and care observers are queried for their perceptions of caring.

The purpose of this study is to describe the inductive development and refinement of a factor-naming theory of the middle range, an empirically derived descriptive theory pertaining to the characteristics of a specified phenomenon (Dickoff & James, 1968; Merton, 1957). The theory, derived from phenomenological studies in three perinatal nursing contexts, provides a definition of caring and the five essential categories or processes that are proposed to characterize caring. Discussion proceeds from a description of the empirical development of the theory, to a contrast of the overall definition of caring with Cobb's (1976) definition of social support and concludes with a comparison of the caring processes, Watson's (1985, 1979) carative factors, and Benner's (1984) description of the helping role of nurses.

THEORY DEVELOPMENT

Overview

Caring was studied in three separate perinatal contexts: as experienced by women who miscarried (Study I) (Swanson-Kauffman, 1986a, 1988b), as provided by parents and professionals in the newborn intensive care unit (Study II) (Swanson, 1990), and as recalled by socially at-risk mothers who had been the recipients of a long-term, intensive public health nursing intervention (Study III) (Swanson-Kauffman, 1988a). The phenomenological method as described by Swanson-Kauffman and Schonwald (1988) was used in all three investigations. Institutional Review Board approval for protection of human subjects was granted for each project, confidentiality was assured, and informed consent of participants was obtained.

Method

Phenomenology involves four basic steps: bracketing, intuiting, analyzing, and describing (Swanson-Kauffman & Schonwald, 1988; Omery, 1983; Oiler, 1986). *Bracketing* is a conscious attempt by the investigator to remain critical and aware of the potential for personal bias and a priori assumptions that may skew the meanings intended by study participants. *Intuiting* is the result of the investigator's remaining open to the meanings attributed to a phenomenon by those who have lived the phenomenon. The investigator need not have experienced the phenomenon per se; however, having solicited many personal accounts of the phenomenon's existence, the investigator experiences the meanings as if the informants' reality were his/her own. Intuiting engages the investigator's self with the existence of those being investigated. *Analysis* involves the methods by which empirical accounts of a phenomenon are elicited (interviews and/or observations), documented (transcribed tape recordings and field notes), coded (sorted by topics addressed), and categorized into essential meaning components or processes (Swanson-Kauffman, 1986b). In the final phase of phenomenology, the phenomenon is described as the investigator has come to understand it. The *description* includes definitions of the essential meaning components (processes) and presentation of sufficient data to support the investigator's conclusions. The findings are internally validated through the quotes of the study participants and externally validated through comparison to the literature. The ultimate test of validity of phenomenological inquiry is concept recognition on the part of research consumers. The valid-ity of the investigation is supported if those who have experienced the phenomenon can recognize their own reality in the phenomenological description.

Study I: Caring and Miscarriage

Study I (Swanson-Kauffman, 1986a, 1988b) began with the question, What are the caring behaviors of others that are identified as helpful by women who have miscarried? Twenty women who had recently miscarried were interviewed on two occasions. About two-thirds of the way through data collection and phenomenological analysis, however, it became apparent that focusing on acts and behaviors was not only premature to understanding the conceptual processes of caring, but also a naive application of the phenomenological method—a method meant to interpret the meaning of lived experiences. Therefore, the research question that ultimately guided analysis was, What constitutes caring in the instance of miscarriage? As summarized in Table 22.1 (first column), the outcome of the miscarriage study was the identification of the five caring processes and their preliminary definitions. These definitions were substantively tied to the clinical context of miscarriage and were awkwardly worded from the perspective of the ones cared for.

Study II: Caring in the Newborn Intensive Care Unit

In Study II (Swanson, 1990), the question posed was, What is it like to be a provider of care in the newborn intensive care unit (NICU)? Data were gathered over the course of one year through participant observation of care provision, attendance at biweekly ethical grand rounds, and a total of 33 interviews with 19 care providers. Care providers interviewed included one nurse administrator, one biomed-

TABLE 22.1.   Definitions of the Five Caring Processes

Study I Women who miscarried[a]	Study II NICU caregivers[b]	Study III At-risk mothers[c]
		Caring Is a nurturing way of re- lating to a valued other toward whom one feels a personal sense of commit- ment and responsibility.
Knowing Identifies the woman's desire to be understood for her experience.	**Knowing** Striving to understand an event as it has mean- ing in the life of the other.	**Knowing** **Striving to understand** **an event as it has** **meaning in the life of** **the other.**
Being with Illustrates the woman's need to have others feel with her—not necessari- ly as her, but with her.	**Being with** Being emotionally present to the other.	**Being with** **Being emotionally** **present to the other.**
Doing for Describes the need to have others do for her (i.e., physical care).	**Doing for** Doing for the other as he/she would do for the self if it were at all possi- ble.	**Doing for** **Doing for the other as** **he/she would do for** **the self if it were at all** **possible.**
Enabling Depicts the need to have her grieving facilitated.	**Enabling** Facilitating the other's passage through life transitions and unfamil- iar events.	**Enabling** **Facilitating the other's** **passage through life** **transitions and unfa-** **miliar events.**
Maintaining belief Focuses on the need to have others maintain be- lief in her capacity to get through the loss and to eventually give birth.	**Maintaining belief** Sustaining faith in the other's capacity to get through an event or transition and face a fu- ture of fulfillment.	**Maintaining belief** Sustaining faith in the other's capacity to get through an event or transition and face a fu- ture with meaning.

NOTE. Underlined = Proposed; Normal = Refined; **Bold = Confirmed**.
[a] n = 20; 40 interviews.
[b] n = 19; 33 interviews.
[c] n = 8; 8 interviews.

ical ethicist, one social worker, five mothers, two fathers, four continuity physicians, and five primary nurses. Each of these informants was either a parent or professional caregiver to at least one of six very low birthweight infants. One of the outcomes of this NICU-based investigation was confirmation of the five caring processes and refinement of their definitions to more generalizable, less context-connected meanings that were worded from the perspective of the one caring. The refined definitions are listed in Table 22.1.

Study III: Caring and the Clinical Nursing Models Project

Interviewed in Study III (Swanson-Kauffman, 1988a) were eight of the 68 young mothers initially enrolled in the Mental Health Intervention Group in conjunction with Barnard's Clinical Nursing Models Project (Barnard, Magyary, Sumner, Booth, Mitchell, & Spieker, 1988). The purpose of the 18-month-long public health nursing intervention was to enable pregnant women who were at high social risk to take control of their lives and ultimately the care of their infants. Despite the highly transient lifestyle of many of these young women, four years after their participation in the intervention protocol, it was possible to contact and interview eight of the mothers. The research question posed was, How do recipients of a long-term intensive nursing intervention recall and describe the nurse-patient relationship four years post intervention? Through this study the five caring processes were confirmed, or in one category (maintaining belief), slightly refined; subdimensions of each process were identified; and ultimately an empirically derived definition of the overall concept of caring was proposed. The processes and overall definition are summarized in Table 22.1 (third column). The subdimensions of the caring processes are listed in Table 22.2.

THE THEORY OF CARING

In the theory's most recent form, caring consists of five categories or processes. They are (a) *knowing*; (b) *being with*, (c) *doing for*, (d) *enabling*, and (e) *maintaining belief*. Although each

TABLE 22.2. Subdimensions of the Five Caring Processes

Knowing	avoiding assumptions centering on the one cared-for assessing thoroughly seeking cues engaging the self of both
Being with	being there conveying ability sharing feelings not-burdening
Doing for	comforting anticipating performing competently/skillfully protecting preserving dignity
Enabling	informing/explaining supporting/allowing focusing generating alternatives/thinking it through validating/giving feedback
Maintaining belief	believing in/holding in esteem maintaining a hope-filled attitude offering realistic optimism "going the distance"

of these categories is presented separately, the categories are not mutually exclusive.

Knowing

Knowing is striving to understand an event as it has meaning in the life of the other. When one is operating from a basis of knowing, the care provider works to avoid a priori assumptions about the meaning of an event; centers on the one cared for; and conducts a thorough, ongoing cue-seeking assessment of the experience of the one cared for. The provider begins with the premise that the desire is to understand the personal reality of the one cared for. Integral to knowing is the provider's philosophy of personhood and the willingness to recognize the other as a significant being. When knowing occurs, the selves of both provider and recipient are engaged.

One of the mothers from the Clinical Nursing Models Project described how the nurse worked with her to get to her true feelings:

> When things weren't right, I could say that things were fine and it was only a matter of time. I mean the nurse would ask certain questions and there would be no way that I could be consistent without telling the truth. And then we would talk, and pretty soon instead of saying it was fine, I would start out with what was really wrong.

In the NICU study, one group of parents described how much they wanted to be recognized for their experience and needs in the NICU. With the birth of their twin sons, the mother and father were in the unit for the third time. On two previous occasions, in the same hospital, they had experienced the deaths of children born prematurely. In the following quote, the father describes how the staff's knowing their experience was essential to meeting their needs:

> They thought at first that we were being like resistive to learning . . . and it wasn't until they found out that this was the third time in three years we've been here . . . [that] they started to figure out that the most important thing we wanted to find out immediately was the major things. We weren't so concerned about movement and that kind of stuff, the major things we were concerned with was the oxygen, the respirators, and how they were doing feeding . . . I was going in there daily. We'd wash up, she'd reach in and touch them first and I'd go right to the charts and start reading.

External validity for the inductively derived category of knowing is found in the philosophical work of Noddings (1984) who examines caring in the contexts of teaching and parenting. In her book, *Caring: A Feminine Approach to Ethics and Moral Education*, she states, "Apprehending the other's reality, feeling what he feels as nearly as possible, is the essential part of caring from the view of the one-caring" (p. 16).

Being With

The second caring process, *being with*, is being emotionally present to the other. It involves simply "being there," conveying ongoing availability, and sharing feelings, whether joyful or painful. Yet, the presence and sharing are responsibly monitored so that the one caring does not ultimately burden the one cared for. Being with goes one small step beyond knowing. It is more than understanding another's plight; it is becoming emotionally open to the other's reality. The message conveyed through being with is that the other's experience matters to the one caring.

A woman from the miscarriage study described how the nurse who cared for her during her dilatation and curettage was able to be with her:

> The male nurse—I think he helped me quite a bit because he tried to comfort me as much as possible . . . he tried to be as gentle as possible . . . he even cried a little bit. He made me feel more like he cared. When they were using the vacuum cleaner, the little suction thing—that hurt quite a bit. I was gritting my teeth, waiting for it to be over, and he tried to comfort me and tell me that it was just about finished . . . He didn't break down and not be able to do his job . . . He just kept saying, "It's a matter of time." You know, he was so sorry. (Swanson-Kauffman, 1986a, p. 42).

In the NICU study, one nurse described how important it was to be with the infants she cared for:

> Barrett was a chronic baby who died recently. I was one of his consistent people. I loved him and I really liked his parents. He went through everything, a terrible lung disease, he was blind, and then he died of SIDS . . . Some of these kids have such a short time and it isn't appropriate to say, "Well, if they make it to two years old, we'll start loving them." They need it now . . . At least before that baby died he knew what it was like to be loved.

Noddings (1984) also provides validation of the *being with* category. She states that presence can occur even in physical absence. Engrossment in the other, regard, and desire for the other's well-being are signs of presence (p. 19).

Doing For

The third caring category is *doing for*. This entails doing for the other what he or she would do for the self if it were at all possible. Care that is doing for is comforting, anticipatory, protective of the other's needs, and performed competently and skillfully. As Larson (1984) and Riemen (1986) have described, clients will oftentimes identify nurses' doing for as those acts which are most appreciated. When a person is in a state of being that requires another to do for them, it can be very embarrassing. Consequently, the caregiver must consciously act to preserve the dignity of the other. As Gadow (1984) states, "Dependence upon another for care of the body constitutes an indignity only when the person cared for becomes an object for the caregiver" (p. 67).

Oftentimes, this type of dignity-preserving doing for must be delivered in an unobtrusive, easily forgotten manner. Bowers (1987) beautifully illustrated the dignity preservation inherent in doing for in her discussion of family caregivers' well-thought-through schemes to maximize their aging parents' capacity to practice self-care. Similar to the subdimensions of doing for, Bowers has identified five categories of caregiving: anticipatory, preventive, supervisory, instrumental, and protective.

The following quote is a description of doing for on the part of a husband whose wife just miscarried. She stated:

> Tim went to the store and got me some sanitary napkins, which I hadn't used in years . . . and he came home with every style that there is out there, it was like every kind in the world. I still have some! I was so hungry. And he was just real sweet . . . fixed me poached eggs, brought them to me in bed. We didn't even really talk about it. We were both thankful I was OK. He said, "All I really care about is that you're all right." (Swanson-Kauffman, 1986a, p. 43).

Once again, support for *doing for* as a caring category may be found in Noddings' (1984) work: "When we see the other's reality as a possibility for us, we must act to eliminate the intolerable, to reduce the pain, to fill the need, to actualize the dream" (p. 14).

Enabling

The fourth caring category, *enabling*, means facilitating the other's passage through life transitions and unfamiliar events. An enabling caregiver is one who uses his or her expert knowledge to the betterment of the other. The purpose of enabling is to facilitate the other's capacity to grow, heal, and/or practice self-care. Enabling involves providing information and explanations as well as offering emotional support in the form of allowing and validating the other's feelings. Enabling often includes assisting the ones cared for to focus on their concerns, generate alternatives, and think through ways to look at or act on a situation.

One mother from the Clinical Nursing Models Project described how the nurse validated her unsure beliefs about parenting:

> Like I said I was really nervous after Tracy was born. So, I called the nurse up several times. My mother did not believe in breastfeeding. We had many heated arguments over it. My husband, he was like, "Nothing's too good for my baby and doctors say that the breast is best." So my mom and husband got into a few fights. But the nurse, she was always agreeable with everything that I felt and she could always back it up with her research.

Mayeroff (1971) supports the importance of enabling another's passage through transition times. He states, "To care for another, in the most significant sense, is to help him grow and actualize himself" (p. 1).

Maintaining Belief

The final caring process, *maintaining belief*, is sustaining faith in the other's capacity to get through an event or transition and face a future with meaning. This definition used to conclude with the words "of fulfillment." In Study III (Swanson-Kauffman, 1988a), however, interviews with women whose lives were riddled with challenges to mere survival revealed that fulfillment may be one step beyond reality for some human experiences. Caring that is *maintaining belief*, involves holding the other in esteem and believing in them. The one caring maintains a hope-filled (as opposed to hopeless) attitude and offers realistic optimism as they "go the whole distance with the other person." In nursing, maintaining belief is a pervasive part of our profession; nurses approach human responses as meaningful aspects of their clients'

realities. Nurses seek to assist clients to attain, maintain, or regain meaning in their experiences of health and illness.

A young mother from the Clinical Nursing Models Project described how the nurse was there with her all the way:

> I was not only pregnant, I felt very unattractive and I had the boyfriend or the partner to prove that you know that he wanted nothing to do with me, and I got a lot of negative feedback from him. All the while I'm trying to keep real positive and yet feeling I'm failing and then Cindy would put me back up and I would keep going. And I did, I kept going.

In maintaining belief, the goal is not to give the other's life meaning. Rather the one caring strives to know, be with, do for, and enable the other so that within the demands, constraints, and resources of the other's life, a path filled with meaning will be chosen. According to Noddings (1984), although we cannot define others' perfection, we must be "exquisitely sensitive" to their ideal of perfection and must act to promote that ideal (p. 102).

CARING: DEFINITION AND DISCUSSION

Through three phenomenological studies, the five caring processes: knowing, being with, doing for, enabling, and maintaining belief were empirically identified and described. Ultimately, the following definition of caring was inductively derived: *Caring is a nurturing way of relating to a valued other toward whom one feels a personal sense of commitment and responsibility.*

Caring as defined through these three perinatal studies is very compatible with Gaut's philosophical analysis of caring. Gaut (1983) has stated that caring, at its very least, involves individual attention to and concern for another, individual responsibility for or providing for at some level, and individual regard, fondness or attachment.

Although caring is most likely an aspect of all socially supportive relationships, not all caring relationships are experienced as social support. The proposed definition of caring may be contrasted with Cobb's (1976) definition of social support, "Information that one is cared for and loved; that one is valued and esteemed; and that one belongs to a network of mutual obligation" (p. 300-301). The caveat between caring, as defined through these investigations, and social support, as defined by Cobb, is at the point of mutual obligation. For example, mutually obligating, socially supportive relationships might include new mothers exchanging babysitting, neighbors borrowing sugar, classmates taking notes for each other, or co-workers sharing rides. In each of these instances, although a sense of caring might motivate the willingness to assist another, the assistance is offered with the implicit or tacit agreement that "you would do the same for me if I needed it." In contrast, if one considers the primary caring relationship—the parent-child relationship—the parent gives to the child from a sense of responsibility and love, not from the expectation that the child will pay back in kind for services rendered. The child may love back; however, the parent does not care with the expectation that the child will reciprocate. Similarly in nurse-client relationships, the nurse cares without obligating the client to reciprocate. As Norbeck (1984) has proposed, it is possible that the reason patients generally do not list health-care providers as members of their social support networks is that patients do not (and should not) feel a sense of mutual obligation when professional caring is provided.

Leininger (1981) claims that "Caring is the central and unifying domain for the body of knowledge and practices in nursing" (p. 3). Yet, caring is not uniquely a nursing phenomenon.

There may, however, be characteristic behavior patterns that are universal expressions of nurse caring. For example, Watson (1985, 1979) has identified 10 carative factors and Benner (1984) has delineated eight dimensions of the helping role of the nurse. The factors and role dimensions are nursing acts that universally cut across client health conditions and developmental levels. The theory of caring, carative factors, and helping role provide cross-validation for each other. Table 22.3 facilitates comparison and contrast among the caring processes, carative factors, and helping role. Because the carative factors and helping role are conceptually grounded in the caring processes, the theory of caring provides a meaning base for why the carative factors and helping role may be perceived as nurturing or helpful by nursing clients. The convergence of the caring processes with Watson's factors and Benner's helping role supports the claim that caring is a central and unifying nursing phenomenon; it does not, however, render the concept of caring as unique to nursing knowledge or practice.

FUTURE DIRECTIONS

A theory of caring has been derived through studies in three perinatal situations; it now needs to be examined for its applicability in other nursing and nonnursing contexts. The congruence of the caring processes with Watson's carative factors and Benner's description of the helping role of the nurse provide evidence that the proposed theory of caring may have validity in nursing beyond the perinatal contexts from which it was derived. Furthermore, the data derived from other health professionals and parents in the NICU study and the congruence of the theory with some of the nonnursing literature (Mayeroff, 1971; Gilligan, 1982; Noddings, 1984) suggest that the proposed theory of caring may generalize to relationships other than those occurring just in nursing.

TABLE 22.3. **Conceptual Cross-Validation of the Caring Processes with Watson's Carative Factors and Benner's Helping Role of the Nurse**

Benner: The Helping Role of Nursing (1984, p. 50)	Caring Process	Watson: Carative Factors (1985, p. 75)
1. Creating a climate for establishing a commitment to healing 2. Providing comfort measures and preserving personhood in the face of pain and extreme breakdown 3. Presencing 4. Maximizing the patient's participation and control in his/her recovery 5. Interpreting kinds of pain and selecting appropriate strategies for pain management and control 6. Proving comfort and communication through touch 7. Providing emotional/informational support to patient families 8. Guiding patients through emotional and developmental changes	**Knowing** Benner Watson 1, 5 1, 3, 10 **Being with** Benner Watson 3, 6, 7 1, 3, 10 **Doing for** Benner Watson 2, 5, 6 4, 8, 9 **Enabling** Benner Watson 4, 8, 7 6, 5, 7, 4 **Maintaining belief** Benner Watson 1, 4 2, 10	1. Humanistic altruistic system of values 2. [Instillation of] faith-hope 3. Sensitivity to self and others 4. Helping-trusting, human care relationship 5. Expressing positive and negative feelings 6. Creative problem solving caring process 7. Transpersonal teaching-learning 8. Supportive, protective, and/or corrective, mental, physical, societal, and spiritual environment 9. Human needs assistance 10. Existential-phenomenological-spiritual forces

At present, a caring-based nurse counseling program for women who miscarry is being developed and tested (National Center for Nursing Research, R29 NR01899-04). Hopefully, this deductive application of the theory of caring will demonstrate the effectiveness of a caring-based intervention on women's health and, ultimately, document the capacity for caring to enhance healing and the potential to find meaning in human experiences of health and illness.

REFERENCES

Barnard, K. E., Magyary, D., Sumner, G., Booth, C. L., Mitchell, S. K., & Spieker, S. (1988). Prevention of parenting alterations for women with low social support. *Psychiatry, 51,* 248-253.

Benner, P. (1984). *From novice to expert.* Menlo Park, CA: Addison-Wesley.

Benner, P. & Wrubel, J. (1989). *The primacy of caring: Stress and coping in health and illness.* Menlo Park, CA: Addison-Wesley.

Bowers, B. J. (1987). Intergenerational caregiving: Adult caregivers and their aging parents. *Advances in Nursing Science, 9*(2), 20-31.

Brown, L. (1986). The experience of care: Patient perspectives. *Topics in Clinical Nursing, 8*(2), 56-62.

Cobb, S. (1976). Social support as a moderator of life stress. *Psychosomatic Medicine, 38,* 300-314.

Dickoff, J., & James, P. (1968). A theory of theories: A position paper. *Nursing Research, 17,* 197-203.

Gadow, S. (1984). Touch and technology: Two paradigms of patient care. *Journal of Religion and Health, 23*(1), 63-69.

Gaut, D. (1983). Development of a theoretically adequate description of caring. *Western Journal of Nursing Research, 5,* 313-324.

Gilligan, C. (1982). *In a different voice.* Cambridge: Harvard University Press.

Larson, P. (1984). Important nurse caring behaviors perceived by patients with cancer. *Oncology Nursing Forum, 11*(6), 46-50.

Leininger, M. M. (1988). Leininger's theory of nursing: Cultural care diversity and universality. *Nursing Science Quarterly, 1*(4), 175-181.

Leininger, M. M. (1981). The phenomenon of caring: Importance, research questions, and theoretical considerations. In M. M. Leininger (Ed.), *Caring: An essential human need* (pp. 3-15). Thorofare, NJ: Charles B. Slack.

Mayeroff, M. (1971). *On caring.* New York: Harper & Row.

Merton, R. F. (1957). *Social theory and social structure* (rev. ed.). New York: Free Press.

Noddings, N. (1984). *Caring: A feminine approach to ethics and moral education.* Berkeley: University of California Press.

Norbeck, J. (1984). Discussion. In K. E. Barnard, P. A. Brandt, B. S. Raff, & P. Carroll (Eds.), *Social support and families of vulnerable infants* (p. 35). New York: March of Dimes Birth Defects Foundation.

Oiler, C. J. (1986). Phenomenology: The method. In P. L. Munhall, & C. J. Oiler (Eds.), *Nursing research: A qualitative perspective* (pp. 69-84). Norwalk: Appleton-Century-Crofts.

Omery, A. (1983). Phenomenology: A method for nursing research. *Advances in Nursing Science, 5*(2), 49-63.

Ray, M. A. (1987). Technological caring: A new model in critical care. *Dimensions of Critical Care Nursing, 6,* 166-173.

Riemen, D. (1986). The essential structure of a caring interaction: Doing phenomenology. In P. L. Munhall, & C. J. Oiler (Eds), *Nursing research: A qualitative perspective* (pp. 85-108). Norwalk: Appleton-Century-Crofts.

Swanson, K. M. (1990). Providing care in the NICU: Sometimes an act of love. *Advances in Nursing Science, 13*(1), 60-73.

Swanson-Kauffman, K. M. (1986a). Caring in the instance of unexpected early pregnancy loss. *Topics in Clinical Nursing, 8*(2), 37-46.

──────. (1986b). A combined qualitative methodology for nursing research. *Advances in Nursing Science, 8*(3), 58-69.

──────. (1988a, July). *Caring as a basis for nursing practice.* Paper presented at the NCAST Institute, Seattle, WA.

──────. (1988b). Caring needs of women who miscarried. In M. M. Leininger (Ed.), *Care: Discovery and uses in clinical and community nursing* (pp. 55-69). Detroit: Wayne State University Press.

Swanson-Kauffman, K. M. & Schonwald, E. (1988). Phenomenology. In B. Sarter (Ed.), *Paths to knowledge: Innovative research methods for nursing* (pp. 97-105). New York: National League for Nursing.

Watson, J. (1979). *Nursing: The philosophy and science of caring.* Boston: Little, Brown and Company.

──────. (1985). *Nursing: Human science and human care.* Norwalk, CT: Appleton-Century-Crofts.

──────. (1988). New dimensions of human caring theory. *Nursing Science Quarterly, 1*(4), 175-181.

23

Nursing and the Next Millennium

MARY H. HUCH, RN, PhD

On March 19, 1993, in Toronto, Canada, at Discovery International, Inc.'s, Biennial Nurse Theorist Conference, five theorists participated in a panel discussion on: caring as an essence of nursing; the value of continuing to develop nursing theory; what constitutes nursing research; the role of advanced practice nurses. The theorists were Imogene M. King, Madeleine M. Leininger, Rosemarie Rizzo Parse, Hildegard E. Peplau, and Martha E. Rogers. Marlaine C. Smith was the moderator and presented the questions to the panel. (Keywords: Advanced practice, Caring, King, Leininger, Nursing knowledge development, Nursing research, Nursing theory development, Parse, Peplau, Rogers.)

Question 1: Is nursing the study of caring in the human health experience?

Dr. Leininger:
Well, I think you already know my answer. Caring is the essence of nursing and I think what Newman, Sime, and Corcoran-Perry did was add caring to the human health experience. So they were really saying, in terms of my theory, that caring is the health experience. But it's more than just the experience, because caring also reveals a lot more about some patterns of behavior and sometimes caring has explanatory value. If you look at the phenomenon of care itself, there's a whole world of knowledge out there to discover. I am pleased that Newman et al. are beginning to see and value caring with the human; this is long overdue. I was stunned when I found out that caring was left out of the metaparadigm in the late 1900s. We had already begun the

caring explication in the 1960s. So, as you know, I have held that caring is the overall concept, and then we have the environmental context. Health flows from care, because if you know care and caring, you then can predict health and well-being. Experience is only one aspect of all this; there's philosophy, there's expression, there are patterns—the linguistic things that you have to examine. And so I say we're moving in the right direction. In our international work we have care as a central, dominant domain of nursing. That's what we're about, and that's what we'll continue to look at until we have established it firmly as the root and the basis. I also take the position that many disciplines are studying health, and health is a unique and important dominant area within nursing. But it is care that will explain health, and that's a different pitch and a very important one.

Dr. King:
If caring is a process, I don't know how it can become a major concept in the nursing meta-

Source: Huch, M. (1995) Nursing and the Next Millennium. *Nursing Science Quarterly* 8(1) 38–44. Reprinted with permission by from Chestnut House Publications

paradigm, because concepts are terms such as perception and health, and they're not processes. And so I have a little problem with that. I also believe that if you use a particular process that leads to a positive outcome, and I think that's what my process and my theory are about, you automatically are caring. We've always had nursing care as part of our literature and history. And what is it? I haven't seen yet in the literature the characteristics that make up care or caring, and I think that's where we have a problem. Maybe I haven't read the right thing.

Dr. Parse:

I think caring is a ubiquitous term; it is not the central phenomenon of nursing. The human-universe-health process is the central phenomenon. The definition of caring is "to be concerned for something or someone," and I think many people in many disciplines are concerned about others. Physicians care, plumbers care, mothers care, and physical therapists care. Caring in the human health experience is not the proper way to state the phenomenon of concern to nursing. That particular phrase forces all the theories and frameworks to take up the issue of caring, and I don't believe that it is a central concept. We talk about human-universe-health process, and we look at the theories and frameworks in relation to that process, and all of the theories do address that. Most of them do not address caring as a central focus. Now, do I think that nurses care or should care? Yes, of course, I do. My disagreement is with elevating the term caring to the conceptual level where we have unitary human being or the human-universe-health process. I would suggest an alternative—that human-universe-health process is the central phenomenon of nursing. That should be our guide—that would be what the theories and frameworks should address—and then our particular practice and research would be guided by those theories and frameworks.

Dr. Peplau:

Up until now it's been pretty much Madeleine Leininger out on a limb all by herself with all the rest of us sawing it off. I don't want to come up the sharpest saw, because Madeleine is a good friend and she does good things for the profession, but I really don't believe that caring is the essence of nursing. I think that the way it's defined, it's a big scrap basket and it covers everything. It's almost a synonym for nursing practice or it's an alternate for the word nursing. I've read some of the caring literature, although I must admit I don't read much of it, but recently I've read a little more than usual. Three men nurses in Scotland have a paper which is about to be published in which they take on the whole concept of caring. They sent it to me for critique and comment and my name is on it, so when it comes out, you'll know I have the saw in hand. I don't know that there's any real benefit to defining what the essence of nursing is, but, if I'm forced to, I would say that it has to do with the nurse and patient in a relationship interacting in such a way that the patient's difficulties are remedied and the patient receives some substantial benefit as a consequence of having this interaction with a professional nurse who is knowledgeable and intellectually competent. I think the one thing that bothers me the most is that nursing has been primarily a woman's profession. We need to move as rapidly as possible to get more men into the profession. The word caring has been associated with women down through the ages and has not been particularly attuned to the behavior of men. And so, in essence, I think when you say caring is the essence of nursing, you are excluding men until the present reformation or transformation or metamorphosis occurs in which men are allowed to be caring individuals who can cry if they want to and hold babies and change diapers and wash dishes and do all of the other things that women do. By the same token, women can get into businesses and be career-oriented and make money and do all the other things that down through the ages men have done so that we have more androgyny in nursing. The percentage of men nurses in the United States has gone up a little bit. I think it's about 3 to 5% now, something like that, but it needs to go up a great deal more because we need a gender mix in order for nursing to reach its full potential. We need the benefits of both men and women. Although I applaud Madeleine's efforts and the efforts of others who have been thinking about caring and have been writing a great deal about it, I do not believe it belongs exclusively to nurses. We have carpet care for instance. We have people who care for your animals. We have all kinds of advertisements on television about how somebody cares for me, my dentist certainly cares, my dental hygienist is a caring person. I have experienced nursing care in a very limited degree in my lifetime experience because I've been phenomenally healthy. But I can't say that the nurses were more caring than the physician I had in that instance or that they were more caring than some of the teachers that I've had in my lifetime or the professional colleagues that I've had down through the years. So I don't think that we should latch onto this one concept and kind of say it belongs to us.

Dr. Rogers:

As far as caring being an effort of any field, it's sort of like the ads. You know mothers love their babies; if a mother cares, she'll give her child Castoria. And if she loves her spouse and cares about him, she'll feed him Nutri-Grain. Now you know, as I have said many, many other times, I happen to believe that everybody ought to care. But any idea that it is an identifying note for nursing is making us look right foolish. Because while we all care, unless there is knowledge that goes before, there is nothing to care with, and I think it's about time that we begin to value knowledge of

some sort. Now, I think this gets into the idea of unique knowledge in nursing. Are we, with our old dependency, going to run off to every other field and say, you tell us what to do and we'll go do it? It's time that we bury the whole idea of caring as the essence of nursing and begin to look at some substance.

Dr. Leininger:

Well, I just want to assure you, it isn't going to be buried. We are moving forward. I feel like I'm in my first seminar with new students. The students come in and say, I don't know what there is to learn about caring. And before we finish and after they get into the body of knowledge, which is really quite substantive, they change their view. As you know, we have over 175 different care constructs. Care is even more important than some of the other things. We have opened a whole body of knowledge that's going to help us in many ways. That people care and banks care is what we call the lay generic perspective. We look at what is professional care. How do we know *that* care? What is it that makes it what it is, and how do we demonstrate it? So I think that when you get into this and begin to systematically study caring, you open some interesting things transculturally and genderwise. As an anthropologist, I know that care has been a part of the male and female world. Margaret Mead proved this very early in her work from 1928 to 1948. I'm not saying care is only exclusive to nursing. I am saying that care is the essence, and I will hold to that. It is the central dominant domain and that must be explicated in this century and into the future. I know other people use care, but I'm saying care has been with us and the least understood and the most ubiquitous because we haven't attended to it. I would gladly refer to nearly 40 some books now on the phenomenon of care and over 2,000 articles. If we get care established as a substrate, this will be one of our major unique contributions to the world at large. I invite you to the International Caring Conferences to really get the substrate. It is exciting to see how it's being teased out and it's not an emotional movement. It is a full substantive knowledge based on care.

Dr. Rogers:

Madeleine, you know I respect you and I love you and I think you've made some major contributions, but I have to ask the critical question when it comes to theory and to theoretical knowledge. What we do is care, but before *we* can *do*, we have to *know*, and that's my point. What do we *know* first before we can exhibit care?

Dr. Leininger:

Caring is the action modality. What you need is to understand what is behind the body of knowledge that is related to care. What all does care mean to you as a professional nurse? What is that knowledge first? You cannot apply and do caring unless you know the phenomenon of care. That's what you have to systematically study.

Dr. Rogers:

I might start off with Patrick Henry. I disagree with everything you say, but I will defend to the death your right to say it! I think as far as research is concerned, whether it's in caring or how to teach or supervise or whatever else, we do need research. Whether one wants to label something care or caring, fine, but that's not the basic knowledge of nursing, and, I think, here again I get concerned when you make the statement about what anthropologists are doing. If nursing is nothing but anthropology, then let's go hire some anthropologists. Give them some manual skills and be done with it. But nursing is no more anthropology than anthropology is physics. Now I'll admit there might be some physical anthropologists who might want to play with physics, but I think we need to give further

thought to how we are using terms. Is there something to know in nursing? Knowledge in another field is not knowledge in nursing.

Dr. Leininger:

I'm not saying it's anthropology; you're missing the point. Knowledge is open to the world—there are no boundaries to knowledge. And just as you are interested in looking at space and energy in physics and that is not nursing, but you can abstract out; you can look at how you use knowledge within the perspective of nursing. It is how we develop the nursing knowledge. We are free to use any knowledge, but it's how we transform it, how we change it to be within nursing, and care is within nursing and has been since the beginning.

Question 2: It has been suggested that the uniqueness of nursing knowledge is not an issue for the next millennium. It may have been an issue in nursing as we struggled for identity as a young discipline, but now as a mature and respected discipline, we can abandon this struggle for identity and work together in interdisciplinary teams to build knowledge around selected phenomena related to health. Meleis offered this view in an article on theory development in the 21st century. So I would like each of you to think about that idea and give your thoughts and opinions.

Dr. Peplau:

Well, the whole notion of uniqueness in nursing has indeed been a 20th-century issue, but I thought it was broader than unique knowledge. Rather, the question is what is unique or what are the unique aspects of nursing per se? From my standpoint, what is unique about any profession are the phenomena which the professional must understand and be able to explain in some theoretical sense and the ability to provide theory-based treatment that will bring about a beneficial outcome. So to me, the issue was never nursing knowledge but rather the broader question of uniqueness. I think there's no doubt that the 21st century is quite likely to be the century of the professional nurse. I think we have come quite a distance now in developing theoretical sophistication, practical know-how, and a good deal of knowledge and information about organizations and networking and publishing and all of that, so that I think we're well on our way.

Whether or not we're going to be on an interdisciplinary team as a participating practitioner or a theory generator or a research assistant or a research participant is a long-standing issue, and I think that issue will continue. But, in terms of our getting away from the theory and moving in that direction totally, I think that would be a great mistake. One of the reasons that I think so comes out of my own experience. In the '40s and '50s I was a member of many important governmental committees which made decisions about government money and where it should go in terms of training grants and research grants and things like that. Additionally, I also was on some World Health Organization consultations in the same vein, and, inevitably, these committees or meetings were interdisciplinary. The one thing that I observed fairly early on was that as nurses we were coming pretty much empty-handed. When it came to talking about what it was that we did, we could always come up with an activity. We could say, we make beds and we pass out medicine and we take temperatures. So we could say what we *did* but not what we *knew*, or what we *understood*, or what the phenomena of nursing were. What were the kinds of phenomena patients presented to nurses about which they were supposed to be knowledgeable and about which they were supposed to provide a beneficial service? When those kinds of questions were raised, we began to stretch it and blow it up and make it up as we went along. I can tick off some of the nurse leaders who,

along with me, would get together afterward and discuss how we did that day. Had we persuaded the boys that we really had this body of knowledge which was called nursing knowledge which, of course, at this point we didn't have? Remember, in the United States we didn't even have a nursing journal until 1952, and then they had to beat the bushes to get articles for it because there was so little research being conducted. That situation has changed. We have a lot of information, a lot of research results and theory development. We have the international theory conferences on a biennial basis now, so that we have many ways to say what it is that nurses know. So when we get into an interdisciplinary meeting we don't come empty-handed. But it would be a grave mistake to say that we know all that we must know. Or that we must stop the development of finding out more in order to get in and work with other disciplines in terms of what we should do, which is the main point of interdisciplinary work in treatment centers, unless you're going to be involved doing the research for them. If you go empty-handed to the interdisciplinary team, you go gravely disadvantaged, and you are then very vulnerable to being put in the position of hand-maiden instead of colleague.

Dr. Rogers:
I think the whole business is still a great deal back at the area of nothing to know in nursing, and I think until we resolve that we're in trouble. Yesterday someone asked who thought should be head of the schools of health sciences in which nursing along with occupational therapy and physical therapy and health education were a part. What did I think of the need for a separate school for nursing? I think that unless we assume our responsibility for a body of scientific knowledge unique to nursing we will be lumped with other professionals. I think that when we get to what is unique, we're dealing with the

uniqueness of any science, the phenomena of concern. One of the problems we've gotten into is we are still so oriented to *doing* that people talk about phenomena as really task-oriented. A few years ago Kellogg paid for a large study by the American Association of Colleges of Nursing. There was this large volume put out about associate degree education and baccalaureate education. They did mention in a couple of sentences the need for a liberal arts base, but the report didn't say much, and then there were pages of numbered lists of activities that all nurses should know how to do. There was not one activity that could be construed as knowledge in nursing. And I am talking about nursing knowledge and the use of nursing knowledge. Now, as long as we operate on that basis, as long as we add up parts and come up with something what we label nursing that is not more nursing than it is any other field, we will not gain the respect of any intellectual or academic group in terms of a knowledge base for nursing. It's interesting that people are very happy to say, well, yes, nursing is concerned with human beings and their environments and as long as you don't define your terms and keep it open, nobody gets into a hassle. But when you begin to define your terms, then, somehow, it looks a little hard. It isn't hard. Either we recognize nursing as a science with its own unique phenomenon of concern and an organized abstract system to underwrite it, or we agree to become a conglomeration.

Dr. Parse:

We, and others like us, have spent our lives carrying out the uniqueness of nursing. And so I think that in the 21st century the carving out of nursing as it grows and develops its theories and frameworks will continue. Nursing is a scientific discipline, just like psychology and physics and sociology. We are all independent; we are separate. And scholars from those disciplines do not give up their identities and do not

stop developing their sciences. No one says to them, well, now you have become sophisticated enough in the development of the phenomena for sociology, so you can move to interdisciplinary groups and you can study phenomena from different perspectives. Sociologists do not study the psychologist's perspective. Psychologists do not study the chemist's perspective or the physicist's. So, I think nursing should stay on the track and continue to evolve the theories and frameworks that we have through research. We need to continue in that way to further specify the discipline. We can move toward much greater specificity. Then we can go to that interdisciplinary table with something in our hands that is very significant. We can be colleagues with scholars of other disciplines and not move into a handmaiden's position. We are unique. We must continue to develop that uniqueness, and in no way would I agree with Meleis where she says that we should leave this theoretical perspective behind and just work on phenomena in general. I think that in coming to an interdisciplinary table, each one brings a different perspective, and I think that nursing's perspective is extremely important there. So, I would encourage all of us to continue to develop the specificity of nursing science.

Dr. King:

This idea just absolutely jarred all the things that I have worked on in the last 30 years. I disagree, but I haven't read Meleis' article. I believe we cannot stop this whole scientific movement called theory development.

Dr. Leininger:

We are still at the beginning of nursing knowledge development, and I think our colleagues have said that. So, we have a whole area ahead of us, and it would be really tragic to shortcut it. That's a lot of foolishness! In any discipline, scholars build, refine, debate, critique, and continue to develop.

Dr. Parse:

I would like to just make a comment that I thought about while Madeleine was speaking. I didn't go through it in the '50s as you did. But I have one major concern about the doctoral programs and the education that our doctoral students are receiving. Many of our doctoral students across the country are invited to do research that is grounded in sociology or psychology or philosophy or in some other area, and they do not utilize the nursing frameworks or theories as guides to research. That is a great concern of mine because I think if we are going to build the discipline, the only way to do it is by building the knowledge of the discipline. If one chooses a framework from outside of the discipline, for example, from a sociological perspective or a psychological perspective, then the research findings enhance that particular discipline. The knowledge, of course, can be used by nurses. We can use any knowledge, the whole world of knowledge. There are very few doctoral programs in this country that require students to utilize nursing frameworks as guides for their research, and that is tragic.

Dr. Leininger:

We ask the question, so what has this got to do with meaning? We already built a body of knowledge. And students have to start right from that base to begin to really systematically examine and study from there.

Dr. Parse:

And I know that you do require nursing theory-based research at Wayne State. But there are many PhD programs that do not. The other concern, too, is somewhat related. It is the way we do research. All of us have spoken in some way about both qualitative and quantitative research. Unfortunately, in many of the doctoral programs if the students want to do qualitative research, there is no one to guide them. Even though you have done it for years,

Madeleine, the first books in nursing on qualitative research were only published in 1985 and 1986. I would encourage doctoral students to go to programs where they can connect with faculty who are working on ideas for research that are of interest to them. When I have my editor's (*Nursing Science Quarterly*) hat on, I sometimes see manuscripts, particularly ones reporting qualitative research, that have weak methodologies. Students are disappointed when their research papers are rejected, because they had assumed their doctoral programs were providing proper guidance for conducting research. We as faculty must be willing to say to students, "Look, this is not my particular area, so I cannot guide it." We have a responsibility to the discipline to educate new scholars properly since these persons will guide and lead the knowledge development in nursing in the next century.

Dr. Peplau:

Well, I just wanted to comment that in essence what Meleis says in that article is enough already on the theory business. Let's go interdisciplinary. And that seems to be a pattern that we've had in nursing. In earlier years when nurses did a research project (and they had to do that in order to get faculty status in academia), they did one itty-bitty little research project and then they said, "Okay, I have done it now; I have done my research." You see the same thing going on in psychiatric nursing, where biomedicalization came in and the biological, biochemical explanations of mental illness got dumped in this "decade of the brain." The nurses pass pills and watch for complications and chart and act as physicians' assistants, as a matter of fact. Then, of course, as Madeleine pointed out, the federal grants office in Washington said that grants must be multidisciplinary, so nurses say, "Okay, if that's where the money is, forget nursing. Let's drop it in a ditch somewhere; after all, we already have all these theories." There's almost a lack of stick-to-it-iveness in nursing. We don't dig very deeply into something. We do it for a little while and then something more interesting comes up or something with money attached to it comes up, and we move on to that. And I find this very ominous. Certainly we don't have enough theory. I could tick off a dozen good research projects where we need theory in order to help nurses to know what to do with a patient who has certain kinds of phenomena. So, I would be absolutely horrified if the nursing population took Meleis seriously on this one.

Question 3: What makes *nursing* research *nursing* research? Must it utilize a nursing framework?

Dr. King:
I wouldn't take a conceptual framework as a basis for a study I wanted to do. I would take a theory and I would test it. To me a conceptual framework is too broad and comprehensive.

Dr. Parse:
Would you agree, Imogene, that the research should be utilizing nursing knowledge? Like in your own system, it would come from the conceptual framework and move into a theory and then be tested. Wouldn't you agree that it has to be nursing knowledge?

Dr. King:
Rosemarie, we've not been at research long enough. We don't have a history of research that tells us that we really have nursing knowledge.

Dr. Parse:
Okay, so you don't think we have nursing knowledge?

Dr. King:
No, because we haven't studied it enough.

Dr. Leininger:
I just want to say another important area that has been growing is the development of theories within the qualitative paradigm. Grounded theory is an example of how you would generate theory from the use of that method. But it is not unique. We now have nearly 20 different distinct methodologies that fall within the qualitative paradigm. Not all theories are tested within the qualitative approach. They are systematically examined to meet the goals and the objectives of the qualitative research project. So, I think there is a lot of opportunity for nurses to do some of these things.

Dr. Peplau:
Well, we have been arguing that for many years. It's nursing research if a nurse does it. It's nursing research if it's done on a nursing service. It's nursing research if it's done on a nursing problem that a patient presents to a nurse. It's nursing research if it uses nursing theory. You know, you could go on down the list. What I wanted to say was that the definition of nursing, which was accepted by the American Nurse Association, and to some extent by the International Council of Nurses, is that nursing is the diagnosis and treatment of human responses to actual and potential health problems. Now, there are a whole bunch of human responses to actual health problems, not to mention potential ones, about which we know nothing as nurses. Some of them I have experienced of late, and I wish somebody would study the exhaustion effect of vigilance. What is the human response to continual vigilance associated with aging, associated with hallucinations, associated with multiple personalities, associated with any number of conditions, strokes, for instance? Now, it seems to me that's something nurses ought to know and know intimately. We have an increasing population of aging people. They are going to have this

problem of vigilance, and they are going to have some kind of response. There's nothing in the literature that I know of on that. We have a whole large area where theory generation is the important thing and then you go and test it. Now you might use a theoretical framework or some kind of theoretical orientation to guide the observation, and I have no problem with that. But I would like to see nurses doing research in which they observe and interview and get patients to describe their own experience, and I am hoping some of that will come out of Parse's theory because she is big on the experiential end. And I am hoping that her students will go and ask people to describe their long-range, long-term experiences, of having a stroke, or whatever. I would like to see a lot of that go on, but I don't expect it will for a long time. I think when you want to go interdisciplinary instead of dealing with more research related to nursing, I think there is going to be less and less of that and we get on to bigger generalizations and bigger generalities and bigger scrap baskets and know less and less about it. But it is in a human response area that we are supposed to know something.

Dr. Rogers:

I think we are doing with research some of the same things we do in talking about nurses when people say a nurse is a nurse, and researchers are researchers are researchers. Everybody is not equipped to do research, everybody doesn't want to, and is there any reason that everybody has to? Certainly people ought to be curious, certainly they ought to read the literature, but we have lots of different kinds of research. Some of the fight over qualitative and quantitative, I think, is like a playback of Descartes and Bacon when they got into the fight over deductive and inductive reasoning. Not too far back, I am sure you all remember, the big hurrah that came up around chaos theory. And it really was a

fancy fad. Fortunately, it is sort of dying away a little bit, but I think it provides an excellent illustration of how we get caught between new realities and changing times and people. When I first got into chaos theory, I read two or three articles that appeared in *Science News* and they didn't bother to include the fine print in there and I thought, oh, boy, with chaos theory, somebody else is believing in the unpredictable besides me. Now, when the chips are down and you begin to get into the whole business, chaos is from an old worldview. There is nothing new about the idea of chaos theory; it had been proposed 30 to 40 years ago and had been worked on then. But what they were saying was, since the human being is not very knowledgeable and he can't possibly know everything, then of course he can't predict everything. Then there was a great big but; but if the human being did know everything, it would all be laid out and he could predict everything. In other words, the same old absolutist philosophy that was supposedly pushed out of the way around the turn of the century when Einstein and some of the others came along. Well, Einstein had trouble with it. At any rate, we are getting into a new reality, a new worldview. I know several of the others on the program here mentioned the idea of emerging worldviews and changing knowledge and that sort of thing. A new worldview that we are moving into now is just as big a shift as when life moved out of the waters onto dry land. Now we are moving into something very, very different. And on an everyday basis, the kinds of things that we have been studying or talking about or wanting to predict about in some distant future simply aren't going to be around to be predicted. Moreover, tools that have been developed out of our old worldviews are not valid for research in new realities. In other words, when one begins to study chaos theory or the idea of unpredictability within a new reality, then it really doesn't matter whether humans know everything or not. In an evolving, continuously changing world, things are unpredictable. There is no absolutism. Now, chaos theory is fading, and I think it will go away because it has perhaps served its purpose. I think it's an excellent example of how we have to recognize that the future cannot be measured according to the past, and that we are not living in the same world. About research, I think we need to be much more specific and recognize what it is that we are talking about and that it's all right for some people not to do research. "Publish or perish" is going to drive all of us crazy yet.

Question 4: There is a move toward the funding of programs for primary care practice or nurse practitioner-type programs. What is your opinion about the movement of primary care or nurse practitioners, and how do you see that related to nursing theory, or does it have any relationship at all?

Dr. Peplau:
Well, it's not hot on my agenda. I suppose you all know that the term now is advanced nursing practice and under that come nurse practitioners and clinical nurse specialists. By my logic, this pulls a specialist down to the level of nurse practitioner, some of whom have graduate degrees, but many of whom have only their RN diploma from a hospital school and maybe four months of training after that. So I find it's a leveling thing. Nobody in nursing can get a little further ahead than anybody else. We can't have specialists and we can't have experts of any kind. Maybe we are at the point where we can't have theorists because they are too smart or they know too much or they know something I don't know. But anyway, we always have this leveling back to a nurse is a nurse is a nurse. So, I have trouble, great trouble, with the advanced practice rubric; however, it's into the political system now and it's in the association's terminology,

so I would guess that it's here to stay. From my viewpoint, every nurse is a practitioner. I mean a nurse practitioner. The attempt to dignify it was originally a political thing. It came at the time in the United States when the American Medical Association began training physician assistants, and nurses were very unhappy at that point. I happened to be the ANA president, so I was the unhappiest of all. And we let it be well-known. As I recall, Martha Rogers called a conference to really deal with this issue, and I was one of the people who helped her deal with it on the podium. In any case, because we were so unhappy about it, our government threw us a bone, gave us money and said, okay, you have this money to train nurse practitioners. So then we had the terrible dilemma of should we take the money and let all those nurses get a little training, however limited, or should we say, keep your money—we will run our own show, which would offend all those politicians and, you know, might have long-term effects. So, anyway, the money was taken and nurse practitioners were turned out in great numbers. They organized. There are more of them than there are clinical nurse specialists. And, as a consequence, they have been running the show. It's one place where money drove the change in practice, and I am sure that has happened many, many times.

Dr. King: At one point, 20 years ago when I met some of the first nurse practitioners, they were in a 3-month training program. And when I saw the first one in a practice setting where this nurse was behaving like a physician, I said to her, "What makes you different from these master's-prepared clinical nurse specialists?" And she said, "Well, I do physical diagnosis." Now that was the behavior. And I said, "Well, I thought that was the basis for the practice of medicine." She said, "No, that's the basis for the advanced practice of nursing." I never saw this nurse ever behave like a nurse. She was like a mini-doctor who teamed up with a couple of doctors and did all of their physical assessments. I don't know why that made me feel negative toward that title. Since then, master's programs have been preparing nurse practitioners. In an attempt to differentiate nurse practitioners from clinical nurse specialists early on, we did say the nurse practitioner extended nursing into medicine and the clinical specialist had an expanded nursing role.

Dr. Rogers:
There is a clear-cut difference between a practitioner of nursing and a nurse practitioner. I think the use of the term nurse practitioner was an old con name to get nurses to accept something that to me is nothing in the world but a physician's assistant. I think Hilda mentioned, that in Washington the bill was set up so anybody who was an RN could take 2 months to 2 years or whatever was needed and be labeled a physician's assistant or a nurse practitioner and be paid for doing it. When it comes to what this means in terms of nursing, I would wonder why in the world nurses want to extend into medicine. I will repeat again, Nightingale said medicine and nursing should never be mixed up. Nurses do not need medicine in order to practice nursing. And if we practiced nursing, we would know that. Now, we certainly ought to learn to work with other groups, and it's a shame that nursing and medicine do not work with each other very well.

Dr. Leininger:
I think a lot of what we're going to see in this next period is what I call partnership care.

How do we work with partners in the community? And how does nursing make its contribution in that partnership?

Dr. Parse:
There was an article in *The American Nurse* which specified that nurses who were moving to advanced nursing practice were very important because patients who met with them said they were friendlier and nicer than physicians and they were cheaper and we could probably be able to pay them better in our health care system. I am very concerned that nurses will be used in that way in the United States, that just because we are cheaper, that we will be asked to practice in ways that will help to decrease the cost of health care.

Dr. Peplau:
That concept that nurses are cheaper is demeaning for nursing, very demeaning, and nurses should be aware of what they are agreeing to be part of in the health care reform.

SUMMARY

This panel discussion among the nurse theorists on key issues related to nursing knowledge development and practice provided the audience with an opportunity to hear various views articulated by leading scholars in the discipline. The diversity of perspectives expressed in dialogues such as this reveals the richness of nursing science.

Part VI

CONTEMPORARY PERSPECTIVES OF NURSING

Over the last decade, several nurse scholars and theorists have shifted from a traditional, logical, positivistic worldview of nursing science to a simultaniety, unitary-transformative paradigm, called the "human science paradigm" in nursing. Martha Rogers' theory of unitary man provided the impetus for this philosophical shift. She challenged her disciples to develop their own theories based on the belief that humans are valued, intentional, free-willed persons engaged in a dynamic, interactive process with others and their environment. Based on this view, the aim of nursing is to guide individuals to explore the meanings their experiences in relation to their past, present, and future and to identify their desired way of being and becoming in life and health. Some renowned nurse theorists whose work is based on the human science paradigm include Rogers, Newman, Parse, and Watson.

In her chapter, "Prevailing Paradigms in Nursing," Margaret Newman describes the ontological, epistemological, and methodological differences that led the movement from logical positivism (reductionistic, objective, cause-effect) to an integrative or summative (body-mind-spirit) worldview, then to the evolving, contemporary, dynamic, interactive human-environment process of humanistic nursing science. She raises relevant questions as to the focus of the nursing discipline and whether nursing should be a single or multiple paradigm discipline. Newman challenges nurses to rethink their values, beliefs, and assumptions about humans, health, and the purpose of nursing interactions with clients.

Humanistic nursing science is based on understanding, valuing, and analyzing the changing life patterns of humans as an ongoing process reflected in the dynamic unity of the "lived experience." In their chapter, "Nursing Knowledge and Human Science: Ontological and Epistemological Considerations," Gail Mitchell and William Cody describe the meaning of human science proposed by Wilhelm Dilthey. They critique the work of several nurse theorists—Paterson and Zderad, Newman, Parse, and Watson—in relation to the "goodness of fit" of these theories with a human science for nursing. This chapter may help nurses to understand the new direction of nursing science and practice.

In her effort to link humanistic nursing science with Carper's "ways of knowing," Dianne Raymond's chapter describes "Esthetic and Personal Knowing through Humanistic Nursing." She begins with a description and critique of Paterson and Zderad's Humanistic Nursing Model, followed by a clinical example. Next, Raymond explains how Paterson and Zderad's phases in a therapeutic nursing relationship are applied as the patient's experience unfolds. The shift in nursing's philosophy of science, and the concomitant changes in research methodology, are described and advocated by this author to expand humanistic nursing science and practice.

Pamela Reed's chapter, "Nursing: The Ontology of the Discipline," introduces the reader to a new conceptualization of nursing. She proposes that nursing is an inherent process of well-being, the substantive focus of the discipline, and cites supporting examples from other nurse scholars. Raymond describes how three characteristics—complexity, integration, and well-being—are manifested in both human and nursing processes. These characteristics are manifested in nursing processes by changes in complexity and integration that generate human's well-being. She advocates including her new definition in the nursing paradigm, and views nursing as creative actions that facilitate human's well-being.

The controversy about whether the nursing discipline should have a single or multiple paradigm continues today. In her chapter, "A Multiparadigm Approach to Nursing," Joan Engebretson examines some discrepancies between holistic nursing theories and biomedical nursing practice, based on diagnostic and outcome classification systems. She discusses some contemporary controversies related to the development and use of nursing theories in practice, and compares cultural differences in holism and healing. Based on her ethnographic work and research, she developed a multiparadigm model to represent a cross-cultural, holistic approach to health and healing. This model consists of four paradigms of healing. The horizontal axis includes mechanical, purification, balance, and supranormal. The vertical axis consists of five types of healing modalities: physical manipulation, applied and ingested substances, energy, psychological, and spiritual. The grid progresses from a positivist to metaphysical science, and from the material or physical to nonmaterial or spiritual therapeutic modalities. Engebretson thoroughly explains each part of her model and provides examples of nursing pratice, theory development, and research.

24

Prevailing Paradigms in Nursing

MARGARET A. NEWMAN, RN, PhD, FAAN

The paradigm issues in nursing need to be sorted out and the focus of nursing as a professional discipline addressed. The challenge is to identify and to agree on the central question and to clarify scientific values and methods.

The variability and ambiguity of things called paradigms, both within and outside nursing, have left me at times feeling very confused. In nursing we often refer to the medical paradigm as opposed to the nursing paradigm, or curing versus caring, or health as the absence of disease versus health as an evolving pattern of the whole.[1] Parse[2] has categorized nursing theories in what she has labeled the totality paradigm versus the simultaneity paradigm. Others speak to a quantitative paradigm versus a qualitative paradigm. These perspectives reflect to some degree various philosophies of science. What is the basis for the naming of a paradigm: the discipline it represents, the subject matter it addresses, the thought processes it reflects, dimensions of time-space, the nature of the data collected, or what? One of the international doctoral students at Minnesota asked me why nursing is so caught up in consideration of paradigms. In answer to her question, my thoughts were that it has something to do with the history of the development of nursing science (eg, our alignment and subsequent disalignment with medicine). When you take a look at the various ways in which we refer to the paradigms, not to mention for the moment

the term *metaparadigm*, it is no wonder that graduate students have difficulty sorting it out.

Nursing is not alone in having to deal with the paradigm issue. Guba's book, *The Paradigm Dialog*,[3] is based on a 1989 conference devoted to this debate in education and related fields. Guba introduced the discussion with an ontologic, epistemologic, and methodologic analysis of four paradigms he identified as relevant: positivism, postpositivism, critical theory, and constructivism. A résumé of the basic belief systems associated with these paradigms (Table 24.1) provides a background for sorting out the paradigm issues in nursing.

EXTANT VIEWS IN NURSING RESEARCH

A wide range of beliefs about what constitutes reality and how to go about finding it is reflected in the research taking place in nursing. Sime, Corcoran-Perry, and I have developed our own version of the scientific paradigms we see at work in nursing research.[4] We pursued this task for the purpose of delineating how the seemingly disparate work of various members of our faculty can indeed relate to a common focus. We tried not to introduce three new labels, but we did not see our categorizations fitting neatly into those already described. Eventually, rather than

Source: Reproduced from Newman, M. A. (1992). Prevailing paradigms in nursing. *Nursing Outlook, 40* (1): 10-13, 32, with permission from Mosby-Year Book, Inc.

TABLE 24.1. Basic Belief Systems of Positivism, Postpositivism, Critical Theory, and Constructivism

	Ontology	Epistemology	Methodology
Positivism	Realist: Reality exists "out there" Driven by natural laws	Objectivist: Inquirer adopts distant and noninteractive posture	Experimental Empiric Controlled Testing of hypotheses
Postpositivism	Critical realist: Same as positivism except cannot be known because of lack of ability to know	Modified objectivist: Objectivity an ideal that can be only approximated Guarded by critical community	Modified experimental Emphasis on critical "multiplism" (elaborated triangulation)
Critical theory	Critical realist: Reality influenced by societal structures	Subjectivist: Values mediate inquiry Goal is to free participants from effect of ideology	Dialogic, transformative Intended to eliminate false consciousness and facilitate transformation
Constructivism	Relativist: Reality is mental construction, socially and experimentally based Many interpretations possible Multiple realities	Subjectivist: Inquirer and respondent are fused into single entity Findings are creation of process between the two	Hermeneutic, dialectic Aims to identify the variety of constructions that exist and bring them to as much consensus as possible

Source: Excerpted from Guba EG. The alternative paradigm dialog. In: Guba EG, ed. *The paradigm dialog*. Newbury Park, Calif: Sage, 1990:17-27.

referring to them as I, II, and III, we succumbed to assigning descriptive labels to depict the key dimensions in each: I—particulate-deterministic, II—interactive-integrative, and III—unitary-transformative. The idea here is that the first of the paired words describes the view of the entity being studied and the second describes the notion of how change occurs.

From the particulate-deterministic paradigm, which holds closely to the positivist view, phenomena are

viewed as isolatable, reducible entities having definable properties that can be measured. These entities have orderly and predictable connectedness to each other. Change is assumed to be a consequence of antecedent conditions—conditions that, if sufficiently identified and understood, could be used to predict and control change in the phenomena. Relationships within and among entities are viewed as linear and causal.[4]

From a particulate-deterministic view, only the most objective, observable manifestations of health, such as physiologic parameters, would be considered suitable subject matter for research. A phenomenon such as caring, considered by some as the essence of nursing, either would have to be removed from its context and given an operational definition or would be considered by some as outside the realm of science.

The interactive-integrative paradigm (similar to postpositivism) maintains allegiance to the need for control and predictability in research but views reality as multidimensional and contextual. It acknowledges the importance of experience and includes both subjective and objective phenomena but holds to the objectivity, control, and predictability of the positivist view. It moves away from linearity and acknowledges that in some instances understanding without predictability is enough. Change is viewed as "a function of multiple antecedent factors and probabilistic relationships."[4] Knowledge is context dependent and relative. From this perspective, nursing phenomena are viewed as both objective and subjective in reciprocal interaction.

The unitary-transformative paradigm presents a significant shift in the view of reality. The human being is viewed as unitary and evolving as a self-organizing field, embedded in a larger self-organizing field.

> It is identified by pattern and by interaction with the larger whole. . . . Change is unidirectional and unpredictable as systems move through stages of organization and disorganization to more complex organization. Knowledge is personal, involves pattern recognition, and is a function of both viewer and the phenomenon viewed. . . . Inner reality depicts the reality of the whole.[4]

Nursing would be studied as a unitary process of mutuality and creative unfolding.

Historically we seem to have moved from addressing primarily the health of the body as affected by environmental factors to interplay

TABLE 24.2. Shift in Emphasis of Nursing Science

Health focus	Science category	Paradigm
Body ‹ environment	Biophysical	Single
Body-mind-environment	Biopsychosocial	Multiple
Unitary field	Human	Emergent

of body-mind-environment factors in health, and, more recently, to health as an experience of the unitary human field phenomenon embedded in a larger unitary field. These three perspectives, biophysical science, biopsychosocial science, and human science relate to different paradigms. The biophysical sciences are single-paradigm sciences with broad consensus among their members, biopsychosocial sciences involve multiple competing paradigms encompassing both objective and subjective phenomena and relating to different views on the nature of human beings and society.[5] Human science embraces a view of the human being as a unitary phenomenon and represents a major paradigm shift from the previous two (Table 24.2).

FOCUS OF THE DISCIPLINE

There is another consideration in nursing science. Nursing science is a professional discipline and as such has a commitment to alleviate the problems of society. The nature of the reality we are dealing with must incorporate knowledge of the process of making things better for society—a knowledge of praxis, "thoughtful reflection and action that occurs in synchrony, in the direction of transforming the world."[6]

What is our commitment then? Some would say "the promotion of health." At least two objections to that focus are that (1) it is phrased in the language of intervention and objectivity and therefore excludes the unitary-transformative paradigm; and (2) it is not an exclusive domain of nursing. Others would say "caring." Similar objections might apply: (1) from a positivist view, caring may not be amenable to scientific study; and (2) it is of a universal nature that is not limited to one discipline.

Sime, Corcoran-Perry, and I found that as we progressed in our exploration of prevailing paradigms, our intent became to identify the unifying focus of nursing as a professional discipline. After much discussion among ourselves and other colleagues and review of the literature, particularly over the past decade, we came to the conclusion that the focus of nursing as a professional discipline can be characterized as "caring in the human health experience."[4] This focus synthesizes the phenomena of nursing at the metaparadigm level and makes explicit the nature of the social mandate of nursing. *Caring* designates the nature of the nursing practice participation. *Human health experience* brings together the focus on *human* health and modifies it to mean the human health *experience*. The experiential dimension characterizes the phenomenon as something beyond the traditional objective-subjective perspective. The whole phrase taken together signifies the social mandate to which nursing has responded throughout our history and circumscribes the boundaries of the discipline.

Each major concept of this focus, taken alone, manifests itself in different ways. Morse and her associates[7] have done a comprehensive review of the variety of ways in which caring has been defined and studied. Their work illustrates the different paradigmatic positions prevalent in nursing today. The same is true for research related to the concept of health. Most of this research emanates from the dominant objective-subjective paradigms.[8] At the same time, research that connects caring and the health experience in a mutual, transformative process is emerging as a powerful force within the explication of our discipline.

ARE WE A MULTIPLE-PARADIGM DISCIPLINE?

This question leads to the question of whether the aforementioned focus can be addressed within the objectivist, interventionist tradition. Benner's answer would seem to be "no." Benner[9] points out that within a social scientific context, caring is "decontextualized" and "operationalized" and becomes just one more therapeutic technique. I take that to mean that this way of viewing caring does not capture the essence of caring.

When we[4] began work on "The Focus of the Discipline" paper, we thought of ourselves as each being representative of one of the three paradigms, but the more we discussed the underlying assumptions of each and came to accept the disciplinary focus of caring in the human health experience, the more each of us became convinced of the necessity of the unitary, transformative paradigm for development of the knowledge of our discipline. We ourselves were transformed in the process. We concluded that knowledge emanating from the first two paradigms is relevant but not sufficient for the full elaboration of nursing science.

Others tend to agree. Pender[10] describes the shift in nursing to human science, which views persons as unified wholes and focuses on the *experience* of health. She calls for a unitary perspective but still uses the language of objectivity in calling for valid and reliable measures. Parse[2] says that a discipline encompasses more than one paradigm to guide inquiry, yet clearly takes her stand in what she calls a simultaneity paradigm, one that embraces mutuality and transformation as the nature of human processes.

We seem to be hedging. Are we afraid to give up the certainty in knowing that the positivist view offers? In discussing the movement to new paradigms, Skrtic[5] points out that the "divorce of science from its contemporary raw empiricist base, and its realliance with judgment, discernment, understanding, and interpretation as necessary elements of the scientific process" means giving up the false certainty of logical positivism and facing the anxiety of less certain forms of knowing.

My original intent was to try to fairly, accurately present each of the prevailing paradigms and to say "Let's agree to disagree and go on about our business." Identifying the paradigms is the easy part. The hard part is acknowledging the pervasive nature of a paradigm, the fact that the values inherent in a paradigm are deeply embedded in the adherents and become normative, indicating what is important and what should be done about it. Paradigms have been compared with cultures in that they represent shared knowledge of what is and what ought to be and *adherents cannot imagine any other way to behave.*[11] This begins to explain some of the uneasiness we experience when an adherent of a paradigm other than our own speaks to the importance of that way of thinking and behaving.

Some argue for accommodation among paradigms; others assert that they have nothing in common. Skrtic[5] takes the position that "the point is not to accommodate or reconcile the multiple paradigms . . . ; it is to recognize them as unique, historically situated forms of insight; to understand them and their implications; to learn to speak to them and through them. . . ." Moccia[12] has described the deeper meaning of what is involved in attempts to accommodate different paradigms: the contradiction of trying to control and not to control, the expectation of being able to predict and at the same time acknowledging the process as innovative.

For almost a decade now, thanks to Munhall,[13] we have been aware of the dis-

crepancies between our values as a profession and our practices as scientists. Now it is important to recognize the inconsistencies within our science, inconsistencies we are passing on to students. Lincoln[14] has experienced the same conflicting values.

I have often told questioners that research training programs should be two-tracked, with training in conventional and emergent-paradigm inquiry models, followed by training in quantitative and qualitative methods both, completed with computer applications for both quantitative and qualitative data.

But with what I have intuitively come to understand about the pervasiveness of the paradigm we use to conduct inquiry, I now think that training in multiple paradigms (at least in more than a historical sense) is training for schizophrenia. If we want to change new researchers' paradigms, we must do more than legitimate those paradigms in the inquiry outlets, such as journals. We have to train people in them, intensively. We probably ought not to be dividing their attention with other than historical accounts of conventional science. We probably ought to recognize the profound commitments people make to worldviews and create centers where such training can go on. . . .[14]

A movement has begun within nursing education to create centers with a particular focus—perhaps to emphasize one paradigm as dominant. The question is, Are we willing to allow, even encourage, that to occur? Or do we want to give all of the paradigms equal time and emphasis in all the programs? Or perhaps a third alternative might be to promote pockets of parallel emphases from different paradigmatic perspectives within a single program.

Some think that positivism is dead—others see it as alive and well and still dominating the scientific community. In graduate curricula, for instance, is it not true that most "basic" research courses emphasize the tenets of controlled, objective science? Does that not say that this is the way it is and anything else is alternative or deviant? And how many of our courses on theory development begin with the isolation of concepts, development of propositional sets, and derivation of causal relationships? If a faculty seeks to convey a different perspective, they would need to examine their basic ontologic and epistemologic beliefs and develop courses that are consistent with those beliefs.

A PARADIGM SHIFT

Evidence of a paradigm shift exists in nursing. Johnson's bibliometric analysis of nursing literature since 1966 depicts a shift from a scientific medical model to a model based on holism.[15] Sarter's analysis of four contemporary nursing theories reveals commonly shared themes, emphasizing holism, process, and self-transcendence.[16] She suggests that it represents an emerging paradigm. The shift perhaps has not been as revolutionary as Kuhn would have predicted. A headline in the *Brain/Mind Bulletin* is apropos: "Can you remember where you were when the paradigm shifted?"[17] Assuming that the shift has occurred, it is incumbent on us to reevaluate the values and structures that shape our discipline.

THE CHALLENGE

The challenge before us is twofold: the need to identify and agree on the central question in nursing, the focus of the discipline, and the need to clarify the scientific values and methods that will address that question.

REFERENCES

1. Newman MA. *Health as expanding consciousness.* St. Louis, Mo.: CV Mosby, 1986.
2. Parse RR. *Nursing science: Major paradigms, theories, and critiques.* Philadelphia, Pa.: Saunders, 1987.
3. Guba EG, ed. *The paradigm dialog.* Newbury Park, Calif.: Sage, 1990.
4. Newman MA, Sime AM, Corcoran-Perry SA. The focus of the discipline of nursing. *ANS* 1991;14(1):1-6.
5. Skrtic TM. Social accommodation: Toward a dialogical discourse in educational inquiry. In: Guba EG, ed. *The paradigm dialog.* Newbury Park, Calif.: Sage, 1990:125-35.
6. Wheller CE, Chinn PL. *Peace & power: A handbook of feminist process.* 2nd ed. New York: National League for Nursing, 1989:1.
7. Morse JM, Solberg SM, Neander WL, Bottorff JL, Johnson JL. Concepts of caring and caring as a concept. *ANS* 1990;13(1):1-14.
8. Newman MA. Health conceptualizations. *Ann Rev Nurs Res* 1991;9:221-43.
9. Benner P. Nursing as a caring profession. Paper presented at meeting of the American Academy of Nursing, October 16-18, Kansas City, Mo., 1988.
10. Pender NJ. Expressing health through life-style patterns. *Nurs Sci Q* 1990;3(3):115-22.
11. Firestone WA. Accommodation: Toward a paradigm-praxis dialectic. In: Guba EG, ed. *The paradigm dialog.* Newbury Park, Calif.: Sage, 1990:105-24.
12. Moccia P. A critique of compromise: Beyond the methods debate. *ANS* 1988;10(4):1-9.
13. Munhall P. Nursing philosophy and nursing research: In apposition or opposition? *Nurs Res* 1982; 31(3):176-7;181.
14. Lincoln YS. The making of a constructivist: A remembrance of transformations past. In: Guba EG, ed. *The paradigm dialog.* Newbury Park, Calif.: Sage, 1990:67-87.
15. Johnson MB. The holistic paradigm in nursing: The diffusion of an innovation. *Res Nurs Health* 1990;13:129-39.
16. Sarter B. Philosophic sources of nursing theory. *Nurs Sci Q* 1988;1(2):52-9.
17. Can you remember where you were when the paradigm shifted? *Brain/Mind Bulletin* 1991; 16(7).

25

Nursing Knowledge and Human Science: Ontological and Epistemological Considerations

GAIL J. MITCHELL, RN, MScN

WILLIAM K. CODY, RN, MSN

This chapter examines the meaning of human science in relation to extant nursing knowledge. The origins of the human science tradition are traced to the philosopher Wilhelm Dilthey, who challenged the dominance of the positivist perspective for generating knowledge of the human lifeworld. Specific ontological and epistemological criteria for human science are proposed. Four nursing frameworks, Paterson and Zderad's humanistic nursing, Newman's model of health as expanding consciousness, Watson's human science and human care, and Parse's theory of human becoming, are found to have consistencies and inconsistencies with the human science tradition. It is proposed that the human science perspective is present in and will continue to be reflected in the evolution of nursing science.

Increasingly, nursing is being referred to as a human science (Connors, 1988; Gortner & Schultz, 1988; Meleis, 1990; Munhall, 1989; Parse, 1981, 1987; Watson, 1985). The meaning of this term as it is used in the literature, however, is not clear. Munhall (1989), Parse (1981) and Watson (1985) refer to human science as distinct from natural science and as bearing specific views, concepts, and methods. Contrary to this position, Connors (1988) and Gortner and Schultz (1988) refer to human science as the fields of biology, psychology, anthropology, and sociology. Is human science inclusive of any inquiry about human beings, or

is it a distinctive philosophical foundation for science? Is nursing currently a human science or is this an ideal to be esteemed and aspired to? The purpose of this chapter is to examine the meaning of human science as originated by Dilthey (1961, 1976, 1977a, 1977b, 1988) and explicated by Giorgi (1970, 1971, 1985) and to compare selected works from nursing's extant theoretical base to the explicit attributes that constitute "human" science.

DEFINING HUMAN SCIENCE

The origins of the term *human science* can be traced to the philosopher Wilhelm Dilthey

Source: Mitchell, G. J., & Cody, W. K. (1992). Nursing knowledge and human science: Ontological and epistemological considerations. *Nursing Science Quarterly, 5* (2): 54-61. Reprinted with permission from Chestnut House Publications.

(1833-1911). The German term for human science, *Geisteswissenschaften*, has also been translated as "human studies." Translators frequently note the linguistic challenge involved in capturing the meaning of freshly coined and esoteric German expressions in English. Also noted in Dilthey's works is his tendency to refer to "psychic" life in a nineteenth-century fashion while writing of the coherent whole of lived experience. Dilthey did, however, describe life as unity, a living nexus. And he consistently referred to individuals as wholes and to human life as interconnected with others and history. The intent of the authors here is to offer an admittedly hermeneutical interpretation of Dilthey's view, in what is believed to be the unitary perspective of human beings that he intended.

Dilthey in the late 1800s was very concerned about what he called a "crisis in science," a crisis of modern consciousness, thought, and values (Ermath, 1978). The industrial society had already concretized the successes of the natural sciences, and the developing science of *Anthropologie*, with no other model, was rapidly abandoning any interest in human consciousness in favor of a crude "mindless" naturalism (Ermath, 1978). Dilthey (1977a) described what he saw as a sterile empiricism that disconnected life from knowledge. His fears were stoked by the growing trend to regard human behavior and culture as susceptible to the methods of natural science, which, he thought, stripped life of human meaning and purpose (Dilthey, 1977a). He proposed that "the deepest problem of modern thought and culture is to understand life as it is lived by man" (Ermath, 1978, p. 17).

Dilthey (1977a, 1977b, 1988) believed that the development of a human science held the only hope for understanding life as it is humanly lived. He proposed that the human sciences required concepts, methods, and theories which were fundamentally different from those of the natural sciences (Dilthey, 1977a, 1988). Dilthey viewed human beings as the preeminent source of knowledge. His philosophy took as its basis the whole of lived experience, the coherent nexus of life as it is humanly lived (Dilthey, 1977a). He wrote about "living" knowledge and "reflective" life. History and culture were, for Dilthey, manifestations of patterns of human life, pervaded with meaning. The natural sciences, concerned with the elaboration of physical laws from observation and experimentation, were, for Dilthey, very different from the concerns a true human science would focus on: meaning, values, and relationships within the coherent texture of humanly lived experience. The subject matter of the human sciences is "the interrelation of life, expression, and understanding" (Dilthey, 1976, p. 175).

Dilthey proposed that the lived experience should be "the basic empirical datum of the human sciences" (Ermath, 1978, p. 97). Further, the researcher, a living being too, is inexorably and unequivocally "in" and "of" what is investigated. There could be no meaningful objective/subjective dichotomy and no analytic reduction beyond experience as humanly lived. Human experience is a coherent whole to which subjectivity is fundamental; objectivity is a human creation. Dilthey maintained that life is a process, a continuous becoming which manifests itself in the dynamic unity of experience (Dilthey, 1976). Human beings were described as individual wholes with intrinsic value (Dilthey, 1977b). Dilthey (1977b) referred to the self as a "life-unity" that is free yet also determined by history. The concept of free will is a fundamental assumption of human science. On free will, Dilthey (1988) wrote, "This is an immediately given actuality. *It cannot be denied* . . . [O]ne *cannot explain* the fact of free will, for it is precisely its hallmark that we cannot break it down in a conceptual system" (p. 270).

More recently, the psychologist Giorgi (1970, 1971, 1985) has reasserted the need for an approach to the human sciences fundamentally different from conventional empirical methods. He proposed to study human beings as persons, as experiencing participants. He challenged the prevailing positivistic methods of psychology, contending that human experience must be understood in the way that it reveals itself, and he maintained that the study of lived experience could be done scientifically (Giorgi, 1985).

According to Giorgi, understanding life experiences requires a focus on meaning within the context of the person's experience of the phenomenon. Human beings cannot be known as objects, nor as separate from their lives. Echoing Dilthey, Giorgi maintained that a person is not "a passive receiver of physical energies, but rather his or her behavior reflects intentionality" (Giorgi, 1971, p. 23). Giorgi also addressed the influence of the researcher in conceptualizing research and the impact of the researcher on study findings. For Giorgi, the most important variable in the human sciences is the meaning of the lived experience for the subject. An exposition of the major thinkers and scholars, such as Gadamer (1976), Geertz (1973), Heidegger (1962), Ricoeur (1974), Schutz (1967), and Winch (1958), who have built on the tradition of which Dilthey is the foremost progenitor, is beyond the scope of this article.

The domination of twentieth-century social science by positivistic approaches in stark contrast to human science philosophy has been well documented (Polkinghorne, 1983) and contributes to the contextual situation in which this article emerges. The philosophical stance of human science outlined here has underpinned or strongly influenced the works of the six seminal scholars mentioned above and many others in the tradition of human science. These scholars have recognized the manifest necessity for the human sciences to explore and understand lived experience, the full complexity of human meanings and values, with no more fundamental reference than the human lives which are the phenomena of concern; indeed this formidable undertaking is the very mission of human science.

Based on the above explications of human science by Dilthey and Giorgi, specific ontological and epistemological attributes emerge as crucial to this approach for nursing science. Human science, in view of its origins and its philosophical foundations, cannot be viewed as a generic term for any and all disciplines studying human beings. It is proposed here that for a scientific discipline to be considered a "human science" logically it must incorporate the ontology and epistemology of its philosophical underpinnings, as described in Table 25.1.

A distinction must be made between a "humanistic" philosophy of science and "human science." According to Webster (1985), "humanism" entails a rejection of supernaturalism and asserts "the essential dignity and worth of man [sic] and his capacity to achieve self-realization through the use of reason and scientific method." Humanism thus is seen to acknowledge human values and potentialities without requiring a critique of "scientific method." Human science, in contrast, unequivocally rejects the methods of natural science (Dilthey, 1976, 1977a, 1988; Giorgi, 1985) and asserts from the outset that lived experience, the world as experienced, meaning, and understanding are all aspects of a unitary process of human life and cannot be adequately described, explained, or analyzed through objectification, measurement, or reduction.

SIGNIFICANCE OF HUMAN SCIENCE FOR NURSING

If nurses embrace the human science paradigm, activities in theory development, re-

TABLE 25.1.   Ontology and Epistemology of the Human Science Paradigm

Ontology	Epistemology
Human beings are unitary wholes in continuous interrelationship with their dynamic, temporal, historical, cultural worlds.	Research and practice focus on the coherent experience of the person's meanings, relations, values, patterns, and themes.
Human experience is preeminent and fundamental and reality is the whole complex of what is experienced and elaborated in thinking, feeling, and willing.	Lived experience is the basic empirical datum, as gleaned from the participant's description free of comparison to objective realities or predefined norms.
Human beings are intentional, free-willed beings who actively participate in life continuously.	The person's coparticipation in generating knowledge of lived experience is respected, and no more fundamental reference than what is disclosed by the person is sought.
The researcher is inextricably involved with any phenomenon investigated.	The researcher seeks knowledge and understanding of lived experience and is cognizant of the other's lived reality as a unitary whole.

Source: Synthesized and condensed from Dilthey, 1961, 1976, 1977a, 1977b, 1988; and Giorgi, 1970, 1971, 1985.

search, and practice will change to reflect the new philosophical perspective. An examination of nursing's philosophical and theoretical body of literature reveals that, in the past decade, such a change has already begun. In order to explore to what extent nurses are incorporating beliefs of the human science paradigm in theory, research, and practice, four nursing frameworks were selected for analysis. These frameworks are Paterson and Zderad's (1988) humanistic nursing, Newman's (1986a, 1990) model of health as expanding consciousness, Watson's (1985) human science and human care, and Parse's (1981, 1987, 1990a) theory of human becoming (formerly man-living-health, 1981). These frameworks were selected because all their authors claim a unitary conceptualization of human beings,

thereby evincing some degree of interfacing with the human science perspective. Further, these authors have publicly renounced the natural science approach and have called for new and different methods more congruent with nursing's philosophical foundations.

Critical to the development of nursing theories underpinned by the human sciences would be the acknowledgment of human beings as individual wholes who are situated in-the-world and who are respected as intentional, free-willed persons. Any theoretical principles and concepts used to structure a theory would need to incorporate these beliefs. Also essential would be approaches which view the individual's lived experience as the focus in both practice and research and which honor the person's lived experience as reality. Researchers and practitioners would be regarded as coparticipants with persons in inquiry and practice in a human science paradigm.

ANALYSIS OF THE NURSING FRAMEWORKS

Inquiry into the four frameworks above revealed a definite commitment to the human science paradigm. Parse's theory of human becoming was found not only to be consistent with the human science beliefs but to clarify, expand, and develop this approach. Consequently, an in-depth analysis of Parse's theory will be offered at a later point. Analysis of the works of Newman, Paterson and Zderad, and Watson illuminated consistencies and inconsistencies in relation to the beliefs of human science. Consistencies and commonalities included affirmation, to varying degrees, of the wholeness of the human being, the significance of subjective experience, and mutual participation in the creation of reality.

The inconsistencies took two main forms. In some instances, the author(s) acknowledged an inability to reconcile traditional objectivist beliefs with beliefs congruent with human science, and consequently they incorporated conflicting beliefs in theoretical conceptualizations. Alternately, the author(s) extended and elaborated on beliefs essential to the human science tradition, leading to significant dissidence with the core philosophy. These two inconsistencies are discussed with specific examples to illustrate logical incongruencies with the human science tradition. The intent here is not to rebuke the nursing theorists for their philosophical obscurities, for obscurity engenders clarification. Rather, the intent is to illuminate the inconsistencies in order to foster clarity and further the development of nursing science.

INCORPORATING DIVERGING BELIEFS

As previously noted, the nursing frameworks revealed both consistencies and inconsistencies with the foundational beliefs of the human science paradigm. Perhaps reflecting the evolutionary nature of knowledge and theory development, several of the authors incorporated diverging beliefs in their work, leaving the reader unclear as to their philosophical underpinnings. The inconsistencies arise in three main areas: the human being's wholeness, the intentionality and free will of the person, and the nature of reality. Each of these will be explored in relation to the works of Paterson and Zderad (1988), Newman (1986a, 1990), and Watson (1985).

Wholeness of Human Beings

Paterson and Zderad (1988) in their humanistic nursing practice propose that "the nurse sees the patient as a whole, a gestalt" (p. 25). Human beings are described as "in-the-world" and nurses are guided to recognize the complexity and uniqueness of each person's relating and experiencing. Paterson and Zderad note, however, that this view of the person as a whole conflicts with the evaluative stance of the conventional nursing process. They address this conflict by positing that "both subject-subject and subject-object relationships are essential for clinical nursing" (Paterson & Zderad, 1988, p. 27) in which focusing on discrete parts rather than the whole person is sometimes necessary. This attempt to incorporate human science beliefs with biomedical traditions leads to conceptual inconsistencies. It is suggested here that nurses cannot switch their very beliefs according to the nature of the practice situation. What seems to be overlooked by Paterson and Zderad is that nurses can live according to human science beliefs and still perform tasks related to the execution of medical orders. There need not be the subject-subject, subject-object dilemma as espoused by these authors. Though Paterson and Zderad reflect on the inadequacy of the labelling process for capturing lived experiences, they accept the linear, causal nursing process and the diagnosing of human responses as necessary evils, required for economic reasons. Paterson and Zderad maintain that the natural science tradition is inappropriate for nursing, yet they do not reconcile the inconsistencies between reductionistic and unitary approaches with human beings.

Newman explicitly expresses a belief in the unitary nature of human beings, yet she also discusses the human being as a "system" made up of physiological structures and functions, such as the immune system and the genetic code, reflecting a natural science orientation. The unity of the human "system," for Newman, is predicated on the idea that "mind and matter are made of the same basic stuff" (1986a, p. 37). It is apparently quite appropriate within Newman's model to discuss the physiological, psychological, and emotional processes of the "human system" in conventional terms, so long as one remembers that everything, from the atom to the human being and beyond, is a manifestation of the implicate order, or "absolute consciousness" (pp. 33-37). Similarly, Watson (1985) maintains that the person is conceptualized as an irreducible whole, yet she repeatedly refers to body, mind, spirit and soul, and physical, emotional, and spiritual spheres. Her definitions of health and illness are dependent on the harmony or disharmony within these aspects. Watson also refers to several selves; the "real self," the "inner self," and the "ideal self" are presented as distinct entities. She refers to the "I" and the "Me" of the person and the potential disharmony of these aspects. It is not consistent to maintain that a person is a unitary whole and then to define the person according

to these separate parts or spheres. Dilthey (1977a) maintained that "we continually experience a sense of connectedness and totality in ourselves" (p. 53). The authors' struggles to incorporate the concept of the unitary human being into nursing theory and practice parallel a long and complex tradition of discourse in the human sciences.

Intentional Free-Willed Beings

Human science conceptualizes human beings as intentional and inherently free-willed; therefore the nurse would seek no more fundamental reference than the lived experience of the person. Paterson and Zderad (1988) address the *nurse's* intention and free will to commit authentically to another. The authors also regard the human being as free-willed, yet they suggest, "The nurse is alert to opportunities for the patient to exercise his [*sic*] freedom of choice within the limits of safe and sound practice" (p. 17). The nurse is guided to monitor the patient's choices and to determine if they are responsible ones. To carry out this monitoring, the nurse would have to rely on some schema of normative standards or beliefs in order to judge what is "responsible," which is an inconsistent practice if the nurse wishes to respect the human science belief that the individual is an intentional being possessing free will.

Newman's (1986a) conceptualization of freedom describes an arclike progression as consciousness expands. Human beings first *lose* freedom as they "come into being," are "bound in time" and "find . . . identity in space," until they reach a stage in which choice is engendered through movement (p. 46). "Restriction of movement forces one into a realm beyond space and time" (p. 62). Thereafter one throws off self-concerns, recognizes one's own "boundarylessness" and "timelessness" and *gains* the freedom of returning to "absolute consciousness" (p. 46). It is essentially the movement toward spirituality that imbues the human being with freedom, which is relative to the extent that consciousness is expanded.

The notion that human freedom underpins human science is quite different, in that freedom is never "lost," and there is no requisite for expanding consciousness to "gain" it. Human beings are believed to be free to choose meaning and direction because they make such choices continuously in living everyday life (Dilthey, 1988). "It is true," writes Dilthey (1988), "that the will depends on intellect, but the will can choose or not choose what the intellect understands . . . in fact the will is free precisely inasmuch as in it the search for a reason ends" (p. 270). Newman's (1986b) proposal for "the diagnosis of pattern" would appear to be hinged on her notion of freedom as relative to expanded consciousness. She states, "The role of the nurse within a paradigm of pattern is to help clients recognize their own patterns," a process in which a "burst of insight" occurs that "opens up" a "pathway of action" (pp. 55-56). From a human science perspective, by contrast, the pathway of action is always open.

Watson (1985) says that human beings are free to self-determine and free to choose. Nurses are guided to hold nonpaternalistic values which respect human autonomy and freedom. Yet this belief is violated in two ways. First, there are references to the nurse's helping, integrating, and "correcting" the patient's condition to increase harmony and to try to find meaning in the situation. Second, Watson maintains that "*ideally* [italics added], a person should have the opportunity for self-determination of the meaning of a health-illness experience *before professionals make decisions* [italics added] about treatments and interventions" (1985, p. 66). Human science philosophy abdicates the position of science as the arbiter of truth; the human scientist is a seeker of truth, a seeker rather than a dispenser of wisdom. Dilthey maintained that "under-

standing constitutes the goal of the human studies in the way that explanation defines the natural sciences" (cited in Makkreel, 1977, p. 7). Knowledge is not used or applied to the person, but rather knowledge enhances understanding for participating with the person in the process of becoming. Dilthey (1976) proposed, "In everything there is the same limitation of possibilities and yet freedom to choose between them, and the beautiful feeling of being able to move forward and to realize new potentialities in one's own existence" (p. 245).

The Nature of Reality

In a human science ontology, human beings and their worlds as experienced cannot be separated. Human science does not distinguish between subjective and objective realities because the focus of scientific activities is the humanly lived experience of the world, in which subjectivity is primal. Paterson and Zderad suggest that "nurses are drawn toward two realities—the reality of the objective scientific world and the reality of the subjective-objective world" (p. 36). The authors' endorsement of the traditional nursing process automatically places the person in the position of object and the nurse in the role of arbiter of truth. Again this reflects the conflicting views proposed with respect to the nurse-patient relationship.

Newman's (1986a) view of the nature of reality draws on Bohm's (1980) theory of the implicate order. All humanly experienced phenomena comprising the explicate order are posited as manifestations of an unseen, unknowable implicate order which comprises the unity of all that is. According to this view, patterns of human experience are reflective of this underlying primary reality. Newman writes, "We need to remind ourselves that our manifest reality is a small portion of the total enfoldment of the pattern in time-space

(1986a, p. 15). Her model theoretically eliminates the subject-object duality, according to its ontology. However, Newman's (1986a, 1986b) view is that neither objectivity nor subjectivity has any validity, since the perspective adapted from Bohm says there are no boundaries to (physical) reality. From a human science perspective, this is still essentially an objectivist reality, founded on the basis of the speculations of physical scientists that the nature of reality is a complex, multidimensional whole. The human being in such a model is defined by what physical science says about matter and energy. By contrast, human science directly asserts that human reality as lived is itself a complex multidimensional whole (Dilthey, 1977a).

The preeminence of the human experience is ostensibly highly valued in Watson's theory. She speaks of developing knowledge about the lived world of human experience and contends that the phenomenological research method is most congruent with her theoretical perspective. However, Watson distinguishes the person's experience of the world (phenomenal field) from the world as it actually is. For example, she proposes that nurses "help integrate the person's subjective experience and emotions with the objective external view of the situation" (Watson, 1985, p. 65). Watson also suggests that there can be incongruencies between the person and nature (world). For example, she states, "If a person does not feel congruent with mind, body, and soul . . . or rejects the self . . . or is obsessed with an ideal self, the person will be dissatisfied and maladjusted" (p. 57). These distinctions reveal a belief in an objective reality separate from the person's experience of it. This essentially dichotomous view is inconsistent with human science philosophy, in which being human means participating in the creation of reality. Human consciousness already is the unity of the person's subjective-objective relationship with the world; it is not some-

thing to be aspired to (Dilthey, 1977a). The use of the conventional subjective-objective constructs speaks to the exigencies of traditional science but is inconsistent with the understanding of humanly lived reality that underpins human science.

EXTENDING ESSENTIAL BELIEFS

In several instances within the frameworks examined, departures from the human science tradition were noted in areas where some congruence might be expected based on the overall presentation and central concepts. Paterson and Zderad (1988) move from focusing on the human being's lived experience to focusing on nurses' lived experiences and their descriptions of human beings. Both Newman (1986a) and Watson (1985) go well beyond the lived experience as the primal foundation of human knowledge by assigning higher order importance to metaphysical concepts.

It is clear that the basic empirical datum in Paterson and Zderad's humanistic nursing is the nurse's experience, "the between" of existentially experienced nursing situations. The authors address the importance of meanings, patterns, values, and themes, but it is not clear whose experiences are paramount, the nurse's or the patient's. Paterson and Zderad contend that nursing must be described phenomenologically, that nurses' descriptions of nursing situations with patients will build the knowledge and "make explicit a science of nursing" (1988, p. 3). This is a description of the practice of nursing, however, not of a nursing science based on the health experience of human beings. Giorgi (1985) proposed that a discipline is not ready-made in the world and simply viewed and studied. Rather, it is created by a unique knowledge base that is housed within its theories. Thus, to study the nursing act phenomenologically as Paterson and Zderad suggest is to study the particular nurse's view of nursing. It is suggested in this article that nursing science focuses on the concepts of human-environment and health, not the nurse's views of the between. To be consistent with the human science approach nurses must rely on the person's description as it is given, and not on what that experience is assumed to be. Paterson and Zderad's focus on the practitioner's experience reflects a serious departure from beliefs related to the practice of a human science, which investigates lived experiences and life expressions of human beings.

Human consciousness is an important concept in human science; it is the origin of all knowledge about lived experience (Dilthey, 1988). The ontology of Newman's theory is largely metaphysical, in that the key concept of "absolute consciousness" is beyond the realm of lived experience. Newman (1986a) ascribes consciousness to atoms, rocks, plants, animals, and unspecified "astral" and "spiritual" entities (pp. 33-37). In human science philosophy there is no way of knowing a more fundamental ground behind or beyond the lived experience of the person. One wonders why Newman (1986a), whose central thesis is "health as expanding consciousness," has completely ignored continental European philosophy and theory on consciousness throughout her work. Instead, Newman cites works of speculative physics as underpinning her theory, even when addressing human experience. Dilthey (1977a) maintained that "consciousness cannot go behind itself" (p. 75). It is the structure of consciousness that sheds light on the coherent unity of human life.

In human science, humanly lived experiences elaborated in thinking, feeling, and willing are the complex whole of reality. Watson emphasizes the significance of human experience as it is lived. However, her emphasis on the metaphysical, spiritual realm clouds

the issue of the primacy of lived experience. Watson (1985) states that "the human soul is more than physical, mental, emotional existence . . . the soul exists for something larger than physical life" (p. 45). She maintains, "The soul, inner self, spiritual self is tied to a higher degree of consciousness . . . that transcends time and space" (p. 46). This soul, which "may be underdeveloped and in need of reawakening" (p. 45), reflects a reality beyond that which is directly experienced by human beings and is in conflict with the purported human science origins of Watson's theory.

Watson explicitly presents her framework as emerging from the human science paradigm. Paterson and Zderad refer to their work as humanistic, a related term but not synonymous with human science. Although the concepts Newman uses are abundantly addressed in human science, the ontology underpinning her theory is derived instead from speculative physics. The selective extraction of inconsistencies with the human science paradigm in these authors' works is not intended to suggest a failing on their part but is intended to foster greater conceptual clarity and is offered in the spirit of scholarly questioning and debate. The purpose of this analysis was to determine to what extent the values and beliefs of the human science paradigm were currently evident in nursing's extant knowledge base. The authors conclude that the human science tradition is present to varying degrees in nursing science.

Of the four theories explored here, Parse's (1981, 1987, 1990a) theory of human becoming remained consistent with the fundamental ontology and epistemology of the human science tradition. The theory can be seen to have expanded and clarified major ideas of the human science tradition. Parse's (1981) work was the first publication in nursing to specify nursing as a human science in Dilthey's traditional sense. Parse's theory is analyzed here with regard to both its adherence to and expansion of the human science tradition.

PARSE'S THEORY OF HUMAN BECOMING

Parse's first chapter begins, "To posit the idea of nursing rooted in the human sciences is to make explicit an alternative to the traditional practice of nursing as a medical model grounded in the natural sciences" (1981, p. 3). Parse describes nursing as a human science focusing on the unitary human being's experience of living and creating health, and she cites Dilthey in her explication of the concepts of her theory. She states that the methodologies of human sciences focus on "uncovering the meaning of phenomena as humanly experienced" and "on understanding the connectedness of life itself," (1981, p. 11). Dilthey (1977b) suggested that explicating human interrelatedness connects that which is universally human with that which is individual.

Parse (1981) synthesized concepts from Rogers' (1970) science of unitary human beings and tenets of contemporary existential phenomenology in such a way that the fundamental notion of human science proposed by Dilthey was brought to fruition for nursing science in the theory of human becoming. The tenets of human subjectivity and intentionality, and the concepts of human coexistence, coconstitution, and situated freedom, drawn from existential phenomenology, reflect the development of ideas germinated by Dilthey and others in the philosophy of human science. The synthesis of concepts from Rogers' work with concepts from existential phenomenology to form a unique, coherent theory of nursing underscores the compelling fit between human science philosophy and nursing as a unique and autonomous discipline. Parse (1987) avoided conceptual inconsistencies by inventing nursing practice and research methodologies which flow directly from the ontological and epistemological foundations of her theory. In this way there is no need to reconcile human science beliefs with biomedical traditions. Parse's theory and her practice and research methodologies express and structure the beliefs which underpin human science in a new way specifically for nursing science.

Parse's (1981, 1987, 1990a) theory of human becoming has three central themes: meaning, rhythmicity, and cotranscendence. Her explication of these themes moves her theory beyond human science as described by Dilthey (1961). Parse describes the human being as an open unity who freely chooses meaning in situations, bears responsibility for choices, and co-constitutes with the environment rhythmical patterns of relating in the process of co-transcending with emerging possibilities. Health is described as a "process of becoming, a cocreated process of living value priorities" (1981, p. 31). Health is the day-to-day living of rhythmical patterns reflecting the person's unfolding and co-transcending with the possibles (the moving onward in life in a chosen way) (Parse, 1981).

The goal of practice in Parse's theory is the quality of life from the person's perspective (1987). Nurses in true presence with people live the practice method, which revolves around the all-at-once of illuminating meaning through "explicating," synchronizing rhythms through "dwelling with," and mobilizing transcendence through "moving beyond" (1987, p. 167). Parse's research method is rooted in phenomenology and is structured to be congruent with the assumptions and principles of the human becoming theory. It focuses on uncovering the structures of universal lived experiences in the human-universe-health interrelationship. The goal of the method is to enhance understanding of lived experiences of health.

CRITIQUE OF THE THEORY OF HUMAN BECOMING

Parse presents her theory as emerging from the human science paradigm and she remains congruent with those philosophical underpinnings throughout her work. The human being is viewed as unitary, mutually interrelating with environment, and there is no reference to human beings other than as living unities. The person's lived experience is clearly regarded as the preeminent ground of human health. The researcher explores universal lived experiences of health, with the goal of enhancing understanding. This is consistent with Dilthey's concern "to understand life as it is lived by man" (Ermath, 1978, p. 17). Both the research and practice methods focus on the lived experience of human beings. There is no subject-object dichotomy; reality is viewed as cocreated with the universe and others while experienced uniquely by the person. Nursing is seen as a scientific discipline in which the concepts of unitary human beings, mutual unfolding, human coexistence, intentionality, free will, and intersubjective sharing of meaning may at last be fully elaborated and incorporated in praxis. Dilthey consistently maintained that all theory was theory for praxis (Ermath, 1978).

Parse suggests that persons "unfold with contemporaries the ideas of predecessors . . . in a continuity that connects past with future" (1981, p. 26). The "way the person lives in interrelationship with others reflects chosen meanings and reveals cherished values" (1981, p. 48). Individuals freely choose the meaning of situations and freely live personal values by choosing ways of being/becoming from among possibilities. Again, this is consistent with Dilthey's (1961) view of human interconnectedness, yet it goes beyond his view.

Guided by Parse's theory, the nurse in true presence with the person focuses on the individual's own meaning without judging, labeling, or trying to change the person. The nurse goes with the person as he or she explores options, images consequences of choices, and plans to live hopes and dreams. In the true presence of the nurse the individual clarifies the meaning of the situation and new meanings are uncovered; new insights generate new possibles, the understanding of opportunities and limitations in light of what is truly valued. The nurse coparticipates with the person in the process of moving beyond the now moment, guided by the theory to understand that the person chooses his or her own way (Parse, 1987). Parse maintains that individuals know their own way, reflectively and prereflectively. The nurse in true presence bears witness to the person's unfolding and becoming (Parse, 1990b). In creating the theory of human becoming, Parse has uncovered the intrinsic relevance of the human science perspective, which is centrally concerned with what it means to be human for the discipline of nursing.

In Parse's (1987) research methodology, the researcher "lives" dialogical engagements with participants. This is described as "an intersubjective being with, in which the researcher and participant live the I-Thou process as they move through an unstructured discussion about the lived experience" (1987, p. 176). The researcher views the participant as the expert on the lived experience being explored and remains focused on the phenomenon as it is revealed by the person. The researcher participates in generating enhanced understanding of the phenomenon by creatively abstracting the structure of the lived experience in the language of science.

In summary, Parse's theory, intentionally structured as a human science theory of nursing, accurately reflects the ontology and epistemology of human science philosophy. Parse's theory lays a foundation for a nursing science that is grounded in the meaning of lived experiences in the human-universe process. The theory focuses on the lived experience of unitary human beings in continuous interrelationship with their worlds. Reality as perceived by the person is not compared to an "objective" reality but is respected, as is the free will of the person, in choosing ways of becoming. Parse's theory is thus congruent with yet goes beyond the ontology and epistemology of human science as posited in this article and is an emergent, a newly created theory for praxis that uncompromisingly incorporates the beliefs of human science into nursing research and practice.

CONCLUSION

Nursing science is currently undergoing change as new views emerge which challenge the traditional methods of natural science-based, biomedical nursing. The human science paradigm is one such view. This perspective is surfacing in nursing at a time when nurse scholars are questioning the precepts of the natural science paradigm and, in doing so, are expressing many of the concerns which led Dilthey to propose a different approach to human science over a hundred years ago. It has been suggested in this article that the human science tradition is not merely any study of human beings, but a particular way of studying human life which values the lived experience of unitary persons and seeks to understand life in all its interwoven patterns of meanings and values.

Nurse scientists are defining boundaries and seeking knowledge which is unique to nursing. This knowledge is currently organized in conceptual and theoretical frameworks, some of which reflect the values and beliefs of the human science paradigm. Of the four frameworks explored here, one, Parse's theory of human becoming. was found not only to be congruent with but to go beyond the human science perspective. The other three frameworks, Paterson and Zderad's humanistic nursing, Newman's model of expand-

ing consciousness, and Watson's human science and human care, demonstrated both consistencies and inconsistencies with the philosophy of human science. Continued explication of the assumptions, values, and beliefs which underpin different theoretical approaches is needed, so that nurses can understand with depth and clarity the foundations of the unique knowledge base of nursing. Only through contemplative consideration of the philosophical basis of the extant body of theory and through open critique and discourse can nurses choose which paths to follow in the quest for knowledge.

REFERENCES

Bohm, D. (1980). *Wholeness and the implicate order*. London: Routledge.

Connors, D. (1988). A continuum of researcher-participant relationships: An analysis and critique. *Advances in Nursing Science, 10*(4), 32-42.

Dilthey, W. (1961). *Pattern and meaning in history: Thoughts on history and society* (H.P. Rickman, Ed. and Trans.). New York: Harper & Row.

———. (1976). *Selected writings* (H.P. Rickman, Trans.). Cambridge: Cambridge University Press.

———. (1977a). Ideas concerning a descriptive and analytic psychology. (Original work published 1894). In R.M. Zaner & K.L. Heiges (Trans.), *Descriptive psychology and historical understanding* (pp. 23-120). The Hague. Netherlands: Nijhoff.

———. (1977b) The understanding of other persons and their expressions of life. (Original work published 1927). In R.M. Zaner & K.L. Heiges (Trans.), *Descriptive psychology and historical understanding* (pp. 123-144). The Hague, Netherlands: Nijhoff.

———. (1988). *Introduction to the human sciences* (R. J. Betanzos, Trans.). Detroit: Wayne State University Press. (Original work published 1883)

Ermath, M. (1978). *Wilhelm Dilthey: The critique of historical reason*. Chicago: University of Chicago Press.

Gadamer, H.G. (1976). *Philosophical hermeneutics* (D.E. Linge. Trans.). Berkeley: University of California Press.

Geertz, C. (1973). *The interpretation of cultures*. New York: Basic Books.

Giorgi, A. (1970). *Psychology as a human science*. New York: Harper & Row.

———. (1971). Phenomenology and experimental psychology: II. In A. Giorgi. W. Fischer & R. von Eckartsberg (Eds.), *Duquesne studies in phenomenological psychology*, (Vol. l, pp. 3-29). Pittsburgh, PA: Duquesne University Press.

———. (1985). Sketch of a psychological phenomenological method. In A. Giorgi (Ed.), *Phenomenology and psychological research* (pp. 8-22). Pittsburgh: Duquesne University Press.

Gortner, S.R., & Schultz, P.R. (1988). Approaches to nursing science methods. *Image: Journal of Nursing Scholarship, 20,* 22-24.

Heidegger, M. (1962). *Being and time* (J. Macquarrie & E. Robinson, Trans.). New York: Harper & Row.

Makkreel, R.A. (1977). Introduction. In R.M. Zaner & K.L. Heiges (Trans.), *Descriptive psychology and historical understanding* (pp. 1-20). The Hague. Netherlands: Nijhoff.

Meleis, A. (1990, September). *Directions for nursing theory development.* Paper presented at the National Nursing Theory Conference, Los Angeles, CA.

Munhall, P. (1989). Philosophical ponderings on qualitative research methods in nursing. *Nursing Science Quarterly, 2,* 20-28.

Newman, M. (1986a). *Health as expanding consciousness.* St. Louis: Mosby.

———. (1986b). Nursing's emerging paradigm: The diagnosis of pattern. In A. M. McLane (Ed.), *Classification of nursing diagnoses: Proceedings of the seventh conference.* St. Louis: Mosby.

———. (1990). Newman's theory of health as praxis. *Nursing Science Quarterly, 3,* 37-41.

Parse, R.R (1981). *Man-living-health: A theory of nursing.* New York: Wiley.

———. (1987). *Nursing science: Major paradigms, theories and critiques.* Philadelphia: Saunders.

———. (1990a, September). [Speaker on] *Panel of nursing theorists.* National Nursing Theory Conference, Los Angeles, CA.

———. (1990b). Health: A personal commitment. *Nursing Science Quarterly, 3,* 136-140.

Paterson, J.G., & Zderad, L.T. (1988). *Humanistic nursing.* New York: National League for Nursing.

Polkinghorne, D. (1983). *Methodology for the human sciences: Systems of inquiry.* Albany: State University of New York Press.

Ricoeur, P. (1974). *The conflict of interpretations: Essays in hermeneutics* (W. Domingo et al., Trans.). Evanston, IL: Northwestern University Press.

Rogers, M.E. (1970). *An introduction to the theoretical basis of nursing.* Philadelphia: Davis.

Schutz, A. (1967). *The phenomenology of the social world* (G. Walsh & F. Lehnert, Trans.). Evanston, IL: Northwestern University Press.

Watson, J. (1985). *Nursing: Human science and human care.* Norwalk, CT: Appleton-Century-Crofts.

Webster's ninth new collegiate dictionary. (1985). Springfield, MA: Merriam-Webster.

Winch, P. (1958). *The idea of a social science and its relation to philosophy.* London: Routledge & Kegan Paul.

26

Esthetic and Personal Knowing through Humanistic Nursing

DIANNE PELLETIER RAYMOND

Carper (1978) discussed four fundamental patterns of knowing in nursing:

1. empirics, the science of nursing;
2. ethics;
3. personal knowledge; and
4. esthetics, the art of nursing.

Paterson and Zderad's (1976) humanistic nursing model offers a methodology for fostering the development of knowledge through personal and esthetic patterns. Empirical science cannot adequately address all phenomena encountered in nursing. Nursing is concerned with such human experiences as suffering, guilt, anger, hopelessness, and fear. The phenomenological approach proposed by Paterson and Zderad (1976) provides the nurse with a method to attend to lived experiences such as these. Phenomenology, however, can neither replace other measures of inquiry in nursing nor account for all its goals (Oiler, 1982). The purpose of this paper is to briefly describe Paterson and Zderad's phenomenological approach, to offer a commentary on McKinnon's 1991 article related to humanistic nursing, to explore a specific nursing situation utilizing the hu-

manistic nursing paradigm, and to advocate use of the model in qualitative research and theory development.

HUMANISTIC NURSING MODEL DESCRIBES LIVED EXPERIENCES

The humanistic nursing model (depicted in the figure "Humanistic Nursing Model"), as proposed by Paterson and Zderad (1976), has its own phenomenological methodology for describing lived experiences. The authors call their approach phenomenological nursology. According to Paterson and Zderad (1976), phenomenological nursology is a medium through which concept and theory development can take place.

Phenomenologic nursology is comprised of five phases. The first four phases involve assessment and the final phase is analogous to the nursing diagnosis. The lived experience as viewed by the patient unfolds through the therapeutic relationship itself. The phases are identified as follows (Paterson & Zderad, 1976):

- Phase I: Preparation of the nurse knower for coming to know (the patient).

Source: Raymond, D. P., (1995) Esthetic and personal knowing through humanistic nursing. *N&HC: Perspectives on community* 16 (6): 332–336. Reprinted with permission by from the National League for Nursing

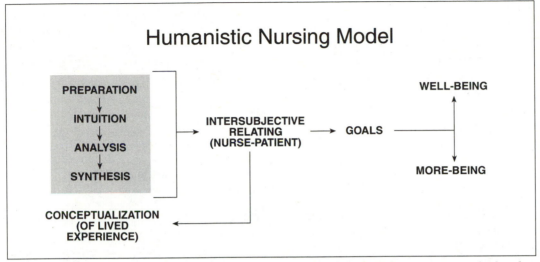

Figure 26-1. Model depicts Humanistic Nursing Framework developed by Paterson and Zderad (1976) as viewed by author.

- Phase II: Nurse knowing the other (the patient) intuitively.
- Phase III: Nurse knowing the other (the patient) scientifically.
- Phase IV: Nurse complementarily synthesizing known others.
- Phase V: Succession within the nurse from the many to the paradoxical one (conclusion).

McKinnon (1991) contended that Paterson and Zderad's model offered neither guidelines for administering patient care nor a means of evaluating its effectiveness. Further, the author stated that a main weakness of the model is its failure to hold the nurse accountable for the quality of patient care. One may argue that the nurse who does not also consider the lived experience of the patient in approach to care may not be totally accountable to the patient. Without a consideration of needs as the patient views it, there is a danger of addressing needs only from an outsider's perspective, which may be narrow or inaccurate. Further, one may argue that fostering the kind of relationship necessary for understanding the world view of

the patient may potentially enhance the quality of patient care delivered. The ethical dictum of phenomenology is the imperative to turn to the people who actually live the experience (Swanson-Kauffman & Schonwald, 1988).

It is important to note that the humanistic model is at a descriptive level in theory development (Brouse & Laffrey, 1989). The aim of the model is to describe the human experience as it is lived by the patient. The model does not attempt to predict or to control nursing phenomena. In other words, the model does not claim to provide all of the guidelines necessary in administering nursing care. According to Brouse and Laffrey (1989), "The phenomenological method is complementary to but operates at qualitatively different levels from empirical science" (p. 207). Empirical science provides a view which is logically deduced, while phenomenology emphasizes the view of the subject (the lived experience). One view should not necessarily discount the other, but may be seen as a complement to the other. Thus, the phenomenological approach attempts to address questions that cannot be answered by empirical science.

The following paragraphs illustrate the application of the humanistic nursing model to a clinical situation in order to demonstrate its usefulness in practice. "Elise" was a patient who I encountered while working as a staff nurse on a psychiatric unit.

CLINICAL SITUATION AS LIVED BY "ELISE"

Elise was a 17-year-old woman of Acadian descent living in a rural community. Elise was referred to the psychiatric unit via the helpline by her mother, who had noted progressive withdrawal in Elise and failing grades in school. Elise lived at home with her mother and her brothers. Her father had died five years prior to the admission. She had been very close to her father. Elise's conversations with her mother were obsessed with thoughts of her father's death and God. She was described as reclusive to her room. Upon admission, Elise made it obvious to all staff that she did not want to be there with much crying and expressions of anger. She experienced auditory hallucinations. Her affect was flat with a mask-like expression on her face. She would sit for hours at a time looking straight ahead, immersed in her own world. Elise was tried on antipsychotic medication with little initial response. After one week on the psychiatric unit, she began to verbalize paranoid delusions of staff wishing to "lock" her up forever and the food being "poisoned." She began to gag on her food and medication and reported nausea. Her appearance further deteriorated.

PHASE I: PREPARATION OF THE NURSE FOR COMING TO KNOW

Through my years of nursing experience and years of education, as well as life experiences, I have prepared myself for coming to know the human condition. Through these experiences, I have developed the ability to empathize—to experience the feelings of another. The key to practice utilizing phenomenology is to have a nurse who is willing to operate in a methodology that mandates an investment of the personal self (Swanson-Kauffman & Schonwald, 1988). The outcome depends on the nurse's ability to engage in another's reality in an empathic sense. I had attended a case review where all the disciplines involved in Elise's care discussed her lack of progress. I was assigned to work with Elise. The most recent subjective data from her chart contained statements such as "I want to go home now!" and "I'm not getting better here." The chart noted that she was only sleeping two or three hours per night. I chose a time when Elise was sitting quietly in the solarium to approach her, respecting her need to maintain the distance between us. I approached her openly, leaving all of the accumulated data base behind—e.g., DSM-III-R diagnosis and increasing distrustful and aggressive behavior. A nurse that can be open provides a model for the patient (Berger, 1977). By approaching Elise openly, I encouraged her to be open with me. I introduced myself to Elise as her staff person for the day.

PHASE II: NURSE KNOWING OTHER INTUITIVELY

After a few superficial exchanges, Elise identified me as an authority figure on the unit and as a person who gave her medication. She proceeded to tell me that she felt that staff was deceiving her. She stated, "They tell me that if I take the medication that I'll get better and then I can go home. I think they tell me that so I'll take it. I don't want to take the medication. It will make me sick." I responded by providing Elise with a brief explanation of her medication and the symptoms that needed to be controlled before discharge was possible.

This was the beginning of an intersubjective relationship with Elise. I intuitively grasped her situation—allowed myself to feel what she must be feeling. Elise was losing her sense of contact with the people and the things in her world. She felt that she was forced into the hospital and forced into strange routines. She was eating unfamiliar food and ingesting medications which she was unaccustomed to taking and had equated to making her feel ill. I allowed myself to experience the situation subjectively through her world view. Hospitalization was an identifiable source of stress for Elise. I experienced the apprehension that arises from being separated from familiar people, personal possessions, and the safety and security of home.

PHASE III: NURSE KNOWING OTHER SCIENTIFICALLY

I reflected on what I knew of Elise intuitively and examined the experience objectively. During our dialogue, I had observed her dilated pupils, her look of bewilderment, her trembling hands, and her guarded, withdrawn manner. I recalled the elevated vital signs and nausea. I analyzed the available data.

PHASE IV: NURSE COMPLEMENTARILY SYNTHESIZING KNOWN OTHERS

I compared Elise's experience with that of other patients with similar symptoms and with what I had read in the literature. I recalled what Gibson described as a "need/fear dilemma" (Berger, 1977). Patients who are out of touch with reality need others desperately to strengthen their inadequate egos. Yet they feel threatened by others and find it hard to main-

tain a clear picture of reality. Thus, they may try to avoid other people to escape their feeling of being engulfed by them, which explains the withdrawal that they manifest (Berger, 1977).

PHASE V: SUCCESSION WITHIN THE NURSE FROM THE MANY TO THE PARADOXICAL ONE

In relating to Elise's experience, I concluded that she was experiencing the phenomenon of fear. Once isolated, the nursing diagnosis of fear can be approached via the nursing process. McKinnon (1991) contended that the humanistic nursing process does not include the development of a plan of care or mutual goal setting with patients of any age. Humanistic nursing practice, however, does call for intersubjective relating where the patient expects to be helped and the nurse expects to give help (Paterson & Zderad, 1976). The plan includes the establishment of a therapeutic relationship which forms the basis of all other treatment that follows. The plan of care utilizing the humanistic model may be supplemented by other theories and approaches. Although phenomenological nursology, an empathic approach, continued to be an important therapeutic approach with Elise, an interdisciplinary treatment approach was critical to her care as well, which included the collaborative efforts between nursing, psychiatry, occupational therapy, social worker, and dietician. The treatment approach focused on reassuring her of her safety.

PLANNING INVOLVES THE PATIENT IN MAKING RESPONSIBLE CHOICES

The effectiveness of the phenomenological approach with Elise was validated through her admission of fear and through direct observation of her behavior. She did not react with hostility. She stated her agreement to continue to take the medication. She acknowledged that she was hearing voices and that she wanted them to go away. Through continued intersubjective encounters with Elise, combined with the other treatment modalities, one could notice a gradual improvement in her mental status. She stayed on the unit for a total of two months. As she was able to relax and to see her own progress; the aggressive behavior disappeared. She began to show trust in staff and to actively involve herself in unit activities. Her affect improved markedly. Although the planning, implementation, and evaluation stages of the nursing process are not directly addressed by Paterson and Zderad, these stages may be inferred. The planning involved eliciting the active involvement of the patient in making responsible choices. The therapeutic relationship that was one of collaboration not only was an important intervention, but facilitated the implementation of other treatment modalities. Evaluation occurred through validation with the patient. The goal of well-being was met through Elise's steady improvement in mental status and her participation in health maintenance behaviors. She was discharged from the hospital and returned to live with her family. As long as Elise can be functional and maintained within the community, there can be continual movement toward the goal of more-being or the maximization of her human potential.

PHILOSOPHY OF SCIENCE AND NURSING THEORY ARE IN A "STATE OF TRANSITION"

Traditionally, logical empiricism with its quantitative methodologies has dominated theory development and testing (Silva & Rothbart, 1984). However, the philosophy of science and nursing theory are in a "state of transition" (Silva & Rothbart, p. 294). According to

Silva and Rothbart (1984), a new philosophy of science known as historicism has emerged. While logical empiricism provides a logical explanation of the nature of scientific knowledge, historicism is a philosophy of science that provides a historical explanation (Silva & Rothbart, 1984). According to Silva and Rothbart, historicists attempt to understand science in terms of research traditions. The authors defined a research tradition as "a broadly based foundation of many theories and [as] an accepted way of viewing fundamental phenomena within a discipline" (p. 295). Further, the authors noted that research traditions are global and changeable within the boundaries of an ontological commitment or nature of being. According to these authors, a methodological commitment which defines the legitimate method of inquiry suitable to a research tradition's ontology is essential. For example, Silva and Rothbart (1984) questioned whether the case study method of inquiry may be better suited to the ontological commitment of holism than a traditional experimental design method of inquiry with its built-in reductionism. Theories based on research traditions view the person as a holistic being as opposed to looking at parts. Thus, according to the authors, the logical empiricists with their deductive approach emphasize science as product, whereas, the historicists place emphasis on science as process.

In addition to the shift in the philosophy of science espoused in the nursing literature, Silva & Rothbart (1984) identified a shift in emphasis from quantitative to qualitative methodologies as another trend. Grounded theory research is an example of a current break from tradition. In grounded theory research, the researcher becomes immersed in the world of the research subject (Bowers, 1988). According to Bowers, the researcher attempts to discover how subjects experience their world. Through bracketing, researchers are able to temporarily relinquish their perspectives and assume the perspective of the research subject (Bowers, 1988). The similarity between grounded theory research and the phenomenological approach proposed by Paterson and Zderad is clearly evident. Moreover, there are other methodologies such as ethnomethodology and ethnography that employ a strategy which allows researchers to apprehend experiences as they are perceived by those who live them (Swanson-Kauffman & Schonwald, 1988).

Further, Silva and Rothbart (1984) suggested that historicism and alternative research methodologies hold promise in helping to bridge the gap to contend with phenomena dealing with humanism and holism. Thus, phenomenological nursology may serve as a valuable tool for qualitative research and for the identification of concepts and further theory development.

Interestingly, Paterson and Zderad published their conceptual framework in 1976, but their model received little attention in the nursing literature (Silva & Rothbart, 1984). Silva and Rothbart (1984) speculated that this may be due to its existential-phenomenological perspective and ontological commitment, which was out of the mainstream of current thinking about philosophy of science at that time. Thus, Paterson and Zderad's humanistic nursing model reflected progressive thinking in keeping with the historicist philosophy.

The humanistic nursing model must not be dismissed due to its unique perspective and nontraditional approach. The model serves as a valuable framework in the development of knowledge through esthetic and personal patterns of knowing. Empathy is an important mode in the esthetic pattern of knowing (Carper, 1978). Further, through the "therapeutic use of self," the nurse develops personal knowledge. Without question, phenomenological nursology is an empathic process which requires the "therapeutic use of self." More-

over, Carper (1978) stated that the more skilled the nurse becomes in empathizing, the more knowledge will be gained in alternative perceptions of reality.

According to Chinn and Kramer (1991), there should be an integration of all patterns of knowing. The authors suggested that there has been little attention given to developing forms of expression for personal and esthetic knowing. Further, they asserted that all patterns of knowing are legitimate sources of knowledge for a collective body of nursing knowledge and for nursing practice.

HUMANISTIC NURSING COMPLEMENTS OTHER APPROACHES IN PATIENT CARE

There is no one theory that serves as a panacea for all nursing problems. All paradigms have their particular strengths and weaknesses. A model is neither all good nor all bad. The phenomenological approach serves as a form of expression for the development of knowledge acquired through esthetic and personal patterns of knowing. The humanistic nursing approach complements other approaches in patient care. It offers a philosophical framework in the therapeutic nurse-patient relationship. Further, the model provides a methodology for qualitative research and for describing human phenomenon derived directly from the lived experiences of patients which is important to clinical nursing practice.

REFERENCES

Berger, M. (1977). *Working with people called patients.* New York, NY: Brunner/Mazel Publishers.

Bowers, B.J. (1988). Grounded theory. In B.S. Sarter (ed.), *Paths to knowledge* (pp. 33–59). New York, NY: National League for Nursing Press.

Brouse, S.H., & Laffrey, S.C. (1989). Paterson and Zderad's humanistic nursing framework. In J.J. Fitzpatrick & A.L. Whall, *Conceptual models of nursing: Analysis and application* (2nd ed.). Norwalk, CT: Appleton and Lange.

Carper, B.A. (1978). Fundamental patterns of knowing in nursing. *Adv Nurs Sci*, 1(1): 13–24.

Chinn, P.L., & Kramer, M.K. (1991). Nursing's patterns of knowing. *Theory and nursing: A systematic approach* (3rd ed.). St. Louis, MO: Mosby-Year Book.

McKinnon, N.C. (1991). Humanistic nursing: It can't stand up to scrutiny. *Nursing and Health Care*, 12(8): 414–416.

Oiler, C. (1982). The phenomenological approach in nursing research. *Nursing Research*, 31(3): 178–181.

Paterson, J., & Zderad, L. (1976). *Humanistic nursing*. New York, NY: John Wiley & Sons, Inc.

Silva, M.C., & Rothbart, D. (1984). An analysis of changing trends in philosophies of science on nursing theory development and testing. In L.H. Nicoll (ed.), *Perspectives on nursing theory* (pp. 293–302). Glenview, IL: Scott, Foresman and Company.

Swanson-Kauffman, K., & Schonwald, E. (1988). Phenomenology. In B.S. Sarter (ed.), *Paths to knowledge* (pp. 97–105). New York, NY: National League for Nursing.

27

Nursing: The Ontology of the Discipline

PAMELA G. REED, RN, PhD, FAAN

The purpose of this article is to contribute to clarifying the ontology of the discipline by extending existing meanings of the term nursing *to propose a substantive definition. In this definition, nursing is viewed as an inherent human process of well-being, manifested by complexity and integration in human systems. The nature of this process and theoretical implications of the new nursing are presented. Nurses are invited to continue the dialogue about the meaning of the term and explore the implications of nursing, substantively defined, for their practice and science. [Keywords: Deconstruction, Knowledge development, Metaparadigm, Ontology, Postmodernism]*

Distinguishing the term *nursing* as a noun from its use as a verb was put forth most profoundly by Rogers (1970), whose vision extended the scholarship of earlier nursing theorists to thrust nursing forward to be recognized as both a scientific discipline as well as a professional practice. It is time, however, to push back the frontier once again, beyond these two important understandings of nursing, by proposing a new meaning of nursing. With this new meaning, the term itself represents the nature and substance of the discipline. In other words, *nursing* is the ontology of the discipline.

The ideas put forth here are done so in the spirit of accepting Watson's (1995) "postmodern challenge" to exploit the climate of deconstruction of nursing (see Rampragus, 1995; Reed, 1995) to extend and, by some degree, reconstruct current understandings of nursing. Smith's (1988a) article outlined the ongoing dialogue about two meanings of nursing, as a verb and a noun. This dialogue is revisited here for the purpose of further clarifying what is the ontology of the discipline, long considered a crucial question by seminal thinkers in nursing (Ellis, 1982; Rogers, 1970; Roy, 1995).

CONTINUING THE DIALOGUE: NURSING AS A PROCESS OF WELL-BEING

It is proposed here that there exists a third and perhaps most basic definition of nursing in which nursing represents the *substantive* focus of the discipline. Disciplines are characterized by their substantive focus: archaeology is the study of the archaeo, or what is ancient and primitive; astronomy is the study of the astro, astronomical phenomena such as the motion and constitution of celestial bodies; biology is a branch of knowledge about biol, or living matter; chemistry deals with the processes and

Source: Reed, P. (1997). Nursing: The ontology of the discipline. *Nursing Science Quarterly.* 10(2):76–79. Reprinted with permission by from Chestnut House Publications.

properties of chemical substances; physics is the study of physical properties and processes; psychology is the study of the psyche, referring to mental processes and activities associated with human behavior; and nursing, the discipline, is proposed here to be the study of nursing processes of well-being, inherent among human systems.

This meaning of nursing, as an inherent process of well-being, derives in part from the root word, nurse, defined as a process of nourishing, of promoting the development or progress of something. The meaning also derives from synonyms of nurse meaning to heal, to foster, to sustain (Laird, 1971; *Webster's New Collegiate Dictionary*, 1979). These descriptions signify that nursing involves a process that is developmental, progressive, and sustaining, and by which well-being occurs.

The Inherent Nursing Process

The theme of human beings' inherent nursing processes as the substantive focus of the discipline is supported in nursing theorists' works from Nightingale in 1859, to the mid-20th century writings of Henderson, to the contemporary turn-of-the-century ideas of Schlotfeldt. Nightingale (1859/1969) wrote about the person's "innate power" and the inner "reparative process." Henderson (1964) eloquently symbolized the power of the nurse within, describing nursing as "the consciousness of the unconscious, the love of life of the suicidal, . . . the eyes of the newly blind, a means of locomotion for the infant, . . . the voice for those too weak or withdrawn to speak" (p. 63). Watson (1985) referred to "self-healing processes," and Schlotfeldt (1994) stressed human beings' "inherent ability and propensity to seek and attain health." In addition, this nursing process is not necessarily based upon a reversal of a disease process, but more upon a moving forward, to

gain a sense of well-being in the absence or presence of disease.

The discipline's understanding of how a nursing process is manifested is shifting away from the mid-20th century mechanistic conception of nursing as a process external to patients and conducted by the nurse, that is, the old nursing process. The process of nursing is viewed now more from a relational perspective, congruent with contextual and transformative conceptions of the world (see Newman, 1992; Pepper, 1942). Nursing is a participatory process that transcends the boundary between patient and nurse and derives from a valuing of what Rogers (1980, 1992) described as human systems' inherent propensity for "innovation and creative change."

"Human systems" refers to an individual or a group of human beings (Rogers, 1992, p. 30). As such, human systems, whether in the form of individuals, dyads, groups, or communities, emanate and participate in nursing processes. Nursing processes may be manifested, for example, in the grieving that an individual experiences, in the caring that occurs among people and their families and nurses, in the healing practices shared by a culture, or in many other as yet undiscovered patterns of nursing. Today, these patterns may be described as intentional or unconscious, automatic or contemplative, relational or chemical, or simply unknown. Nevertheless, with continued nursing research, education, and practice, nursing processes can be learned and knowingly deployed to facilitate well-being. Murphy's (1992) visionary book, for example, addresses some of these possibilities. He proposes a future wherein people are more aware of their innate healing potential and employ it to more purposefully enhance health.

Nightingale did not invent nursing, described here in terms of an inherent propensity for well-being. Just as earthquakes existed before geologists and photosynthesis before botanists, nursing processes existed in human beings, ultimately described by Nightingale (1859/1969) as that which nurses were to facilitate by placing the patient in the best situation possible. It follows, then, that nursing does not belong exclusively to certain groups of people, such as "well" persons or professional nurses; it belongs to human nature.

Defining the substance of the discipline of nursing in terms of a well-being process inherent among human beings does not negate the importance of knowledge of factors that interface with nursing to influence well-being and healing. Examples of these factors, often the focus of study in ancillary professions and disciplines, include the environmental, financial, cultural, surgical, and pharmacological. However, any sense of well-being involves, most basically, a nursing process. The quest for nursing is to understand the nature of and to facilitate nursing processes in diverse contexts of health experiences.

The Nature of Nursing Processes

What is the nature of nursing processes that distinguishes them from other human processes? It is proposed that the intersection of at least three characteristics—complexity, integration, well-being—distinguishes human processes as nursing; specifically, nursing processes are manifested by changes in complexity and integration that generate well-being. Importantly, other distinguishing characteristics of nursing processes may be identified as the dialogue continues beyond this article.

This new understanding of the nature of nursing processes derived from various theorists' work, such as von Bertalanffy's (1981) systems view of human beings; Rogers' (1970, 1992) science of unitary human beings; Lerner's (1986) developmental contextualism; and complexity theory (see Kauffman, 1995; Waldrop, 1992). While the translation of these theorists' ideas may not be entirely congruent

with those presented here, their ideas nonetheless can help inform development of a new nursing ontology.

Human beings are viewed as open, living systems and not as passive but intrinsically active and innovative. As an open system, human systems are capable of self-organizing, where *self* refers to the system as a whole. Self-organization is an inherent capacity for generating qualitative change out of ongoing events in the life of a system and its environment.

In his seminal work on development, Werner (1957) explained this process of qualitative change as his "orthogenetic principle," which posits that living organisms change over time from lower to higher levels of differentiation and integration. Werner (1957) called this change "development," in contrast to mechanistic processes of change, which are not developmental.

Similarly, Rogers' (1980) principles of homeodynamics describe the inherent innovative patterning of change that occurs in open systems, both environmental and human. Her three principles of helicy, resonancy, and integrality together depict the nature of qualitative change in human beings in terms of ongoing movement from lower to higher levels of diversity.

Complexity theorists (for example, Kauffman, 1995; Waldrop, 1992), and developmentalists (for example, Lerner, 1986; Werner, 1957) in particular have clarified a distinction between quantitative and qualitative change, both of which are necessary for development; contrasting terms such as complexity and order, and differentiation and organization, depict this distinction. Similarly, two distinct forms of change can be identified in Rogers' (1980, 1992) works, namely diversity and innovation (Reed, 1997).

Because of the articulation between quantitative and qualitative change, human systems are not simply complex systems (SCS) but rather are complex innovative systems

(CIS) (see Stites, 1994). In the context of nursing, then, nursing processes entail at least two forms of change, complexity and integration.

Complexity.   Complexity refers to the number of different types of variables that can be identified in a given situation. A variable is simply something that varies (*Webster's*, 1979). Complexity occurs when human systems experience or express variables (for example, life events, physiologic events) as parts, separated from the whole, rather than as patterns of the whole. So, for example, complexity is evident when loss of a loved one or chronic illness introduces many new and seemingly disconnected variables into an individual's life, on various levels of awareness. Increasing complexity means change in quantity (size or number) not change in quality of the whole; this would become chaotic were it not accompanied by corresponding changes in integration.

Integration.   Integration refers to a synthesizing and organizing of variables such that there is a change in form, not just change in size or number of events. A certain level of complexity is needed for integration to occur. Integration is evident, for example, when people construct meaning or identify a pattern in the variables or events experienced. Integration may also occur on levels of awareness that are not yet so readily apparent. Integration is trans*form*ative, involving qualitative change in form.

Well-Being

While changes in complexity and integration may be used to explain many facets of human development and systems' changes, this process may also be used to understand health, healing, and well-being. The rhythm between complexity and integration is proposed here to be a means by which innovative change occurs, as a manifestation of the underlying process called nursing. Thus, well-being may be explained in part by changes in complexity that are tempered by changes in integration. Complexity provides life with diversity, specialization, and depth in experiences, whereas integration provides organization, coherence, and breadth.

Examples of nursing processes are abundant. For example, groups incorporate new attachments or children into an organization called family. Persons with spinal cord injuries develop different pathways that link together shattered parts of life and bodily functions. Premature infants' behaviors become more innovative as they organize the complexity of their environment. Adults reminisce to integrate past life events and inevitable death. Healing after the loss of a loved one or the occurrence of chronic illness requires an integration of what seem like disjointed events and experiences, including memories of the past, future dreams, altered rhythms and routines, physical pain and other bodily symptoms, sadness, anguish, and self-doubt. Further, Sachs (1995) depicted what can be called nursing processes, through his stories about people with various maladies, such as a colorblind painter and a surgeon with Tourette's syndrome. These people were able to create a new organization that fit with their altered needs and world. These health events, in all their initial complexity and heartbreak, gave way to metamorphoses and innovation. Regardless of whether there is a "cure" that can reverse a particular ailment, well-being occurs when the particulars of a life experience are brought together and synthesized in a coherent way. Any less, and people risk feeling disintegrated, dis-associated, dis-organized.

While the centrality of well-being as a focus in nursing has been established, other disciplines also may be concerned with well-being and its correlates. However, promoting well-being based upon a perspective of the inherent process of complexity and integration is distinctly nursing.

CHALLENGING THE STATUS QUO: NURSING RECONSTRUCTED

The definition of nursing proposed here is that of an inherent process of well-being, characterized by manifestations of complexity and integration in human systems. The substantive focus of the discipline, then, is not how *nurses* per se facilitate well-being but, rather, how *nursing processes* function in human systems to facilitate well-being. The focus is, in a very basic sense, how nurses can facilitate nursing.

Refocusing the Lens

This new construction of nursing provides another lens of focus for nursing researchers and practitioners. Smith (1988b) wrote metaphorically about three different camera lenses used to view human wholeness. One in particular, the motion lens, focuses on process and rhythmic flow, and requires a "creative leap" to identify this process. Nurses typically encounter people in motion, in dynamic flow with their environment, whether in life-threatening experiences or perceived memory loss, chronic illness or acute pain.

The creative leap necessary for formulating the motion lens of nursing inquiry may be to address the rhythmic processes of complexity and integration that enhance well-being across these health experiences. From premature infants to dying adults and their families and communities, it is proposed that human systems have nursing processes, that is, inherent resources for well-being based on a capacity to integrate their complexities.

Debates on holism and on what represents the critical focus of nursing may be enlivened by including a new ontology of nursing—an ontology that transcends debates about part versus whole, person versus environment. Nursing processes are not necessarily bound by dimensions such as biologic, environmental, or social. Instead, the lens is focused on any human process that manifests complexity and integration related to well-being. Looking through this new lens, researchers and practitioners may identify a myriad of human manifestations of wholeness, whether they be labeled physiologic, phylogenic, or philosophic, that are integral to well-being.

NURSING AS A METAPARADIGM CONCEPT

Given this reconstructed view of nursing, as a substantive focus of the discipline, the term *nursing* should be a central concept in the nursing metaparadigm. In the past, for good reason, some have suggested the elimination of the term nursing from the metaparadigm (Conway, 1985). However, rather than remove the term nursing from the metaparadigm, this fin-de-siècle may be the time in nursing history to consider renaming the discipline to something other than a verb, to better distinguish the disciplinary label from the substantive focus of the science and practice.

To help clarify this distinction, a term such as Paterson and Zderad's (1976) "nursology," or another disciplinary label with the "nurs" prefix could be developed, while reserving the term nursing as the *process* word and verb that it is, for the metaparadigm. By identifying nursing as a substantive, metaparadigm concept, nurses can better claim their unique focus and clarify the ontology of their discipline.

APPROACHING THE FRONTIER

Rogers (1992) explained that one could not push back the frontier of knowledge until one approached it. This article has not been about maintaining the status quo, but about approaching a frontier so that others might join in a dialogue that pushes back the frontier a bit more. In this era of healthcare reform, the discipline must define nursing as nurses truly envision it and not necessarily as others would have it be defined. Nurses may decide against renaming the discipline as was suggested here. Nevertheless, within a broadened and partially reconstructed view of the discipline that embraces nursing at its most fundamental meaning, new understandings that blend with the old can emerge to present a fuller picture of the discipline.

Nursing (as practice and praxis) is a way of doing that creates good actions that facilitate well-being. Nursing (as syntax and science) is a way of knowing that creates goods in the form of knowledge. And nursing (the substance and ontology) is a way of being that creates patterns of changing complexity and integration experienced as well-being in human systems.

Nurses are invited to try on the substantive definition of nursing to see how it fits within the context of their practice and science. Ongoing philosophic dialogue about the ontology of the discipline will help ensure that nurse theorists are theorists of nursing in its fullest sense, and likewise, that nurse researchers are researchers of nursing, and nurse practitioners are practitioners of nursing.

REFERENCES

Conway, M. E. (1985). Toward greater specificity in defining nursing's metaparadigm. *Advances in Nursing Science, 7*(4), 73–81.

Ellis, R. (1982). Conceptual issues in nursing. *Nursing Outlook, 30* (7), 406–410.

Henderson, V. (1964) The nature of nursing. *American Journal of Nursing, 64* (8), 62–68.

Kauffman, S. (1995). *At home in the universe: The search for laws of self-organization and complexity.* New York: Oxford University Press.

Laird, C. (1971). *Webster's new world thesaurus* (rev. ed.). New York: Simon and Schuster.

Lerner, R. M. (1986). *Concepts and theories of human development* (2nd ed.). New York: Random House.

Murphy, M. (1992). *The future of the body: Explorations into the further evolution of human nature.* New York: J.P. Tarcher.

Newman, M. (1992). Prevailing paradigms in nursing. *Nursing Outlook, 40,* 10–13.

Nightingale, F. (1969). *Notes on nursing: What it is and what it is not.* New York: Dover (Original work published 1859)

Paterson, J. G., & Zderad, L. T. (1976). *Humanistic nursing.* New York: Wiley.

Pepper, S. P. (1942). *World hypotheses: A study in evidence.* Berkeley: University of California Press.

Rampragus, V. (1995). *The deconstruction of nursing.* Brookfield, VT: Ashgate.

Reed, P. G. (1995). A treatise on nursing knowledge development for the 21st century: Beyond postmodernism. *Advances in Nursing Science, 17* (3), 70–84.

Reed, P. G. (1997). The place of transcendence in nursing's science of unitary human beings. In M. Madrid (Ed.), *Patterns of Rogerian knowing* (pp. 187–196). New York: National League for Nursing Press.

Rogers, M. E. (1970). *Introduction to the theoretical basis of nursing.* Philadelphia: F. A. Davis.

Rogers, M. E. (1980). A science of unitary man. In J. P. Riehl & C. Roy (Eds.), *Conceptual models for nursing practice* (2nd ed., pp. 329–337). New York: Appleton-Century-Crofts.

Rogers, M. E. (1992). Nursing science and the space age. *Nursing Science Quarterly, 5,* 27–34.

Roy, C. L. (1995). Developing nursing knowledge: Practice issues raised from four philosophical perspectives. *Nursing Science Quarterly, 8,* 79–85.

Sachs, O. (1995). *An anthropologist on Mars: Seven paradoxical tales.* New York: A. Knopf.

Schlotfeldt, R. (1994). Resolving opposing viewpoints: Is it desirable? Is it practicable? In J. F. Kikuchi & H. Simmons (Eds.), *Developing a philosophy of nursing* (pp. 67–74). Thousand Oaks: Sage.

Smith, M. J. (1988a). Nursing: What's in a name? *Nursing Science Quarterly, 1,* 142–143.

Smith, M. J. (1988b). Perspectives of wholeness: The lens makes a difference. *Nursing Science Quarterly, 1,* 94–95.

Stites, J. (1994). Complexity research on complex systems and complex adaptive systems. *Omni, 16* (8), 42–50.

von Bertalanffy, L. (1981). *A systems view of man* (P.A. La Violette, Ed.). Boulder: Westview Press.

Waldrop, M. M. (1992). *Complexity: The emerging science at the edge of order and chaos.* New York: Simon and Schuster.

Watson, J. (1985). *Nursing: Human science and human care.* Norwalk, CT: Appleton-Century-Crofts.

Watson, J. (1995). Postmodernism and knowledge development in nursing. *Nursing Science Quarterly, 8,* 60–64.

Webster's new collegiate dictionary. (1979). Springfield, MA: G. & C. Merriam Co.

Werner, H. (1957). The concept of development from a comparative and organismic point of view. In D. B. Harris (Ed.), *The concept of development* (pp. 125–148). Minneapolis: University of Minnesota Press.

28

A Multiparadigm Approach to Nursing

JOAN ENGEBRETSON, DrPH, RN

Nursing theory development has made good progress in differentiating the domain of nursing from medicine; many of these theories are categorized as holistic theories. Nursing classification systems are also being developed to organize extant nursing practice. The dissonance between the two has been one of the most difficult contemporary issues for the leadership of nursing. A framework is proposed that would account for these disparate approaches. This proposed framework for the domain of healing is in keeping with the metaparadigm of health and uses a multiple paradigm approach. Nursing interventions are discussed in relation to the framework. It invites a dialogue in keeping with the scholarship of holism. Practice and scholarship implications are discussed. [Keywords: Classification systems, Culture, Holism, Paradigm, Theory]

Nursing theory has, since the 1960s, sought to define the profession of nursing and to differentiate its scope of practice from that of biomedicine.[1] This search has led to some discrepancies between theory development that differentiates nursing action from biomedical nursing practice, the latter of which uses many nursing actions derived from biomedicine. Differentiating autonomous nursing practice was a necessary step, because historically many nursing functions were derived from biomedicine, since nurses have practiced in biomedically dominated settings.

One primary differentiating feature was holism, which was contrasted with biomedical reductionism. The movement to declare nursing holistic is now well accepted; however, a holistic framework must be inclusive of, not only differentiated from, biomedicine. In alignment with holism, the appropriate construct for the nursing profession is healing. Health is a derivative of healing, or making whole, and part of the metaparadigm of nursing.

Another element of professional evolution is the development of diagnostic, intervention, and outcomes classifications systems. These are often grounded in nursing practice and thus reflect both nursing activities as well as predominant sociocultural ideologies. There is often a disjuncture between the differentiating and defining theories and the more pragmatic classifications systems.[2] In an effort to reconcile grand conceptual models and practice, this article presents a conceptual framework for discussion as a step toward the consolidation of a holistic approach to nursing. The intent is to support both unique autonomous actions and to incorporate medically derived actions. Using the construct of healing, a multiparadigm model is presented to incorporate both

Source: Engebretson, J. (1997). A multiparadigm approach to nursing. *Adv Nurs Sci* 20(1):21–23. Reprinted with permission by from and copyright © 1997 Aspen Publishers, Inc.

the medical model and other cultural healing models on which nurses may ground their actions. This integration is at the level of paradigm, which allows the incorporation of and expansion beyond the biomedical model and avoids the pitfalls of the derivative–differentiation polarity.

Nursing has over the past 30 years made great strides in the development of nursing theories and conceptual models. These activities have been necessary to define the professional domain to its members and to society at large. Theory guides the practice and the activities that are unique to the profession, informs research efforts, and provides direction for future development.[3]

CONTEMPORARY CONTROVERSIES

Despite the progress made, the use of nursing theories in practice has been a matter of controversy. One area of controversy is the dichotomy between medicine and nursing, with many theories focusing on unique nursing functions and in some cases redefining actions associated with medical models. This position has often still held the medical model as the orthodox standard against which nursing defined itself by negation or differentiation, thereby maintaining dependence on the medical model.

Closely related to the nursing–medicine dichotomy is the rupture between academia and practice. Academia and much of theory development focused on the autonomous nature of nursing, differentiating it from medicine. Extant nursing practice often eschewed the nursing theories learned in school, and practicing nurses functioned in a more pragmatic manner reflective of the medical model.[4] Many times the praxis of nursing is covertly, if not overtly, aligned with the medical model. This

alliance with the medical model is understandable considering the hegemony of the medical bioscientific model in U.S. culture. Barnum[4] noted that normative theory evolves from practice rather than academic theory development and that inconsistencies develop when practice (theory) is not intellectually analyzed and scrutinized according to logical coherence.

A third, related problem area is the disjuncture between nursing theories and the diagnosis, intervention, and outcome classification systems. The two strongest competitors in the theory business are holistic theories and nursing process,[1,4] which often represent opposing philosophies regarding content, methodology, and interpretation. Holistic theories are global, espouse a transcendental view of humans, and are committed to not viewing subject matter as an accumulation of parts.[4]

Nursing process approaches are much more concrete and practice based and have focused on nursing action and classification systems.[5] The International Council of Nurses,[6] the Omaha Project,[7] the Iowa Project,[8] and separate projects by Grobe[9] and Saba[10] have recently developed nursing classification systems.

Recent debates in nursing have also reflected controversies over the usefulness of a unified theory vs multiple theories. Reed[11] proposed an approach that links science, philosophy, and practice in the development of nursing knowledge. She advocated a metanarrative that involves a dialogue of practice and philosophy. This metanarrative provides an excellent format for the development of nursing theory that is holistic in nature and can integrate multiple paradigms from the patient's perspective and from the nurse. It is in this spirit of inviting a dialogue and providing a format for a dialectic discussion between paradigms that the author presents the multiparadigm model.

HOLISM AND NURSING

Grand theory, or the concept level of theory development, has evolved into a metaparadigm with four propositional statements related to the concepts person–health, person–environment, health–nursing, and person–environment–health.[12] The global level defines the frameworks within which the more restricted structures develop.

Consistent with the concept heal–health, the related ideologies for nursing theory development would come from healing, rather than be restricted to medicine. Healing and health stem from the root word *hale*, or to make whole.[13] This etymology grounds the concept heal–health in holism. Barnum[4] identified holistic theories as the fastest growing trend in nursing. Holistic concepts in nursing have been evident since the time of Florence Nightingale and evolved in nursing theories through the influence of Teilhard de Chardin, Jan Smuts, and Ludwig von Bertalanffy.[14] Anthropology, another discipline based on holism, provides another source of information on healing that can inform nurses in the development of holistic theory. Traditionally, in many cultures, healers, shamans, and medicine people reflected the broader concept of healing rather than the science-based concept of cure.

Holistic health has recently become very popular among both lay and professional groups. Characteristics of holistic health have been described in many studies.[15–19] Two common mistakes occur in the analysis of holism from a modernist perspective based in a scientific or reductionistic paradigm. Alster's[15] analysis of holistic health is an example of such an attempt; it reaches the syllogistic conclusion that holistic health cannot be studied scientifically because it is not scientific.

The opposite pitfall is to romanticize traditional or primitive healing systems and unfavorably compare science and biomedicine.

This antiscience position is often seen in lay literature that attributes all social ills to scientific–rational thinking while extolling a holistic framework as the alternative. A consistent holistic framework incorporates science but does not hold that paradigm as sufficient for explaining the human experience or for bringing about health or healing. The model proposed in this article recognizes the holistic nature of nursing and expands the domain from disease treatment to the broader concept of health by incorporating several paradigms and their adjunctive ideological perspectives on humans, health, and therapeutic actions.

HISTORICAL CONTEXT OF WESTERN MEDICINE

Healing systems reflect and influence the cultural values of the parent culture. Contemporary biomedicine has been informed by and influential in the development of modernism. Modernity had its philosophical origins in the 17th century with the emphasis on rationality by the protagonists Galileo and Descartes.[20] Kuhn[21] described the shift of vision that enabled people to see and think about phenomena in a different manner and that he labeled a "paradigm shift." Modernity is characterized by the development of science and technology, the valorization of reason and humanity's dominion over nature. The scientific paradigm of modernity has dominated medicine and health care.

The establishment of the scientific model as the foundation for biomedicine paralleled the development of modernity. The scientific paradigm is characterized by philosophical dualism between the material and nonmaterial, and the corresponding designation of matter as the subject of science and the nonmaterial or metaphysical as the domain of religion. Descartes is often credited with conceptualiz-

Positivist ⟵———————————————————————————⟶ Metaphysical

	Modalities	Mechanical	Purification	Balance	Supranormal
Material	Physical manipulation	Biomedical surgery	Colonics Cupping	Magnetic healing Polarity	Drumming Dancing
	Applied and ingested substances	Pharmacology	Chetation	Humoral medicine	Flower remedies Hallucinogenics plants
	Energy	Laser Radiation	Bioenergetics	Tai chi Chi gong Acupuncture Accupressure	Healing touch Laying on of hands
	Psychological	Mind-body	Self-help (confessional type)	Mindfulness	Imagery
Nonmaterial	Spirtual	Attendance at organized religious functions	Forgiveness Panance	Meditation Chakra Balancing	Primal religious Expedence Prayer

Figure 28.1. A Multiparadigm approach to healing.

ing the mind–body dualism and the corresponding value of the mind–soul as the superior demarcation of the human.

Throughout the following centuries, especially in England, increasing cultural value was placed on the scientific, material, rational, and technical.[22,23] Metaphysical and nonmaterial issues associated with religion were progressively devalued, especially among intellectuals.[24] Medicine, which historically had been based in a metaphysical model and supported by religion, became the domain of science and was severed from its metaphysical and religious roots. This split allowed medicine to make unprecedented technological advances through the application of scientific reason. But a contemporary surge of public interest in alternative healing modalities suggests that the biomedical scientific approach by itself is insufficient for healing.

DEVELOPMENT OF THE MULTIPARADIGM MODEL

The multiparadigm model was developed from the author's ethnographic work with healers and nurses. Field work, including participant observation, long interviews, free list-

ing, and pile sorts, was used in a study exploring and comparing the conceptual frameworks of health and healing between nurses and healers.[25] A matrix of healing modalities that incorporated biomedicine and examples of alternative models emerging in the United States in the late 1980s and early 1990s was developed to focus the study on healers using healing touch[26] and used to orient nurse practitioners to alternative healing modalities that their clients might be using.[27]

This matrix was then developed into the Heterodox Explanatory Paradigms Model for health practice that incorporated multiple healing modalities.[28] The philosophical coherence of the model and the related positioning of modalities was presented as a framework for developing integrated health care models. Because nurses and healers have similar conceptual frameworks of healing,[25] this model could be adapted for nursing as a possible framework toward a more holistic model.

Philosophical Design

The multiparadigm model (Fig. 28.1) developed from the author's previous work[25–28] represents a multiparadigm approach to healing. Philosophical dualism between the material and nonmaterial is represented on both axes. Four paradigms of healing are incorporated and philosophically arranged from the most material to the most nonmaterial along the horizontal axis, which represents a philosophical continuum from logical positivism to metaphysics. Consistent with the positivist–metaphysical continuum, the mechanical paradigm is on the extreme left, reflecting the logical positivism of its philosophical scientific foundation. The paradigms are progressively more nonmaterial, ending in the most metaphysical paradigm, supranormal, at the extreme right. The vertical axis represents the Cartesian body–mind dualism in healing activities. Activities that are most material or physical are at the top. Moving down, activities become progressively less material and more psychological or spiritual.

Horizontal Axis

The four paradigms are mechanical, purification, balance, and supranormal. The mechanical paradigm is best represented by examples from biomedicine, which is primarily a mechanistic, materialistic paradigm exemplified by the focus on discovering explanatory mechanisms to understand a healing activity. The positivist philosophy bases knowing on objective, material data perceived by the senses.[29] It is characterized by determinism, mechanism, and reductionism. Disease is assumed to be reducible to disordered body functions and a disease-specific etiology.[30] Treatment and intervention are disease specific.

The purification paradigm has examples cross-culturally and throughout Western history. This paradigm is characterized by healing actions that cleanse or purify. The name of the prestigious English medical journal *Lancet* is a remnant of the bloodletting and purges that dominated Western medicine before technical advances in surgery and antibiotics in the 20th century. Health and healing activities related to cleanliness or purification either physically or symbolically have been documented in many ritual practices.[31] The hygienic health reform movement of the late 19th century[32,33] incorporated many practices that were understood as cleansing and keeping the body pure.

The balance paradigm is best represented by Eastern or humeral systems. In Eastern systems health–healing is viewed as the proper balance of yin and yang and unimpeded flow of Chi (or Ki or Qi).[34] Humeral medicine, or the balance of vital forces or humors, is evident in Hippocratic, Galenic, and Ayurvedic medicine.[35] Nineteenth-century vitalism also incorporated this approach. Health is attained or maintained by creating a balance in daily living through types of foods, activities, temperature, and so forth. Personality types, environment, and circumstances are considered in determining the corrective balance. One example is the hot and cold classification in Mexican folk medicine. The balance paradigm is on the right half of the model and therefore cannot be fully understood through a materialist mechanistic paradigm.

The supranormal paradigm incorporates all magicoreligious and psychic phenomena used to promote health or create healing. Spiritual, symbolic, and other nonmaterial understandings of healing are in this column. The supranormal paradigm is philosophically the most metaphysical, going beyond physics, sense experience, or any discipline and involving ultimates.[36] This paradigm incorporates psychic, spiritual, and other types of healing such as prayer, distant healing, and other spontaneous healing that cannot be explained by mechanistic models or one of the other paradigms.

Vertical Axis

The vertical axis describes types of healing activities that progress along the continuum from body to mind–soul, from material to nonmaterial. The first row contains physical manipulations, and examples are given for each paradigm. Physical manipulation may be performed either by the patient or on the patient by a healer.

In row 2 applied and ingested substances are listed according to each paradigm. Such substances include all foods, herbs, and pharmaceuticals that are ingested, inhaled, or topically applied.

Using energy, the third activity, is a concept that is poorly understood in biomedicine but important in other paradigms. Many healing activities are understood and conducted as an active manipulation of energy. The concept of energy, or the transfer from matter to energy to matter, has been proposed by some scientists (eg, Bohm, Capra[37]) as the basis for quantum physics and as a possible link in understanding the material and nonmaterial worlds. This could be a promising area in linking the material, physical body with nonmaterial thought, spirit, and so on. The concept of energy has been proposed by some nurses as the basis for understanding the benefits of touch therapies.[38-40]

Psychological activities deal with functions of cognition and of the mind. Mind to body medicine has been a rapidly growing area of research. With the discovery of neurotransmitters and hormonal–neural pathways, mechanisms have been discovered by which thoughts and feelings can manifest in physiological changes.[41] Theory has been developed and researched regarding the association of personality characteristics with illness, in particular hostility and heart disease.[42] Psychoneuroimmunology is another promising field where theory is developing. Associations have been demonstrated between various personality characteristics and mortality and morbidity.[43,44]

Spiritual activities are at the polar opposite of the continuum from physical manipulation. Spiritual actions are distinct from cognitive activities. Spirituality, being the most distant from the physical or material, is the least understood from a modernist perspective. Some studies have found that attendance at religious activities is related to improved health or healing.[45] Attendance at religious activities represents a mechanistic conceptualization of spiritual activity, whereas a primal spiritual experience as described by Cox[46] would be a more metaphysical approach.

The model has, at present, four paradigms, but others could be added along the continuum. Restriction to a two-dimensional format is often interpreted as containing mutually exclusive cells. A more appropriate geographic conceptualization would be as general areas on a double-axis continuum, with no specific boundary between areas. Modalities in the model are examples only, and many other modalities could fit in each location. The modalities describe healing activities only. An individual practitioner–healer could, and often does, use many modalities.

The positioning of modalities according to philosophical continuums also reflects the degree of passivity or activity of the healer. Starting from the upper left corner, where the modalities are most material, the healer is most active and the recipient most passive. Moving diagonally down and across, the person who is healing is progressively more active and the role of the healer increasingly that of facilitator, consistent with healing philosophy, which posits that real healing is done by the "healee."

One area that is a vital part of the nursing metaparadigm and other healing systems is the environment, especially social relationships. Although not specifically addressed in the model, an additional line at the bottom could be added to address social activities.

Positivist ←——→ Metaphysical

	Modalities	Mechanical	Purification	Balance	Supranormal
Material	Physical manipulation	Positioning Exercise therapy Joint mobility	Bathing	Exercise promotion	Intuitive body work†
	Applied and ingested substances	Medication administration	Wound and bladder irrigation Leech therapy	Nutritional counseling	Homeopathic remedies
	Energy	Laser precautions	Phototherapy	Acupressure Acupuncture†	Therapeutic touch
	Psychological	Cognitive restructuring	Active listening†	Counseling*	Simple guided imagery
Nonmaterial	Spiritual	Activity therapy*	Forgiveness and purification rituals	Meditation	Spiritual support*

*NIC listed intervention that could be developed with understanding of the paradigm
†No NIC listing and should be considered as a potential referral or potential development for nursing action

FIGURE 28.2. Nursing activities and interventions.

APPLICATION TO NURSING

The multiparadigm model is holistic and avoids the medicine–nursing and practice– academia dichotomies by placing the Western biomedical model in context with other paradigms of healing. It speaks to the domain of healing, which is the stated domain of nursing. This model can provide a framework for nursing diagnoses and interventions that easily integrates biomedical model functions with complementary functions that either are autonomous nursing activities or might constitute appropriate referrals. The model also incorporates paradigms that can be useful in understanding cross-cultural healing practices and systems.

IMPLICATIONS FOR PRACTICE

Operating from a multiparadigm model allows nurses to adapt whatever paradigm or modality fits the situation. This flexibility is helpful in working with patients who practice health- and healing-related activities from other para-

digms. A multiparadigm approach that incorporates models of health–healing can help providers better understand beliefs and practices of patients that may be poorly comprehended in the biomedical model.

Most health practices originate in the popular sector,[47] which includes family and social networks. This sector has beliefs about health maintenance and hierarchies of resort that direct types of health–healing activities, healer consultants, and adherence to treatments. The orientation of the popular sector often incorporates other paradigms than the scientific–mechanistic approach of biomedicine. By understanding the explanatory paradigm of health practices, the practitioner is better able to communicate and collaborate with the client and family in the management of health–healing.

Many interventions listed in the various nursing classification systems may be positioned in this model. Examples from one of these systems, the Nursing Interventions Classification (NIC),[8] have been identified in Fig 28.2, along with other modalities that could be referral sources for the client. Examples are easily placed in the mechanistic and purification paradigms but more difficult to place in the balance and supranormal paradigms. Thus, the model can display areas where nursing has developed actions and where referrals are more appropriate. It is important to note that a holistic paradigm is impossible to implement in its entirety by any one person or discipline; therefore, nurses should be able to understand how other providers fit into an overall plan of care.

By understanding these modalities through the appropriate paradigm, practitioners may select whatever modality is appropriate for the client, either by interventions or referral to other providers. For example, existing NIC actions in the mechanical paradigm for physical manipulation could incorporate positioning, exercise therapy including range of motion, and ambulation. Applied and ingested substances include medication administration of all types. Although energy is poorly understood in the mechanical model, it is present on the NIC as laser precautions. Energy, if better understood, could have potential for much broader use.

Psychological interventions in the mechanical (medical) model include cognitive restructuring and reality therapies. Spiritual interventions may include assisting a patient with religious practices such as attending chapel or praying. This is not specifically listed in NIC but is covered under activity therapy.

Examples of nursing actions in the purification paradigm using physical manipulation include bathing and other hygiene activities. Wound and bladder irrigations are good examples of applied and ingested substances. Many medications have cleaning or purification action, such as emetics, expectorants, and purgatives. Psychological and emotional catharsis are examples of psychological purification. These are not specifically listed, although could be covered under the NIC active listening.

Spiritual purification includes a number of rituals that serve to purify and cleanse the individual, such as confession, seeking of forgiveness, ritual bathing, and use of incense. These would need to be developed or referred because there is no NIC entry related to this.

Nursing interventions are being expanded into the balance and supranormal paradigms through the work of nurses who have expanded their individual practice and those who are using many of the more recent nursing theories, such as Rogers,[48] Watson,[49] Parse,[50] or Newman,[51] to direct their practice. Exercise promotion is listed in NIC and could be expanded and developed with a better understanding of the balance paradigm. Nutritional counseling is based on providing a balance of nutrients and could also be expanded to incorporate use of some herbs for the promotion of health. Approaching these from the perspective of balance rather than mechanical cure allows for an expansion into health and attention to individual life systems. Acupuncture or acupressure are not on the NIC but could be a source of referral. While currently not part of the balance paradigm, counseling, simple relaxation therapy, or self-modification assistance have the potential for development into that paradigm. Meditation also has potential for development.

Nursing interventions in the supranormal paradigm cluster in the nonmaterial areas. Intuitive body work, if not done by a nurse, could constitute a referral. Likewise, activities using homeopathic remedies or flower essences are included as they are understood to work through the spiritual level.

Therapeutic touch is well developed in nursing and is understood as a supranormal use of energy. Guided imagery is a supranormal psychological technique that is listed in the NIC. Spiritual support, including prayer, could be further developed to fully express this paradigm.

IMPLICATIONS FOR RESEARCH AND SCHOLARSHIP

By constructing a paradigm map with health–healing activities, nurses can determine appropriate paradigms to guide their understanding and research of particular modalities. Locating it on the model can serve as a guide for better understanding a particular modality; it also provides a direction for further scholarship and research. An exploration of both axes can enhance understanding. For example, nursing actions in the mechanical paradigm are often best understood by a better comprehension of the medical–scientific model, and research using the positivist philosophy is often appropriate. Many of the NIC classifications can be understood from this paradigm.

Working with a modality such as guided imagery could be enhanced by exploring both the supranormal paradigm and the psychological literature. Healing touch, a modality with a rich history in nursing, is located at the nexus of energy and the supranormal, the two axes least understood by biomedical science. Nurses who have conducted research using this modality or the existential psychological theories can attest to the frustration in conducting research without documented material and measurable mechanisms of action that are compatible with the mechanical paradigm. Research in these areas can be enhanced by learning more about the approaches of anthropology, theology, some psychology, and other humanity disciplines consistent with the supranormal paradigm. Investigation of energy through quantum physics (energy) and Eastern healing are also proximal areas that can illuminate the understanding of touch therapies.

The model can serve as an agenda for research and scholarship. In some modalities, links have been or can be developed that en-able more mechanistic studies. In others, their position invites more qualitative or naturalistic methodologies of inquiry. Nursing theories may develop links that connect modalities for practice. For example, some of the developmental theories may have links across paradigms on the psychological axis. Although methods may be successfully combined, caution must be taken in attempting to link paradigms. Many paradigms are based on contradictory beliefs that are impossible to adhere to simultaneously.[52]

The multiparadigm model provides a holistic approach to bridging the gulf between holistic theories and biomedical nursing praxis. The dialectic method is appropriate scholarship for holistic frameworks.[4,53] In this approach, the whole is seen as governing relationships and providing coherence to the parts. The dialectic process would describe a nursing issue from one position—for example, the mechanical paradigm—and then counter that description with an oppositional position, the supranormal. After debate and dialogue, a third position emerges. This position can, in similar fashion, be refined by the same process. Placing the polar opposites in one model invites a dialectic methodology, appropriate for holistic nursing scholarship. The challenge remains for nurses to continue to develop theory that links modalities and explanatory paradigms. These links are being developed along nursing themes of health, environment, and individual potentials for healing. The model could help to provide a geographic map to locate these dialogues.

REFERENCES

1. Chinn PL, Kramer MK. *Theory and Nursing: A Systematic Approach*. St. Louis, Mo: Mosby; 1995.
2. Fitzpatrick JJ, Whall AL. *Conceptual Models of Nursing Analysis and Application*. 3rd ed. Stamford, Conn: Appleton & Lange; 1996.

3. Newman MN. *A Developing Discipline: Selected Works of Margaret Newman.* New York, NY: National League for Nursing Press; 1995.

4. Barnum BJS. *Nursing Theory: Analysis, Application, Evaluation.* Philadelphia, Pa: Lippincott; 1994.

5. Snyder M. Defining nursing interventions. *Image J Nurs Sch.* 1996;28(2):137–141.

6. International Council of Nurses. *Nurses' Next Advance: An International Classification for Nursing Practice.* Geneva, Switzerland: ICN; 1993.

7. Martin KS, Scheet NJ. *The Omaha System: Applications for Community Health Nursing.* Philadelphia, Pa: W.B. Saunders; 1992.

8. McCloskey JC, Bulechek GM. *Nursing Interventions Classification (NIC).* St. Louis, Mo: Mosby; 1996.

9. Grobe SJ. The nursing lexicon and taxonomy: Implications for representing nursing care data in automated patient records. *Holistic Nurs Pract.* 1996;11(1):48–63.

10. Saba VK. The classification of home health nursing. *Caring.* 1992;11(3):50–57.

11. Reed, PG. A treatise on nursing knowledge development for the 21st century: Beyond postmodernism. *ANS.* 1995;17(3):70–84.

12. Fawcett J. *Analysis and evaluation of nursing theories.* Philadelphia, Pa: F.A. Davis; 1993.

13. *Webster's Ninth New Collegiate Dictionary.* Springfield, Mass: Merriam-Webster; 1990.

14. Owen MJ, Holmes CA. Holism in the discourse of nursing. *J Adv Nurs.* 1993;18:1688–1695.

15. Alster, KB. *The Holistic Health Movement.* Tuscaloosa, Ala: University of Alabama Press; 1989.

16. English-Lueck JA. *Health in the New Age: A Study in California Holistic Practices.* Albuquerque, NM: University of New Mexico Press; 1990.

17. Gordon, JS. The paradigm of holistic medicine. In: Hastings AC, Fadiman J, Gordon JS, eds. *Health for the Whole Person.* Toronto, Ontario: Bantam Books; 1980.

18. Lowenberg JS. *Caring and Responsibility.* Philadelphia, Pa: University of Pennsylvania Press; 1989.

19. Mattson PH. *Holistic Health in Perspective.* Palo Alto, Calif: Mayfield; 1982.

20. Toulmin S. *Cosmopolis: The Hidden Agenda of Modernity.* Chicago, Ill: University of Chicago Press; 1990.

21. Kuhn T. *The Structure of Scientific Revolutions.* Chicago, Ill: The University of Chicago Press; 1972.

22. Tarnas R. *The Passion of the Western World: Understanding the Ideas That Have Shaped our World View.* New York, NY: Ballantine Books; 1991.

23. Lavine TZ. *From Socrates to Sartre: The Philosophic Quest.* New York, NY: Bantam; 1984.

24. Johnson P. *Intellectuals.* New York, NY: Harper Perennial; 1988.

25. Engebretson J. Comparison of nurses and alternative healers. *Image: J Nurs Sch.* 1996;28(2):95–100.

26. Engebretson J. *Cultural Models of Healing and Health: An Ethnography of Professional Nurses and Healers.* Houston, Tex: University of Texas-Houston, School of Public Health; 1992. Dissertation.

27. Engebretson J, Wardell D. A contemporary view of alternative healing modalities. *Nurse Practitioner.* 1993; 18(9):51–55.

28. Engebretson J. Models of heterodox healing. *Alternat Ther Health Med.* In press.

29. Andrews MM, Boyle JS. *Transcultural Concepts in Nursing Care.* 2nd ed. Philadelphia, Pa: Lippincott; 1995.

30. Freund PES, McGuire MB. *Health, Illness and the Social Body: A Critical Sociology.* Englewood Cliffs, NJ: Prentice-Hall; 1991.

31. Douglas M. *Purity and Danger: An Analysis of the Concepts of Pollution and Taboo.* London, England: Ark Paperbacks; 1989.

32. Brown PS. Nineteenth-century American health reformers and the early nature cure movement in Britain. *Med History.* 1988; 32:174–194.

33. Whorton JC. *Crusaders for Fitness: The History of American Health Reformers.* Princeton, NJ: Princeton University Press; 1982.

34. Kaptchuk TJ. *The Web that Has No Weaver: Understanding Chinese Medicine.* New York, NY: Congdon and Weed; 1993.

35. Helman CG. *Culture, Health and Illness: An Introduction for Health Professionals.* 3rd ed. Wolburn, Mass: Butterworth-Heinemann; 1994.

36. Reese WL. *Dictionary of Philosophy and Religion: Eastern and Western Thought.* Atlantic Highland, NJ: Humanities Press; 1991.

37. Horgan J. *The End of Science, Facing the Limits of Knowledge in the Twilight of the Scientific Age.* Reading, Mass. Addison Wesley; 1996.

38. Dossey BM, Keegan L, Guzzetta CE, Kolkmeier LG. *Holistic Nursing: A Handbook for Practice.* Gaithersburg, Md: Aspen Publishers; 1995.

39. Slater VE. Toward an understanding of energetic healing, part 1: Energetic structures. *J Holistic Nurs.* 1995;13:209–224.

40. Slater VE. Toward an understanding of energetic healing, part 2: Energetic process. *J Holistic Nurs.* 1995;13:225–238.

41. Rossi E. The *Psychobiology of Mind-Body Healing.* New York, NY: W.W. Norton; 1993.

42. Orth-Gomer K, Schneiderman N. *Behavioral Medicine Approaches to Cardiovascular Disease Prevention.* Hillsdale, NJ: Erlbaum; 1996.

43. Dreher H. *The Immune Power Personality.* New York: Dutton; 1995.

44. Schneiderman N, McCabe P, Baum A. *Perspectives in Behavioral Medicine: Stress and Disease Processes.* Hillsdale, NJ: Erlbaum; 1992.

45. Larson DB. Religion and spirituality—the forgotten factor in public health: What does the research share? Presented at the 12th annual meeting of the American Public Health Association, November 18, 1996; New York, NY.

46. Cox H. *Fire from Heaven.* Reading, Mass: Addison-Wesley; 1995.

47. Kleinman A. *Patients and Healers in the Context of Culture.* Berkeley, Calif: University of California Press; 1980.

48. Rogers ME. *An Introduction to the Theoretical Basis of Nursing.* Philadelphia, PA: F.A. Davis; 1970.

49. Watson J. *Nursing: Human Science and Human Care: A Theory of Nursing.* New York, NY: National League for Nursing.

50. Parse RR. *Man—Living—Health: A Theory of Nursing.* New York, NY: Wiley; 1981.

51. Newman MA. *Health as Expanding Consciousness.* 2nd ed. New York, NY: National League for Nursing; 1984.

52. Nagle LM, Mitchell GJ. *Theoretic Diversity: Evolving Paradigmatic Issues in Research and Practice.* Gaithersburg, Md: Aspen Publishers; 1991.

53. McKeon ZK. *On Knowing the Natural Sciences.* Chicago, Ill: University of Chicago Press; 1994.

Part VII

INTERRELATIONSHIPS AMONG NURSING THEORY, RESEARCH, AND PRACTICE

Ideally, nursing theory develops from practice, is tested and validated by research, then is used to change or modify nursing practice. However, this ideal cycle rarely occurs in the nursing arena. Although the interrelationships of theory, research, and nursing practice have been debated for years, the advancement of nursing science depends on generating nursing theory, testing theory in practice, and modifying practice based on theory. Hopefully, as more graduate nurses learn the value of nursing theory and research and take leadership positions in practice they will utilize nursing theories and research more consistently.

In "A Nursing Perspective on the Interrelationships between Theory, Research, and Practice," Steven Pryjmachuk discusses the meaning and relevance of each process to nursing and proposes a model illustrating a learning cycle for the acquisition of knowledge. He acknowledges the knowledge gap between theory and nursing practice and suggests using both formal and informal research to close the gap. Pryjmachuk also compares levels of knowledge acquisition to Benner's levels of nurses' expertise and their role in research. He concludes that continued development of nursing's body of knowledge depends on encouraging nurses to use theories and models to guide their practice and to test and refine them in practice.

Gayle Acton, Barbara Irvin, and Barbara Hopkins also expressed concern about the lack of empirical validation of nursing models in "Theory-testing Research: Building the Science." These authors identify some problems and constraints that have limited testing nursing theories and propose 15 criteria for determining whether a research study tests a theory. They apply their criteria to six research studies to determine its usefulness, and conclude with recommendations for continured development of nursing science.

29

A Nursing Perspective on the Interrelationships between Theory, Research and Practice

STEVEN PRYJMACHUK RMN, MSc

This paper is concerned with the interrelationships between the three concepts of theory, research and practice. In the course of discussing the interrelationships between these concepts, research is identified as the link between theory and practice on both a formal (explicit) and informal (tacit) level. The role of formal and informal research in the development of nursing expertise is also given some consideration.

THEORY, PRACTICE AND RESEARCH IN NURSING

Most nurses have some familiarity with the concepts of 'theory', 'research' and 'practice'. Many, however, find clarification of these concepts somewhat difficult, in that they lack a true understanding of the importance of theory, research and practice to the continuing development of nursing as a profession. Moreover, and more significantly, most nurses perhaps fail to acknowledge the importance of interrelationships between the three concepts.

What of these interrelationships? With regard to the theory–research diad, there appears to be some, albeit tentative, evidence for the existence of a relationship, in that academics view theory development and research as mutual, coexisting activities. With regard to the theory–practice diad, the fact that much

has been written about the so-called 'theory–practice gap' implies that, at the very least, a relationship between these two concepts *should* exist. The evidence for a relationship between research and practice is, however, rather less clear.

Nonetheless, when the three concepts are examined in detail, explicit interrelationships between the three concepts are found to be manifest. It is possible, moreover, to illustrate the nature of these relationships by means of a model. Such a model is proposed by the author later in this paper.

To begin the discussion, there is a need to consider one of the concepts in detail. A logical choice is 'theory'.

What is 'Theory'?

'Theory', like most terms, has a number of different meanings. Whilst various taxonomies of its meanings are available (see McCaugherty 1992a, for a taxonomy of its meanings within nursing), a simple consideration of its formal

Source: Pryjmachuk, S. (1996). A nursing perspective on the interrelationships between theory, research and practice. *Journal of Advanced Nursing* 23, 679–684. Reprinted with permission by Blackwell Science Ltd.

TABLE 29.1   Descriptions of the 'formal' and 'informal' arenas

Formal	Informal
Public	Private, personal
Academic	Practical
Explicit	Implicit, tacit
'Macro'	'Micro'
Exogenous	Endogenous
External	Internal

and informal meanings will suffice for the purposes of this discussion.

Used informally, theory describes an idea or hunch, a hypothesis, about the world. More formal interpretations of the term, on the other hand, tend to see a theory as a set of ideas, hunches or hypotheses that provides some degree of prediction and/or explanation of the world. (Formal definitions of theory within nursing can be found in Dickoff & James, 1968a; Stevens, 1984, and Chinn & Jacobs, 1987.)

The Formal and Informal Arenas

Reference was made above to formal and informal theories. These terms have significance throughout this paper (a significance which stems from the applicability of the proposed theory–research–practice model to both the formal and the informal arenas). To help the reader gain a better understanding of what is meant by the terms 'formal' and 'informal', some qualities of both arenas are listed in Table 29.1. All of the concepts discussed in this paper (including concepts introduced at a later point, such as 'learning', 'knowledge' and 'education') have both formal and informal connotations.

THEORY AND PRACTICE

Given that theory has undergone some degree of clarification, its relationship to practice and research can be considered.

Its relationship to practice appears to have some substance, in the formal arena at least. (Formal practice is the collective, public actions of a specific discipline; informal practice merely our day-to-day actions.) Disciplines with an established body of formal knowledge (broadly speaking, the sciences) frequently seek out practical applications for that knowledge: every pure science has its applied counterpart. Moreover, it is the theories of the pure scientists that dictate the actions of those in practice, the applied scientists. Though the relationship between theory and practice appears to exist, it seems somewhat unidirectional in nature.

Further evidence for a unidirectional relationship comes from the activities of the practice-based disciplines. Of the practice-based disciplines that have sought out theoretical justifications for their actions, most (and nursing has to be included here) have merely borrowed theories from other (usually more powerful, scientific) disciplines, using those theories to define their practices.

There are, however, some practitioners, notably social workers (Howe 1987), who argue the converse: that in a practice-based discipline foreign theories cannot dictate practice; if theory is to have any relevance, it has to be extracted from practice.

There is, as such, some justification in assuming that the relationship between theory and practice is, in the formal arena at least, bidirectional. If a bidirectional relationship between theory and practice exists in the formal arena, is such a relationship evident in the informal arena? Is there a relationship between informal theory (thought) and informal practice (action)? To answer this question, the discussion has to enter the realms of cognitive

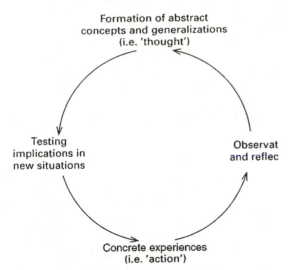

FIGURE 29.1 Kolb's learning cycle (adapted with permission from Kolb *et al.*, 1991 *Organizational Behavior: An Experiential Approach* 5th edn. Prentice Hall, New Jersey, p. 59).

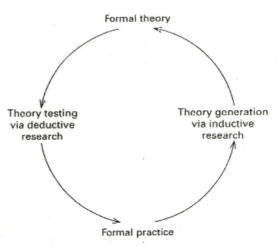

FIGURE 29.2 A learning cycle for the acquisition of formal knowledge.

psychology. Learning theorists, in particular, have something to say on the matter.

Kolb's Learning Cycle

One leading learning theorist, Kolb (see, for example, Kolb *et al.*, 1991), has not only speculated on the interrelationships between thought and action, he has also addressed the nature of these interrelationships. Consider Kolb's model of learning, adapted in Figure 29.1.

Learning is, according to Kolb, a cyclical process; a continual dialogue between thought and action that is effected via two processes: testing and reflection. Preconceived ideas, i.e., thoughts, about the world are tested against reality (ideas are put into practice; action is taken), after which the relative successes or failures of these actions are reflected upon. These reflections, in turn, lead to the refinement and development of our thoughts about the world.

Because Kolb's learning cycle considers the relationships between thought and action, rather than theory and practice, it is essen-

tially a model of informal learning; it is a model depicting the acquisition of informal (personal, implicit, 'micro') knowledge.

Though Kolb uses the terms 'testing' and 'reflection' to describe the processes linking thought and action, these processes can be described using a single word, 'research'. This comment becomes all the more meaningful if an analogous learning cycle for the formal arena is considered (see Figure 29.2).

A Universal Model of Knowledge Acquisition

Given that knowledge is acquired in the same manner in both the formal and the informal arenas, it is possible to delineate a universal model of knowledge acquisition. Such a model, as proposed by the author, is depicted in Figure 29.3.

Several points need to be made about this model. Firstly, the model stresses the importance of experience ('applying') in the acquisition of knowledge. Secondly, it acknowledges that knowledge has both cognitive and practical dimensions: it is both a model of theory (thought) development and of practice

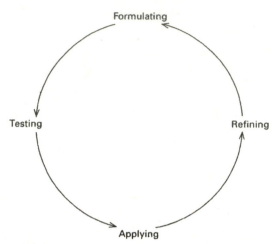

FIGURE 29.3 A learning cycle for the acquisition of knowledge.

TABLE 29.2   A Typology of 'research'

'Testing'	'Refining'
Analysing	Interpreting
Experimentation	Reflecting (I)
Deducing	Inducing
Deductive research (F)	Inductive research (F)
Quantitative research (F)	Qualitative research (F)
The scientific method (F)	Phenomenological research (F)
Theory/hypothesis testing	Theory generation
'Assaying' (Dickoff & James 1968b)	'Divining'; 'heuristic' research (Dickoff & James 1968b)

F, a term employed mainly in the formal arena.
I, a term employed mainly in the informal arena.

(action) development. It is, as such, a holistic model of knowledge acquisition. Thirdly, it sees the acquisition of knowledge as a dynamic process. Finally, learning is only complete when formulating and applying fuse, that is when there is no 'theory–practice gap'. (This point is discussed in more detail later.)

Research as the Link Between Theory and Practice

Research plays a key role in the acquisition of both formal and informal knowledge: testing and refining are the links between formulating and applying. In other words, learning cannot occur without research.

Though the author has labelled the two types of research 'testing' and 'refining', a variety of terms have been employed to describe these two processes. These are summarized in Table 29.2.

It is worth remarking that the universal model of knowledge acquisition proposed has striking similarities to Lewin's model of action research (see, for example, Lewin's 'change spiral' in Lewin, 1958). These similarities, however, are to be expected, as learning is an inherent part of 'change', a key concept in Lewin's work.

THE THEORY–PRACTICE GAP IN NURSING

The notion of the theory–practice gap has caused much debate within nursing (Vaughn, 1989, Lindsay 1990, Cook, 1991, McCaugherty 1991, McCaugherty, 1992b, Nolan & Grant, 1992). Two interrelated factors appear to be at the centre of this debate: (a) the necessity of a theory–practice gap if learning is to commence, and (b) its attenuation if learning is to progress.

The necessity of a theory–practice gap in nursing has been recognized by several authors (Lindsay, 1990; Cook 1991). As such, these authors argue that those (like Vaughn, 1989) who propose 'solutions' for the theory–practice gap are barking up the wrong tree.

Nevertheless, knowledge development, both formal and informal, can by definition only occur if the theory–practice gap narrows.

As such, much of the debate on the theory–practice gap (both within and outside nursing) has centred on the factors thought to hinder the narrowing of this gap. The major hindrance appears to be the cultural dominance of 'technical rationality' (Schön 1988).

The Dominance of Technical Rationality

Technical rationality is an objective approach to the discovery of 'truth'; an epistemology that unashamedly sees the relationship between theory and practice as unidirectional; theory precedes practice. Theory is, as such, afforded a greater status than practice or, to use the framework of the universal model of knowledge acquisition, formulating is afforded a greater status than applying. Technical rationality, furthermore, prides itself in its objectivity: testing (deductive experimentation) is seen as the superior research method, whereas refining (reflection and inductive research) is derided because of its subjective nature.

The dominance of technical rationality is evident in the organization of higher education and in a consideration of the professions. Those disciplines with a well-established body of theoretical knowledge (obtained largely from experimentation) are afforded the greatest status. Similarly, those disciplines distinguished enough to be called a profession are usually grounded in science. Consider, for example, the status of the pure sciences over the social sciences, and the status of medicine over nursing and social work.

Technical rationality, however, gives a very biased and artificial view of the world. Appleyard (1992) writes:

> . . . scientific knowledge is fundamentally paradoxical . . . all of science's 'truths' about the 'real' world are based upon the most flagrant distortion. In cre-

ating an understandable universe, we have committed ourselves to the most gross and obvious oversimplification. We have excluded the understanding mechanism, the self. (p. 208)

Schön (1988) suggests that this paradox can be resolved by acknowledging the importance of subjectivity in the acquisition of knowledge; for example, by reflecting on our actions, and by granting inductive research an equal status with deductive research. He calls for

> . . . an epistemology of practice which places technical problem solving ['science'] within a broader context of reflective enquiry . . . (p. 76)

Theory–practice gaps fail to narrow, therefore, because technical rationality denies subjectivity a place in the acquisition of knowledge. For knowledge to be acquired effectively, both forms of research—testing and refining—need to be in place. Adherence solely to technical rationality or, indeed, to its converse, reflective inquiry, serves only to deflect the acquisition of knowledge.

APPLICATION OF THE MODEL TO NURSING

Three messages become apparent when the universal model of knowledge acquisition is applied to nursing.

Firstly, a theoretical component is essential if a practice-based discipline, like nursing, is to develop. Nursing only really develops if improvements in patient care become manifest. As such, Nolan and Grant (1992) are justified in making the salient point that the ultimate benefit of theory in nursing is the improvement in patient care.

Secondly, research, being the link between theory and practice, is the key to the development of a discipline. Research should, furthermore, be carried out on both a formal and an informal level. Whilst informal research (putting ideas into practice and reflecting on them) is the key to individual development, the qualities of individual practitioners will also be reflected in the make-up of the discipline as a whole. And whilst formal (deductive and inductive) research is the key to the development of a discipline as a whole, the outcomes of such research (a change in formal theory and/or practice) will, in turn, influence the individual members of that discipline.

Thirdly, the research process has to be bidirectional. There is indeed a need for reflective skills and for formal, deductive research in nursing. Refining, however, has to coexist with testing; if nursing is to develop, it has to be both a science and an art.

From Novice to Expert: Nurse Education

In order to discuss the relevance of the universal model of knowledge acquisition to nurse education, a brief consideration of the work of Benner is required.

In her seminal book *From Novice to Expert*, Benner (1984) examines the acquisition of 'expertise' in nursing. She argues that there are five levels of nursing proficiency: novice, advanced beginner, competent, proficient and expert. Given that these levels are hierarchical, a continuum of nursing expertise is implied.

In her glossary, Benner defines expertise as a hybrid of theoretical and practical knowledge. Given that the universal model of knowledge acquisition is essentially a model of the acquisition of theoretical and practical knowledge (the two are, after all, intrinsically linked), the model can be incorporated into

THE NURSING EXPERTISE CONTINUUM

Novice Advanced beginner Competent Proficient Expert

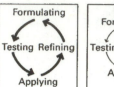

FIGURE 29.4 The universal model of knowledge acquisition and the transition from novice to expert in nursing.

Benner's theoretical framework with relative ease (see Figure 29.4).

In the novice, the gap between formulating and applying (theory and practice) is understandably and necessarily wide. The gap reduces as expertise develops, to the extent that the gap no longer exists when expertise is attained. At this point, the boundaries between theoretical and practical knowledge become blurred: action effectively becomes intuitive.

The thickness of the arrows in the novice learning cycle indicates that the cycle is highly active; novice nurses have a lot to learn. As the novice progresses towards expertise, the learning cycle becomes less active (hence the thinner arrows) until, when expertise is achieved, it grinds to a halt (hence the absence of arrows).

This is not to say that experts cannot learn. Expertise develops only in certain discrete areas of nursing; the cycle of learning must recommence whenever the expert is faced with new situations. It could, as such, be argued that expertise is never truly achieved.

The Role of Research

Though not making explicit reference to the role of research in the acquisition of expertise, Benner does nevertheless imply the necessity of research. She writes:

Expertise develops when the clinician *tests* and *refines* propositions, hypotheses, and principle-based expectations in actual practice situations. (p. 3; emphasis added)

Though informal research is the key to developing the personal expertise of a practitioner, note that formal research can play a similar role in developing the expertise of a discipline as a whole.

USES AND ABUSES OF NURSING MODELS

Novice nurses literally have no idea of how to practice. Whilst the novice nurse may well have informal theories (that is, ideas) of how to act in a particular situation, the nurse cannot feasibly test those theories (and indeed reflect on them) because of the risks to patients if the nurse blunders.

Novice nurses, therefore, require some guidelines for practice. This is where the value of formal models (such as hospital rules, standard procedures, the nursing process, nursing models and models borrowed from other disciplines) comes into play. Gordon (1984) writes:

For the individual lacking mastery, formal models can serve as *a substitute for personal knowledge and experience.* (p. 230)

She adds:

Let formal models . . . be regarded as training wheels, essential for the first safe rides, unnecessary and limiting once replaced by greater skill. (p. 243)

This latter quote from Gordon has a far-reaching implication for nursing, namely that expert nurses need only their own informal, internalized, personal theories to guide prac-

tice (subject, of course, to ethical and legal constraints). This remark may alarm those in the nursing profession who believe in the sanctity of one or other of the many nursing models, but it is concurrent with Benner's notion of an expert as an intuitive practitioner.

The Nursing Process

Whilst expert practitioners in other disciplines (in the medical profession, for example) enjoy the autonomy granted by informal theories, there is a need to ask why nurses continue to be passive and rule-bound. Take the nursing process, for example. As a simple set of rules for systemizing nursing care, it provides a particularly useful guide for the novice nurse. However, the nursing process soon becomes internalized in most nurses (most reasonably experienced nurses intuitively carry out the nursing process), so why does the nursing profession insist on documentation under discrete titles like 'assessment', 'plan' and 'evaluation' and why does every nursing action have to be rigidly recorded?

Why nurses are passive and rule-bound is a complex question, for which there are no immediate answers, though Meleis (1991) speculates that historical and cultural paternalism are largely to blame. Meleis suggests, furthermore, that the passivity of nurses has hindered theory development in nursing, because theory development (and, indeed, practice development) are, as we have seen, part of the same active process.

CONCLUSION

If the body of knowledge, both theoretical and practical, of a practice-based discipline is to develop, then research has to play a key role. Furthermore, if individual practitioners are to develop expertise, they too must undertake research, even if on an informal, personal level.

The successful education (and continuing education) of nurses is, as such, dependent on the opportunity both to test and refine, and to experiment and reflect. Nurse educators may well need to provide novice nurses with a range of formal models and theories to guide practice initially, but they equally need to encourage nurses to test and refine those models and theories so that they might develop their own personal models of practice.

As a final comment, the author urges nurses to heed the advice of Lindsay (1990), who notes that:

> Each nurse needs to recognize that the theorist, researcher . . . and practitioner exist to some extent in all of us. (p. 35)

REFERENCES

Appleyard B. (1992) *Understanding the Present: Science and the Soul of Modern Man*. Pan, London.

Benner P. (ed.) (1984) *From Novice To Expert: Excellence and Power in Clinical Nursing Practice*. Addison-Wesley, Menlo Park, California.

Chinn P.L. & Jacobs M.K. (1987) *Theory and Nursing: A Systematic Approach* 2nd edn. C.V. Mosby, St. Louis.

Cook S.H. (1991) Mind the theory/practice gap in nursing. *Journal of Advanced Nursing* 16, 1462–1469.

Dickoff J. & James P. (1968a) A theory of theories: A position paper. *Nursing Research* 17, 197–203.

Dickoff J. & James P. (1968b) Researching research's role in theory development. *Nursing Research* 17, 204–206.

Gordon D.R. (1984) Research application: Identifying the use and misuse of formal models in nursing practice. *In From Novice to Expert: Excellence and Power in Clinical Nursing Practice* (Benner P. ed.), Addison-Wesley, Menlo Park, California, pp. 225–243.

Howe D. (1987) *An Introduction to Social Work Theory: Making Sense in Practice*. Wildwood House, Aldershot.

Kolb D.A., Rubin I.M. & Osland J. (1991) *Organizational Behavior: An Experiential Approach,* 5th ed. Prentice-Hall International, London.

Lewin K. (1958) Group decision and social change. *In Readings in Social Psychology* 3rd ed. (Maccoby E., Newcomb T.M. & Sanford N. eds), Henry Holt, New York, pp. 197–211.

Lindsay B. (1990) The gap between theory and practice. *Nursing Standard* 5(4); 34–35.

McCaugherty D. (1991) The use of a teaching model to promote reflection and the experiential integration of theory and practice in first-year student nurses: an action research study. *Journal of Advanced Nursing* 16, 534–543.

McCaugherty D. (1992a) The concepts of theory and practice. *Senior Nurse* 12(2): 29–33.

McCaugherty D. (1992b) The gap between nursing theory and practice. *Senior Nurse* 12(6): 44–48.

Meleis A.I. (1991) *Theoretical Nursing: Development and Progress,* 2nd ed. Lippincott, Philadelphia.

Nolan M. & Grant G. (1992) Mid-range theory building and the nursing theory-practice gap: A respite care case study. *Journal of Advanced Nursing* 17, 217–223.

Sch{auo}n D.A. (1988) From technical rationality to reflection-in-action. *In Professional Judgement: A Reader in Clinical Decision Making* (Dowie J. & Elstein A. eds), Cambridge University Press, Cambridge, pp. 60–77.

Stevens B.J. (1984) *Nursing Theory: Analysis, Application and Evaluation* 2nd edn. Little Brown, Boston.

Vaughn B. (1989) Two roles—one job. *Nursing Times* 85(11), 52.

30

Theory-testing Research: Building the Science

GAYLE J. ACTON, RN, MSN

BARBARA L. IRVIN, RN, MN

BARBARA A. HOPKINS, RN, MSN, CNAA

Lack of emphasis on the empirical validation of nursing models has hindered the development of nursing science. This chapter explores issues concerning theory development in nursing and criteria for evaluating theory-testing research. From a comprehensive review of the literature on theory testing, 15 criteria are identified as essential for evaluating theory-testing studies. The criteria are applied to selected research reports, and recommendations for future use of criteria are suggested.

The paucity of reported research that specifically tests nursing models is a deterrent to the development of the scientific base for nursing. Further, the lack of attention to criteria for evaluating theory-testing research has led to the inadequate use of nursing models for guiding the design and analysis of many nursing studies. We will address problems related to theory-testing research and offer criteria that the authors hope will prove useful for advancing the science of nursing.

BACKGROUND OF THE PROBLEM

To establish nursing as distinct and separate from other health-care professions, we nurse scientists must identify and validate that body of knowledge that is uniquely ours. Essential to this task is the establishment of a solid theoretic base upon which to develop knowledge, conduct research, and guide practice. The lack of such a base has been identified as an important problem facing nursing today.[1] To overcome this problem, support for theory in the form of testing must be demonstrated.[2]

Nursing is in the early stages of developing its science. Typical of a young science are theoretic gaps and inconsistencies. These inconsistencies are usually the result of newly discovered concepts and relationships that do not fit into or are not addressed by existing theories, thereby creating theoretic gaps.[3] Such gaps exist in nursing today, although theory development has been a goal since the 1950s. It has only been in the last decade that nursing has been able to agree on a universal definition of nursing. With the publication of the *ANA Social Policy Statement*,[4] the focus of nursing changed from the disease process to the identification of human responses to health

Source: Acton, G. J., Irwin, B. L., & Hopkins, B. A. (1991). Theory testing research: Building the science. *ANS, 14* (1): 52–61. Reprinted with permission from and copyright © 1991 Aspen Publishers, Inc.

and illness. This focus created new concepts and relationships to be discovered and explored. Testing of both new and established concepts and relationships, however, has not earned priority status.

Nurse leaders have called for increased theory validation for the past 30 years. Evidence that unique theories are being developed is provided by Moody,[5] who compiled a list of 11 established and 30 emerging nurse theorists. However, few authors responded in 1984 when Chinn,[6] as editor of *ANS*, called for manuscripts reporting theory-testing research. Further, Moody's analysis of nursing research from 1977 to 1986[7] showed that, of 720 studies described in six research journals, only 3% tested theory, concepts, or hypotheses from an explicit conceptual or theoretical framework. Silva[8] also reported that only 9 of 62 research reports identifying a specific nursing theory fell into the category of theory testing. One can conclude from these analyses that the nursing profession has been more concerned with the development of theory than with its testing. Yet theories for nursing are only as strong as their tests of accuracy.[9,10]

Theory-testing research seeks to develop evidence about hypotheses derived from a theory. Thus, deductive reasoning forms the basis for theory testing. Deductive reasoning begins with broad theoretic concepts and narrows to specific observations. That is, it explains and predicts what will be observed, thus converting theory into relational statements, propositions, and hypotheses that can be tested by appropriate research methods.[11]

The question, "Can nursing theory be tested?" was both raised and answered by Jacobs, who responded, "Yes and no, perhaps."[12(p39)] This apparent ambivalence results from the problem of directly testing nursing theory. Tests of the grand theories are problematic, because the abstract theoretical constructs do not lend themselves to empirical measurement. Regardless of this dilemma,

however, Fawcett[13] stressed that nursing must continue to work on theory development. She emphasizes the need to create conceptual-theoretical-empirical structures that will allow for theory testing. Such structures identify and describe nursing conceptual model constructs, including propositions, that result in theory-level concepts and propositions that can be empirically measured and tested.

Despite the emphasis on testing, theories cannot be proven or disproven. Theories are dynamic and, at best, tentative. They attempt to explain what has been observed in reality and to predict what will be observed in research.[11] Theory-testing research evaluates how well the explanations and predictions that evolve from the theory hold up and thus refines theory into a clearer and more useful depiction of reality.[9,14]

Through scientific research, a theory may be validated, refuted, or modified. Typically, several studies are necessary to test a theory adequately, and the more rigorous the test, the more valuable the theory becomes. Therefore, it is only when theories are tested and refined repeatedly that their worth can be evaluated.[10,15]

REVIEW OF LITERATURE

To identify criteria for evaluating theory-testing research, a comprehensive search of the nursing literature, as well as a review of theory-testing literature in the social sciences, was conducted. The articles reviewed were primarily those published between 1986 and 1990. Potential sources were obtained by searching titles, abstracts, and keyword indices using the terms *theory*, *testing*, and *research*. Studies for this article were not restricted to any particular nursing model, unlike the search by Silva[8] that was limited to five nursing models. In fact, an effort was made by the authors to include new nursing models that are examples of developing mid-range theories.

In her now classic article, Silva[8] addressed the pressing need for the development and testing of nursing theory to establish the scientific base for nursing. She pointed out the lack of clarity about what constitutes theory testing, particularly with regard to nursing theory. Silva identified the degree to which empirical research explicitly tested nursing theory by using specified evaluation criteria. She evaluated and reported three exemplary cases of empirical research that tested theoretic constructs or propositions derived from a nursing grand theory. In addition, Silva discussed various implications for nursing theory, practice, and research, including factors that impede and enhance the testing of nursing theory.

One of the major flaws identified by Silva[8] is that many researchers have mistakenly labeled their work as theory-testing research. In fact, most authors merely use an identified model or theoretic framework for organization of the study or structuring of instruments. Because of this Silva classified the 62 studies she analyzed into three categories: minimal, insufficient, and adequate use of models to constitute theory testing. Of these studies, 24 fell into the minimal category, 29 into the insufficient category, and only 9 into the adequate category.

As a result of these findings, Silva[8] determined that an expressed purpose of a theory-testing study is to examine the underlying validity of the assumptions or propositions of a selected nursing model. She also stated that a nursing model must be explicitly identified as a theoretic framework for the research. The model must be discussed comprehensively enough for the connection of the hypotheses or purposes and the model to be clear.

Other criteria identified by Silva[8] are that the hypotheses or purposes must be empirically tested in an appropriate manner, and that, as a result of this test, indirect evidence exists of the validity (or lack thereof) of the designated assumptions or propositions. Silva also stated that authors should present a discussion of the extent to which the evidence explains, supports, or refutes the relevant aspects of the model or theory.

Walker and Avant[16] adapted Silva's criteria to make them more specific and concise. They also added the following criterion: "The hypotheses used to test a specific theory are designed to put the theory at risk for falsification by virtue of their specificity and compatibility with only a limited set of events."[16(p199)] These authors argued that "the more specific the predictions that can be made from a theory, the more readily it can be falsified and the narrower the range of data that will support the theory."[16(p199)] They further stated that a theory can be judged as valid and falsifiable when the results of testing highly specific hypotheses yield data that closely fit predictions.

In a comparative discussion of theory-testing versus theory-generating research, Chinn and Jacobs[14] articulated theory-testing criteria. These authors asserted not only that the portion of the theoretic framework under study must be described explicitly and summarized, but also that the literature review must describe previous studies based on the theory and must trace how the study has been conceived. The research problem may be stated in question form, but it must clarify how the research is to be accomplished, clarify the variables or events to be studied, and reflect possibilities for operationalizing abstract concepts.[14]

Chinn and Jacobs[14] also discussed the importance of the theoretic adequacy of instruments and approaches to assessing changes that can be expected on the basis of the theory. "The problems of reliability and validity of both direct and indirect observations . . . are also important in theory-testing research."[14(p161)] Further, these authors state that sample selection should be such that subject responses will support or refute the theory. Obviously, this statement assumes that the requirements for statistical analysis will be met.

Chinn and Jacobs[14] asserted that testing relationships between variables requires deliberate manipulation of circumstances so that what was hypothesized can be assessed. Accordingly, the design must be consistent with the theoretic basis for the study. In addition, data analysis "must be consistent with the purposes of the research as well as the research design."[14(p163)] The analysis should yield enough quantitative and qualitative evidence to answer the research question or to support or reject the hypotheses. An interpretive analysis of the results as they pertain to the theory should be included in the study conclusions. In addition, the conclusions should address the theoretic significance of the research.

To supplement the above discussion, it is worth noting a few observations by other authors. Nieswiadomy,[17] for example, stressed that hypotheses or research questions must be based on a propositional statement or statements from the theory. Polit and Hungler added that hypotheses are "predictions about the manner in which variables would be related, if the theory were correct and useful."[18(p92)]

Serlin[19] noted that scientists must state in advance what outcomes will be accepted as falsification of the theory under test, agreeing that no ad hoc appeals to unaccounted factors should be made. Looking toward the future, Serlin argued for "the appraisal of theories and the detection of progress if science is to take on an historical character, replacing the pitting of two theories against each other with a competition between research programs."[19(p369)]

It should be noted here that the substantive use of structural equation modeling has been growing in psychology and other social sciences and is beginning to find some acceptance in nursing as well. One reason is that these confirmatory methods provide researchers with a comprehensive means for assessing and modifying theoretic models.[20]

In describing the findings of a study, Nieswiadomy[17] stressed the need to focus on explanations provided by the theory being tested. Further, she stated that any implications for nursing must be based on "the explanatory power of the theory."[17(p102)] The ability of a theory to explain study findings, or conversely, its inability to hold up as expected, is important in the determination of its value for clinical practice.

The preceding discussion has addressed some of the issues related to theory-testing research. From this review of the literature concerning theory-testing, 15 criteria were identified by the authors as essential for evaluating theory-testing studies. No attempt was made to include all criteria necessary for a comprehensive research critique. As Silva stated, just "because a study has met the evaluation criteria for theory testing does not necessarily guarantee that the study is sound. Other evaluation criteria, in addition to those related to theory testing, are important in assessing the overall quality of a study."[8(p4)] The criteria proposed by the authors and the rationale for the selection of each criterion follow.

CRITERIA FOR EVALUATING THEORY-TESTING RESEARCH

Criterion 1

The purpose of the study is to examine the empirical validity of the constructs, concepts, assumptions, or relationships from the identified theoretic frame of reference.

Rationale. It is important for the investigator to explicate the purpose of the study as being the testing of specific aspects of a theory or theoretic framework. Doing so assists the reader in determining that the investigator really did test a theory and did not just use it to organize the study or guide instrument selection. Readers need to know if the underlying tenets of the theory are valid, to avoid erroneous interpretations of data.

Criterion 2

The theoretic frame of reference must be explicitly described and summarized.

Rationale. Making explicit the tenets of a model or theoretic frame of reference accomplishes two purposes. First, readers can become familiar with the model and/or validate their perceptions of it. Second, readers can follow the logic (or illogic) of the author through the remaining steps of the report. Potential consumers must be able to determine a clear relationship between the model and the hypotheses to be tested.

Criterion 3

The constructs and concepts to be examined are theoretically defined.

Rationale. Theoretic definitions communicate the general meaning of the concept and permit the identification of empirical indicators.[14] The researcher must define the concepts or constructs on the basis of the theory so that accurate and valid measures will be obtainable.[17] Appropriate instruments are sometimes hard to find, and the researcher may elect to adapt a conceptual definition; however, this decision must then be explicated for the reader.

Criterion 4

An overview of previous studies that are based on the theoretic framework, or that clearly show

the derivation of the concepts being tested, must be included in the review of the literature.

Rationale. The researcher must present evidence that he or she has conducted an extensive search of the literature for studies based on the theoretic frame of reference. The reporting of this research demonstrates that the investigator is thoroughly familiar with and understands previous theoretic work. Studies reported in the review of the literature should provide a logical base for the present study. In addition, Polit and Hungler[18] noted that the researcher should evaluate the theory before using it as the basis of a study.

Criterion 5

The research questions or hypotheses are logically derived from the definitions, assumptions, or propositions of the theoretic frame of reference.

Rationale. Research questions or hypotheses should be "explicitly formulated . . . to show, with the maximum exactness possible, relationships between the theory base for the research and the particular research study being conducted."[14(p156)] Theory-testing research permits the investigator to ascertain how accurately the theory is able to predict events in the empirical world. To determine the accuracy, the researcher poses hypotheses derived from the theoretic relationships that can be empirically tested and states them as questions or hypotheses.[21]

Criterion 6

The research questions or hypotheses are specific enough to put the theoretic frame of reference at risk for falsification.

Rationale. The goal of theory testing is to refute or falsify hypothetical relationships derived from the theoretical framework. "When a hypothesis states a relationship between empirical indicators, all assertions about that relationship must be testable."[22(p59)] "A falsifiable hypothesis must be sufficiently precise so that incompatible empirical results can be easily identified."[22(p60)] The findings must provide support for potential confirmation or disconfirmation of the theory.[18] Hypotheses must also be justifiable, that is, they must be derived from the theoretic frame of reference and their relationships supported by prior research findings.[18,23,24]

Criterion 7

The operational definitions are clearly derived from the theoretic frame of reference.

Rationale. To test a theory empirically, concepts must be clear and empirically observable.[22] If the purpose of the study is theory testing, then the operational definition of the concepts must be derived from the theory.[17] According to Jacobs,[12] one variant of testing theory is the selection of conceptual linkages from the parent framework for testing. The need for theoretically derived operational definitions is particularly important to this process.

Criterion 8

The design is congruent with the level of theory described in the theoretic frame of reference.

Rationale. To use the empirical approach, one must determine what sort of evidence will validly test the theory and must rule out competing hypotheses.[3] The evidence needed will be based on the extent to which the theory is developed. If all phenomena have not been clearly described, then the theory-testing task would be to describe one or more phenomena. If the phenomena are described, but all relationships are not established, then the researcher's task would be to explore relationships among the phenomena. Once these relationships are known, theory testing would seek to validate them. Often, the theory-testing design is experimental, quasi-experimental, or correlational.[18,25]

Criterion 9

The instruments must be theoretically valid and reliable.

Rationale. To validate or refute theory, measurement of the theoretic concepts and their relationships must be made. Measurement via empirical instruments is fundamental to the testing of theoretic concepts and their relationships. Evidence of instrument validity and reliability for the concepts under study must be included in the research report. Such information permits the reader to determine whether the concepts of the theory were indeed measured correctly.[26]

Criterion 10

The theoretic frame of reference guided the sample selection.

Rationale. If one is conducting research to validate or falsify theory, selection of the sample must be theoretically guided. "Theory must determine in what ways the sample should be representative."[19(p366)] If the sample is not representative of the persons to whom the theory applies, the researcher will not have put the theory at risk for falsification.

Criterion 11

The statistics used are the most robust possible.

Rationale. The purpose of theory-testing research is to validate or falsify the theory; therefore, the strictest possible test must be used. Experimental, quasi-experimental, or exploratory designs are commonly associated with theory-testing research, and they necessitate the use of inferential statistics. Causal or structural equation modeling is the most stringent statistical test, because it allows the researcher to assess and modify the model.[3] However, the developmental level of the model will dictate the design and, accordingly, which statistic is the most robust for the study.

Criterion 12

The analysis of data must provide evidence for supporting, refuting, or modifying the theoretic framework.

Rationale. The empirical validity of a model must be determined so that one may use the theory upon which the study is based.[8] The analysis of data must also be congruent with the aims of the theory for appropriate interpretation of the data to occur.[14] Reynolds stated that "there are three possible outcomes for any research: either it supports the theoretical statement, it does not support the theoretical statement, or it is inconclusive."[15(p118)] The purpose of the analysis of data is an attempt to produce one of these outcomes. Data analysis, therefore, presents evidence to accept or reject the proposed hypotheses that allows a researcher to make conclusions regarding the validity of the model.

Criterion 13

The research report must include an interpretive analysis of the findings in relation to the theory being tested.

Rationale. For the reader to evaluate the theory in question, the researcher must provide an interpretive analysis of the data in relation to the explanations provided by the theory. Theory is only as strong as its tests of confirmability; therefore, the research report must present conclusions supporting, or failing to support, the theoretic relationships.[10,15]

Criterion 14

The significance of the theory for nursing is discussed in the report.

Rationale. Reynolds[15] stated that substantive significance is usually more important than statistical significance. The researcher must report the implications for nursing on the basis of the support provided by the explanatory power of the theory.[17] Without such information, the reader is unable to determine the potential usefulness of the theory for practice.

Criterion 15

Ideally, the researcher makes recommendations for further research on the basis of the theoretic findings.

Rationale. Although this is not really an essential criterion for theory-testing research, it is a vital step in the research process. First, the researcher should now be thoroughly familiar with the theory in question and therefore expert in the research needed to further its validity. Second, the researcher is most familiar with the data generated by the study and best able to ascertain directions that might prove fruitful for further investigation. Failure to report these recommendations could hinder future efforts to provide support or rejection of the theory,

Study Author	1. Purpose	2. Theory	3. Construct/concept	4. Review of literature	5. Question/hypothesis	6. Specificity	7. Operational definitions	8. Design	9. Instruments	10. Sample	11. Statistics	12. Analysis	13. Interpretation	14. Significance	15. Recommendations
Braden	+	+	+	+	+	+	+	+	+	+	+	+	+	+	+
Frey	+	+	+	+	+	+	+	+	+	+	+	+	+	+	–
Frey & Denyes	+	+	+	–	+	–	+	+	+	–	+	+	+	–	–
Leidy	+	+	+	+	+	+	+	+	+	±	+	+	+	+	+
Mishel & Braden	+	+	+	+	+	+	+	+	±	+	+	+	+	–	–
Smith	+	+	+	+	+	+	+	+	+	+	+	+	+	+	+

FIGURE 30.1. Evaluation of the usefulness of the identified theory-testing criteria, using six selected studies.

+ = criterion met; – = criterion not met; ± = criterion partially met

thereby retarding the development of nursing science. Therefore, the authors have elected to make this an essential criterion.

APPLICATION OF EVALUATIVE CRITERIA

A number of studies were examined to evaluate the usefulness of the identified theory-testing criteria. Of these, six[27-32] were selected for critique, so as to demonstrate the application of the 15 criteria. These studies represented well-known nursing models and differed in design and statistical analyses. Figure 30.1 presents the studies examined during the process of determining the adequacy of the criteria.

The research reports selected for critique were representative of research explicitly testing theory. Each used a nursing theory or conceptual model to provide the framework from which concepts and propositions for testing are derived. Four of the reports[27-29,32] explicitly stated that they were testing concepts or propositions from a nursing theory or conceptual framework. Braden,[27] Kline-Leidy,[30] and Smith[32] demonstrated fulfillment of all 15 identified criteria. Each of these reports is an excellent example of theory-testing research. While Frey,[28] Frey and Denyes,[29] and Mishel and Braden[31] did not fulfill each of the 15 criteria, they are to be commended for research aimed at expanding the knowledge base for nursing.

RECOMMENDATIONS

First, researchers should identify theory-testing studies in their abstracts, publication titles, and library retrieval keywords. This strategy was initially proposed by Silva[8] to remedy the difficulty that investigators face in locating studies that have tested nursing models. By specifying the model or theorist in the title or abstract, the author will facilitate the dissemination of information about the validity and use of specific methods.

Second, investigators should continue to study and refine theory-testing criteria. Through systematic effort to identify, apply, and evaluate criteria used in theory-based research, nurse scientists will accelerate development of the nursing database.

Third, nursing scholars should consider theory-testing criteria in relation to their individual research programs as well as to the research priorities for the nursing profession as a whole. Decisions about nursing versus interdisciplinary models, methodology, and level of theory development affect the quality of the research outcomes as well as the focal variables for study.

CONCLUSIONS

The authors have examined the concept of theory testing and some issues concerning theory testing in nursing. In addition, they have identified from the literature 15 criteria that are proposed as essential for evaluating theory-testing research. To demonstrate the value of the criteria, the authors applied them systematically to six studies in which concepts deducted from nursing models were tested.

This builds on the work of Silva[8] and others[14,16-20] who have explicitly delineated formative evaluation criteria. The authors put forth this effort in the spirit of challenge and hope that nurse scientists will continue to improve the quality of theory-testing research.

REFERENCES

1. Engstrom JL. Problems in the development, use and testing of nursing theory. *J Nurs Educ*. 1986;23:245-251.

2. Schlotfeldt RM. Resolution of issues: An imperative for creating nursing's future. *J Prof Nurs*. 1987:136-142.

3. Hanley C. A problem of theory testing. *Int Rev Psycho-Anal*. 1983;10:393-405.

4. *ANA Social Policy Statement*. Kansas City, Mo: American Nurses Association, 1980.

5. Moody LE. *Advancing Nursing Science Through Research*. Newbury Park, Calif: Sage, 1990.

6. Chinn PL. From the editor. *ANS*. 1984;6:ix.

7. Moody LE, Wilson ME, Smyth K, Schwartz R, Tittle M, Van Cott ML. Analysis of a decade of nursing practice research: 1977-1986. *Nurs Res*. 1988;37(6):374-379.

8. Silva MC. Research testing nursing theory: State of the art. *ANS*. 1986;9(10):1-11.

9. Thomas BS. *Nursing Research. An Experiential Approach*. St. Louis, Mo: Mosby, 1990.

10. Treece EW, Treece JW. *Elements of Research in Nursing*. St. Louis, Mo: Mosby, 1986.

11. Seaman CHC. *Research Methods. Principles, Practice and Theory for Nursing*. Norwalk, Conn: Appleton & Lange, 1987.

12. Jacobs MK. Can nursing theory be tested? In: Chinn PL, ed. *Nursing Research Methodology*. Rockville, Md: Aspen Publishers, 1986.

13. Fawcett J. Conceptual models and theory development. *J Gynecol Neonat Nurs*. 1988;17(6):400-403.

14. Chinn PL, Jacobs MK. *Theory and Nursing. A Systematic Approach*. St. Louis, Mo: Mosby, 1987.

15. Reynolds PD. *A Primer in Theory Construction*. New York, NY: Macmillan, 1971.

16. Walker LO, Avant KC. *Strategies For Theory Construction in Nursing*. 2nd ed. Norwalk, Conn.: Appleton & Lange, 1988.

17. Nieswiadomy RM. *Foundations Of Nursing Research*. Norwalk, Conn: Appleton & Lange, 1987.

18. Polit DF, Hungler BP. *Nursing Research. Principles and Methods*. Philadelphia, Pa: Lippincott, 1987.

19. Serlin RC. Hypothesis testing: Theory building, and the philosophy of science. *J Counseling Psychol*. 1987;34(4):365-371.

20. Anderson JC, Gerbing DW. Structural equation modeling in practice: A review and recommended two-step approach. *Psychol Bull*. 1988;103(3):411-423.

21. Woods NF, Catanzaro M. *Nursing Research, Theory and Practice*. St. Louis, Mo: Mosby, 1988.

22. Fawcett J, Downs FS. *The Relationship of Theory and Research*. Norwalk, Conn: Appleton-Century-Crofts, 1986.

23. Phillips LRF. *A Clinician's Guide to the Critique and Utilization of Nursing Research*. Norwalk, Conn: Appleton-Century-Crofts, 1986.

24. Wilson HS. *Research in Nursing*. Menlo Park, Calif: Addison-Wesley, 1985.

25. Campbell DT, Stanley JC. *Experimental and Quasi-experimental Designs for Research*. Boston, Mass: Houghton Mifflin, 1963.

26. Rew L, Stuppy D, Becker H. Construct validity in instrument development: A vital link between nursing practice, research, and theory. *ANS*. 1988;10(4):10-22.

27. Braden C. A test of the self-help model: Learned response to chronic illness experience. *Nurs Res*. 1990;39(1):42-47.

28. Frey MA. Social support and health: A theoretical formulation derived from King's conceptual framework. *Nurs Sci Q*. 1989;2(3):138-148.

29. Frey MF, Denyes MJ. Health and illness self-care in adolescents with IDDM: A test of Orem's theory. *ANS*. 1989;12(1):67-75.

30. Kline-Leidy N. A structural model of stress, psychosocial resources, and symptomatic experience in chronic physical illness. *Nurs Res*. 1990;39(4):230-236.

31. Mishel M, Braden C. Finding meaning: Antecedents of uncertainty in illness. *Nurs Res*. 1988;37(2):98-103, 127.

32. Smith M. Testing propositions derived from Rogers' conceptual system. *Nurs Sci Q*. 1988; 1(2): 60-67.

Part VIII

APPLICATION OF
THEORY IN ADVANCED
NURSING PRACTICE

Theory-based nursing is the application of theories, models, and principles from medical, behavioral, humanistic, and nursing disciplines to professional nursing practice. Knowledge of various theories, models, and principles, and critical thinking skills are essential for nurses to determine the congruence, or "goodness of fit," between a client's health experience and appropriate theories and models. Advanced nurses practitioners need to understand each theorist's definitions of her major concepts, the underlying assumptions and beliefs, and the interrelationships of the concepts of a variety of theories and models before deciding which ones to use with individual or family clients.

In her chapter, "Critical Thinking and Theory-based Practice," Ellen Birx emphasizes the importance of using both analytical and synthesis skills to identify clients' patterns and select appropriate theories to guide nursing practice decisions. She discusses ways that nurses use both metacognition and metatheory in theory-based practice. Birx believes that critical thinking fosters nurses' empowerment through inquiry, reflection, exploration of creative alternatives, and articulation of nurses' insights, which leads to effective theory-based practice and high quality nursing care.

Although many nurses are unfamiliar with or do not know about theory-based nursing practice, in her chapter, "The Nature of Knowledge and Theory in Nursing," Madelon Visintainer beautifully illustrates how each practice discipline uses different theories and frameworks to identify and treat clients' problems. Based on a case study, she shows how different medical specialists inaccurately diagnose a toddler's problems based on their narrow theories or "maps." Then Visintainer explains how a nurse applied several theories to correctly diagnose the child's problems and select appropriate interventions, aptly demonstrating the relevance of theory-based nursing practice.

The last chapter in this book, "Theory-based Advanced Practice Nursing," by the editor, Janet Kenney, is based on many years of teaching graduate students to apply theories in their nursing practice, and her textbooks, *Nursing Process: Application of Conceptual Models*, fourth edition. Kenney explains why and how theories are essential to provide rationale, holistic, systematic, individualized professional nursing care compared to rote, cookbook, medical-dependent technical nursing care. She describes the broad knowledge base of theories, types of theories from various disciplines, and the critical thinking skills nurses continuously use for effective theory-based practice. Guidelines for choosing appropriate theories, congruent with individual client's health problems and lived experiences are provided, along with related suggestions from other nurse scholars. Theory-based practice enhances nurses' autonomy, creativity, and effectiveness and is based on nursing knowledge and science.

31

Critical Thinking and Theory-based Practice

ELLEN CLARK BIRX, PhD, RN

Critical thinking is an essential and ongoing process in using theory to guide nursing practice. Theory involves seeing patterns that bring order to chaos. Chinn and Kramer define theory as "a systematic abstraction of reality that serves some purpose."[1(p20)] This definition emphasizes the idea that theory is an abstraction and not reality itself. From a different perspective or for a different purpose an alternate theory might be developed and found to be useful. The purpose of nursing theory is the description, explanation, and prediction of phenomena within the domain of nursing with the ultimate aim of guiding nursing practice.

A key question in using theory to guide nursing practice is, "What theories are useful in particular nursing situations?" Critical thinking on the part of each nurse is required to select or develop theories to guide practice in diverse clinical settings. While theories can be useful in organizing and guiding our practice, they can also be blinders that limit us from seeing things as they are. Critical thinking helps us gain awareness of how we are viewing and creating our world of practice.

There is a large body of literature in the fields of psychology, education, and nursing about critical thinking, what it is, how it is learned, and how it is applied in practice. The National League for Nursing (NLN)[2] mandates that nursing programs emphasize the development of critical thinking and independent decision making. However, there is a lack of clarity about just what critical thinking entails. In a national survey of 470 deans or directors of NLN-accredited nursing programs, 51% of whom responded, Jones and Brown[3] found that most of the respondents conceptualized critical thinking as an objective, rational, linear problem-solving process similar to the nursing process. They concluded that most of the sample defined critical thinking in a rather narrow way, excluding aspects of critical thinking like imaginative speculation.

Experts have defined critical thinking in various ways. Ennis defines critical thinking as "reasonable reflective thinking that is focused on deciding what to believe or do."[4(p10)] While this definition includes reasoning and decision-making processes, it is not limited to these. It also incorporates reflective thought and creative thinking processes.

Smith[5] views critical thinking within the context of thinking in general. Smith describes thinking as "a single, continual, all-embracing operation of the mind, powered by an imagination that never rests, not a collection of disparate skills . . ."[5(p124)] Smith's holistic view of critical thinking as inseparable and overlapping with other natural thinking processes resonates with nursing's holistic world view. It is also consistent with the current trend in nurs-

Source: Birx, E. C. (1993). Critical thinking and theory-based practice. *Holistic Nurse Pract.* 7(3):21– 27. Reprinted with permission by from and copyright© 1993 Aspen Publishers, Inc.

ing toward integrating multiple types of thinking or patterns of knowledge—empirical, ethical, aesthetic, and personal—to guide clinical decision making.[6]

Smith's[5] emphasis on the role of imagination in our thinking processes is also especially pertinent. Critical thinking not only involves rational, linear thinking processes, but also intuitive, imaginative thinking processes. The ability to imagine an alternative leads us to question the current system and move toward more humanistic health care environments and relationships.

Viewing or defining critical thinking in a broad way, rather than limiting it to linear problem-solving processes encompasses the many aspects of critical thinking that are needed to select or develop theories to guide nursing practice. Increasing our awareness of various critical thinking processes facilitates our ability to use these processes in the complex world of practice.

ATTITUDE OF INQUIRY AND OPENNESS

Smith[5] suggests that critical thinking is facilitated by an attitude of doubt. An attitude of doubt involves questioning what is happening within and around us and a comfort with uncertainty or not knowing. According to Smith, "Thought flourishes as questions are asked, not as answers am found."[5(p129)] An open and inquiring mind is needed to question the way things are in our clinical practice and to be open to new possibilities.

Through research and theory development, the profession is engaged in developing knowledge on which to base our clinical practice. The knowledge on which we base our practice is not just an accumulation of facts and theories, but also a dynamic, ongoing process of awareness, inquiry, investigation,

integration, imagination, and openness to realities and possibilities. Our knowledge base is not static; it is constantly evolving.

KNOWLEDGE OF THE DISCIPLINE OF NURSING

Critical thinking involves both process and content. We must have something to think about. In a practice discipline like nursing, we have a body of knowledge gleaned from our literature and the direct experience of clinical realities from our everyday practice to think critically about. While the undergraduate student and beginning nurse are able to think critically at a beginning level with freshness of vision, the graduate student and experienced nurses are able to think critically at an advanced level due to an expanded familiarity with nursing literature and a rich background of clinical experience.

Most of the nurses in the graduate course in nursing theory that the author teaches are currently practicing nurses from diverse clinical settings. Two major objectives of the course are to familiarize the students with a broad range of nursing theories in as interesting a manner as possible and to encourage critical thinking about the relevance of these theories to their own clinical practice. Students often comment that they were not looking forward to taking a course in nursing theory and expected it to be dry and tedious. However, by the end of the semester, they express much enthusiasm for the course and find it to be a real eye-opener. They state that they have become more aware of the theories that, whether they realized it or not, have been guiding their clinical practice; they are able to critique and select useful theories to improve their practice; and they are inspired to imagine what new theories are needed to guide practice in their specialty area.

METACOGNITION AND METATHEORY

Another type of critical thinking process used in selecting or developing theories to guide clinical practice includes metacognition and metatheory. These terms refer to the processes of thinking about thinking and thinking about theory, respectively. Metacognition involves the awareness of the thought processes we are using and the ability to select appropriate thinking strategies to accomplish our task.[7] Metatheory focuses on philosophical and methodological issues related to nursing theory, such as questioning the type of theory needed in nursing, critiquing nursing theories, and analyzing nursing theories to identify recurring themes and trends.[8] Both of these critical thinking processes require that we step back from our clinical practice and reflect about the theories we need to guide our practice and the thought processes we need to use to select or develop these theories.

Metatheory involves asking questions such as

- "What are the values of the nursing profession?"
- "What are the assumptions we are making when we approach nursing situations in a particular way?"
- "What are characteristics of nursing's world view?"

The ability to identify underlying values, assumptions, and perspectives is an essential critical thinking skill.

INTEGRATING MULTIPLE LEVELS OF THEORY

Selection of theory to guide nursing practice involves multiple levels of theory, including metatheory, grand theory, and midrange theory. Grand theory "deals with broad goals and concepts representing the total range of phenomena of concern within a discipline."[1(p199)] Midrange theory is more specific and limited in scope, dealing with a single phenomenon or a limited number of phenomena within the domain of nursing.

The use of theory to guide clinical practice involves selecting, adapting, or developing a grand-level nursing theory or conceptual framework. This conceptual framework then guides the selection, adaptation, or development of midrange theories that are specific enough to guide nursing actions. The conceptual framework is like the two-by-fours that frame in a house, outlining where walls, windows, and doors will go. The midrange theories complete the house with various wall finishings and varieties of windows and doors. We first select the overall house plan, and then we select fixtures, colors, flooring, and so forth. Even when the house is finished, we are open to the possibility of remodeling to update or improve the house in various ways.

An example of this process is the use of Levine's[9] grand nursing theory to guide clinical practice in a neonatal intensive care unit. Levine's Conservation Principles provide a useful conceptual framework for organizing nursing care in this complex setting. The four conservation principles, (1) conservation of energy, (2) conservation of structural integrity, (3) conservation of personal integrity, and (4) conservation of social integrity, guide the nurse in providing holistic and comprehensive care for the neonate and family.

In addition to selecting this broad nursing conceptual framework, additional midrange theories must be selected to provide the specific knowledge to guide nursing action. Levine's conservation of energy principle guides the nurse in selecting or developing physiological theories and nursing theories related to temperature regulation, oxygenation, nutrition, fluids and electrolytes, and rest and activity aimed at conserving the energy of the neonate for growth and healing. The principle of conservation of structural integrity guides the nurse in selecting or developing theories related to immune response, positioning, range of motion, wound healing, and skin care. The principle of conservation of personal integrity guides the nurse in the selection of nursing theories and the adaptation of theories from related disciplines dealing with early psychological development. The principle of conservation of social integrity guides the nurse in the selection or development of nursing theories and the adaptation of theories from related disciplines, such as sociology and anthropology, to guide nursing care for neonates within the context of their family, community, and culture. Examples of midrange theories that are useful in neonatal intensive care that can be integrated within Levine's broad nursing conceptual framework are the synactive theory of infant development,[10] crisis intervention theory,[11] attachment theory,[12] and maternal role attainment theory.[13] A wide range of theories from nursing and related disciplines are organized within Levine's conceptual framework to provide theory-based care that is congruent with nursing's holistic, caring world view.

Cromwell proposes a definition of critical thinking as "the ability to apply disciplinary frameworks in personal, academic, and professional settings and to monitor and evaluate that activity."[14(p40)] As the nurse engages in metatheoretical inquiry, and in the evaluation of nursing conceptual frameworks and midrange theories for use in clinical practice, he or she is engaged in critical thinking. Critical thinking is an ongoing process in clinical practice as the nurse monitors and evaluates the usefulness of the theories he or she has applied. Critical thinking is a creative process as nurses identify areas within their clinical practice where new theories need to be developed.

In that critical thinking is both a rational and a creative process; the selection and application of theory to guide clinical practice is not performed in a mechanical way. It is a reflective, creative process. Johnston and Baumann[15] discuss a process for selecting and tailoring nursing models to meet the needs of particular clinical settings. Among the steps in the process they outline are reflection on the nurse's own values and ideas about person, environment, health, and nursing; categorizing the attributes of the client population served; and identifying effective intervention used on the unit. This is followed by the selection or development of a nursing conceptual framework that fits well with these considerations and that allows for collaboration with other disciplines practicing on the unit. Johnston and Baumann suggest selecting conceptual frameworks to guide practice at the unit level rather than at the level of an agency or institution as a whole. This allows the selection and development of theory that is most useful in guiding nursing practice in particular clinical settings.

PERSPECTIVE TAKING

A critical thinking process that is especially pertinent to the development of theory-based practice is the ability to view a situation from multiple perspectives. The discipline of nursing has a rich tradition of valuing not only the nurse's perception of a situation, but also the client's perception of the situation; of valuing subjective realities; and of valuing multicultural perspectives.[16-18] In addition, nursing practice requires consideration of multiple historical, philosophical, economic, and political viewpoints. Engaging in dialogue with nursing colleagues, colleagues from other disciplines, health care consumers, and families enhances perspective-taking ability.[19] Through critical dialogue, nurses can move toward a synthesis of multiple perspectives.[20]

Gebser[21] describes and predicts the evolution of human consciousness beyond the synthesis of multiple perspectives to an integral or aperspectival consciousness. According to Gebser, humankind has evolved through archaic, magical, mythical, and mental stages and is now on the verge of evolving to a stage of integral or aperspectival consciousness. He describes the awareness of a person in aperspectival consciousness in the following way: "For him them is no longer heaven or hell, this world or the other, ego or world, immanence or transcendence; rather beyond the magic unity, the mythical complementarity, the mental division and synthesis is the perceptible whole."[21(p543)] Aperspectival consciousness is characterized by integration rather than synthesis.

Lassalle emphasizes that in integral or aperspectival consciousness, "thinking is not determined solely by reason; in it intelligence, feeling, will, spirit, and the body play equally important roles."[22(p63)] In this new thinking, previous stages are not eliminated, rather they are integrated and brought into balance in an awareness of the whole. Ultimately, this level of holistic thinking is desirable to guide nursing practice.

EMPOWERMENT

A further consideration regarding critical thinking and theory-based nursing practice is empowerment. Smith[5] encourages examination of the extent to which individuals are allowed to be critical thinking in hierarchical, bureaucratic systems. He contends that a necessary ingredient in critical thinking is that people be given the authority to be independent thinkers. This he refers to as empowerment.

Empowerment that fosters critical thinking in nursing practice involves communicating to nurses that they have the authority, ability, and responsibility to think critically about their practice. The authority to think critically is conveyed by eliciting, listening to, and valuing the views and experiences of nurses engaged in clinical practice. Authority, is conveyed through an atmosphere of collaboration and equality with other disciplines. The ability to think critically is cultivated through role-modeling. Nurses grow in their ability to think critically when they work with and observe other nurses engaged in inquiry, critical reflection, exploration of creative alternatives, and articulation of what they are seeing.

Theory-based practice is not just a matter of latching onto the latest theory. It goes far deeper than this. We must critically reflect on the theories, whether implicit or explicit, we are using to guide our practice. As nurses, we have not only the authority and ability, but also the responsibility to question and work toward better health care systems.

While the present emphasis on critical thinking as the use of problem-solving skills in nursing practice is necessary, it is not sufficient or representative of the broad range of critical thinking processes required for theory-based clinical practice. An attitude of openness and inquiry, knowledge and clinical experience in nursing, metacognition and metatheoretical reflection, the integration of multiple levels of theory, perspective taking, and empowerment are all important critical thinking processes.

In addition to taking a holistic approach to critical thinking, it is important to view critical thinking as an ongoing process in using theory to guide clinical practice. As the nurse engages in clinical practice, there is the need to continually question, "What is going on here?" "Are the theories I am using to guide my practice really helpful or are they limiting my authenticity, creativity, and compassion in helping this person?" "What new theories need to be developed in this practice setting?" Through critical thinking, we continually become more open, more inquiring, more knowledgeable, more experienced, more reflective, more integrated, more sensitive to multiple perspectives, and more empowered to refine and develop theory to improve clinical practice. Critical thinking creates theory-based practice that is nursing at its best.

REFERENCES

1. Chinn PL, Kramer MK. *Theory and Nursing: A Systematic Approach*, 3rd ed. St. Louis, Mo: Mosby; 1991.
2. National League for Nursing. *NLN Self-Study Manual*. New York, NY: NLN; 1989.
3. Jones SA, Brown LN. Critical thinking: Impact on nursing education. *Journal of Advanced Nursing*. 1991;16:529–533.
4. Ennis RH. A taxonomy of critical thinking dispositions and abilities. In: Baron JB, Sternberg RJ, eds. *Teaching Thinking Skills: Theory and Practice. New York, NY*: W.H. Freemonk; 1987.
5. Smith F. *To Think*. New York, NY: Teachers College Press; 1990.
6. Carper BA. Fundamental patterns of knowing in nursing. *Advances in Nursing Science*. 1978;1(1):13–23.
7. Beyer BK. *Practical Strategies for the Teaching of Thinking*. Boston, Mass: Allyn & Bacon; 1987.
8. Walker LO, Avant KC. *Strategies for Theory Construction in Nursing*. Norwalk, Conn: Appleton-Century-Crofts; 1983.
9. Levine ME. The conversation principles: Twenty-years later. In: Riehl-Sisca J, ed. *Conceptual Models for Nursing Practice*. 3rd ed. Norwalk, Conn: Appleton & Lange; 1989.
10. Als H. Neurobehavioral development of the premature infant. In: Avery ME, First LR, eds. *Pediatric Medicine*. Baltimore, Md: Williams & Wilkins; 1989.
11. Aguilera DC, Messick JM. *Crisis Intervention: Theory and Methodology*. 5th ed. St. Louis, Mo: Mosby; 1986.
12. Klaus MH, Kennel JH. *Parent-Infant Bonding*. 2nd ed. St. Louis, Mo: Mosby; 1982.
13. Mercer RT. *First-Time Motherhood: Experiences from Teens to Forties*. New York, NY: Springer; 1986.
14. Cromwell LS. Assessing critical thinking. In: Barnes CA, ed. *Critical Thinking: Educational Imperative*. San Francisco, Calif: Jossey-Bass; 1992.
15. Johnston N, Baumann A. Selecting a nursing model for psychiatric nursing. *Journal of Psychosocial Nursing*. 1992;30(4):7–12.
16. Orlando I. *The Dynamic Nurse-Patient Relationship*. New York, NY: Putnam; 1961.
17. Watson J. Nursing: *Human Science and Human Care: A Theory of Nursing*. New York, NY: National League for Nursing; 1988.
18. Leininger M. *Transcultural Nursing: Concepts, Theories, and Practices*. New York, NY: Wiley; 1978.
19. Chaffee J. Teaching critical thinking across the curriculum. In: Barnes CA, ed. *Critical Thinking: Educational Imperative*. San Francisco, Calif: Jossey-Bass; 1992.
20. Lorensen M. Response to "Critical theory: A foundation for the development of nursing theories." *Scholarly Inquiry for Nursing Practice*, 1988;2(3):233–236.
21. Gebser J. *The Ever-Present Origin*. Athens, Oh: Ohio University Press; 1985.
22. Lassalle HE. *Living in the New Consciousness*. Boston, Mass: Shambhala; 1988.

32

The Nature of Knowledge
and Theory in Nursing

MADELON A. VISINTAINER, RN, PhD

The formulation of nursing as a discipline is under way. Work on theory develop-
ment, concept clarification, and the development of a knowledge base is spurred by the
creation of new doctoral programs and the emphasis on nursing research. As nursing
establishes itself as an inventor of theory, the contrasts and similarities between its ex-
istence as both a practice profession and academic discipline come into sharp focus. As
nursing strives to understand itself both as a user-applier and discoverer-inventor of
knowledge and theory, it provides a model for other practice professions and academic
disciplines to explore such questions as, What is the nature of theory in practice? What
is the role of application in the formulation of theory? This chapter examines the char-
acteristics of theoretical constructs as they apply to the practice of nursing, the use of
theory in that practice and the limitations of theory in application.

The formulation of nursing as a discipline is under way. Nursing is establishing its place as an inventor of theory, discoverer of knowledge and educator of its disciples. With this new development, it is interesting to examine the course of growth, the consequences of decisions, and the change through evolving selection. With nursing, this examination is particularly interesting because of its two separate yet dependent existences: its life as a practice profession and its life as an academic discipline.

The purpose of this chapter is to examine the task facing nursing as a practice discipline—the task of selecting and developing knowledge to inform its work and direct its research. To clarify, this is not a paper defining nursing or the theory base for nursing; nor is it a paper about the philosophy of science or the conduct of inquiry. Rather, it addresses the interface between a knowledge or theory base and its application. Selected characteristics of theoretical constructs are examined as are the use of theory in nursing and some limitations of theory in application.

MAPS AND MAPMAKERS

Reichenback (1968) defines the development of knowledge in terms of category construction:

> The essence of knowledge is *generaliza-*
> *tion*. That fire can be produced by rubbing
> wood in a certain way is a knowledge de-

Source: Visintainer, M. A. (1986). The nature of knowledge and theory in nursing. IMAGE: *Journal of Nursing Scholarship, 18* (2): 32-38. Reprinted with permission from Sigma Theta Tau International.

rived by generalization from individual experiences; the statement means that rubbing wood in this way will *always* produce fire. The art of discovery is therefore the art of correct generalization. What is irrelevant, such as the particular shape or size of the piece of wood used, is to be excluded from the generalization; what is relevant, for example, the dryness of the wood, is to be included in it. The meaning of the term "relevant" can thus be defined; that is relevant which must be mentioned for the generalization to be valid. The separation of the relevant from the irrelevant factors is the beginning of knowledge. (p. 5)

This simplification of knowledge development is a useful point from which to examine differences among theoretical perspectives and among disciplines. The definition of a knowledge base for a discipline begins with the separation of that knowledge which is important to the discipline and that which is not: the kernel from the chaff, the essential from the trivial, the main effects from the random error.

Right from the start there is a rub: Who shall define that which is relevant? And what does relevancy mean? Is relevancy inherent, universal, and certain so that once what is relevant is defined there is no need ever to reexamine the position, no need to sift once more through the chaff to be sure that some grain of relevance was not overlooked? The answers to these questions lie in examining the purpose for which the relevancy was established: What is relevant for one purpose may be irrelevant to another, while what is irrelevant for the first may become the essence of the matter for the next.

The "definer" of the relevancy is the one who asks the questions and sets the purpose. The "one" is often a discipline formed by a collection of scientists, scholars, practitioners, philosophers or artists who share a common purpose and a common perspective on the empirical world. Side by side the disciplines examine the same real world for a variety of purposes, from many different vantage points, each producing a different perspective that is no more or less "true" than the other.

To examine the impact that the division of the world into the relevant and the irrelevant has on thinking, consider the analogy of maps. We can begin with a geographic territory. There are many kinds of maps that can be used to describe any given region of the world: There are weather maps outlining air currents, temperature maps, maps of rainfall, road maps, maps of air-traffic patterns and maps of the geology and mineral distribution. Although all of these maps represent the same spot on the earth, they differ in what they represent to be the relevant aspects of the territory. They direct our attention to those aspects of the environment that will provide the most information relevant to the purpose of the observation.

It is obvious from this very partial list of maps that there is so much to know about a place that if all available information were to be included, without the relevancies highlighted, the maps would be useless in directing attention to aspects appropriate for any one purpose. However, as Bateson (1961) cautioned, the map is not the territory but rather an invented representation that serves a particular perspective; therefore the question, Which map is best? is not an appropriate formulation. The accuracy, or "bestness," of the map depends on which purpose is being served or which question is being asked.

The maps of a discipline operate in a way similar to that of maps of a geographic region. They provide a framework for selecting and organizing information from the environment. In studying a discipline, one learns the maps and through mastery of the maps learns what to ask about, what to observe, what to focus on, what to think about. The maps enable the user to zero in on the kernels of relevancy appropriate to the domain of the discipline. They enable the user to focus on the essential aspects in a sea of variables.

In addition to guiding our thinking along already charted routes of knowledge, maps of theory serve as a framework to which new knowledge can be added and through which new discoveries can be plotted. Theories are dynamic inventions against which observations and predictions can be examined, thereby determining a temporary "truth." The continual exchange between the representation and the phenomenon serves to add detail, precision, and validation within a particular perspective.

Because maps guide observations and serve as blueprints for the construction of additional knowledge, they assure that any new knowledge developed will reflect the specific domain of the discipline. The knowledge developed will bear the hallmark of the particular perspective through selective jargon, a style of questions, and specific methodology. Indeed the maps provide the guide for the socialization of one into a particular discipline, its language, interest, and view of the world.

In summary, the theoretic perspectives that serve as the basis for "knowing" about our existence grow out of many different examinations of that existence. The collection of knowledge specific to a particular perspective and the subsequent discoveries resulting from that perspective provide the basis for a discipline. These collections—these maps—guide the user in selecting from the environment information relevant to the specific domains that the maps represent. The maps further provide a dynamic blueprint for adding new information and directing discovery of information that will fit into the domain of the maps.

MAPPING THE DOMAIN OF NURSING

Practice professions have in common the goal of manipulating phenomena: medicine curing disease, education increasing knowing, and nursing improving the level of health and functioning of humans. With the purposes of manipulation and change being fundamental to their disciplines, the practice professions differ from the basic sciences that have as their purposes the explanation of phenomena and the extraction of order. Each of the practice professions uses knowledge and explanations invented by other disciplines. The current vernacular is that the practice professions "apply theory," with the associated implication that practice professions do more borrowing of knowledge and less developing of it. In fact, whether applied disciplines develop knowledge at all causes great debate.

This particular question is of interest to nursing as a practice and a discipline. The domain of nursing is often described as the delivery of care. Care is defined in a number of ways but always involves a number of individual-focused activities that deal with support, nurturance, improvement of function, and so on. As an example, consider Leininger's (1984) comprehensive and explicit definition:

> Care in a generic sense refers to those assistive, supportive, or facilitative acts toward or for another individual or group with evident or anticipated needs to ameliorate or improve a human condition or lifeway. (p. 4)

Such a definition attempts to capture the enormous chunk of phenomena that the task of caring carves out of the world. What is striking about this definition of caring and others like it (Watson, 1985) is that it does not immediately call to mind a particular base of knowledge. That is, on hearing the definition, we do not say, "Ah, yes, we will be borrowing the knowledge of chemistry or physics or psychology or physiology," as we might when we read the definition of engineering or of teaching. The definition of caring does not delimit the knowledge that is required to accomplish that which falls under its domain.

This lack of specificity is not a problem with the definition, however. It is in the very nature of care that the relevant knowledge needed to accomplish it is situation dependent. The delivery of care is a complicated goal for a profession to have. It is not apparent from the myriad of tasks that nurses perform, for example, that the application of any one theory predominates over the application of any other. And when one theory does dominate over others in providing the basis for particular interventions, we often criticize the performer as not being holistic enough.

With what theory base does nursing identify? Many will argue that the discipline has its own base: nursing theory. But how should we characterize that theory in terms of the knowledge it creates? And what is the relationship between that knowledge and the knowledge that nursing borrows to carry out its caring function? Is the fact that nursing is so amorphous in its base of information an indication of its nonscientific nature?

Perhaps rather than a limitation of the discipline, the lack of a specific scientific base may indicate something about the domain of nursing and its perspective on the empirical world. Nursing is interested in improving the condition of persons through the application of care behaviors. Those behaviors depend on what condition needs improvement and what improvement means to specific individuals. A nursing perspective on a situation looks at function, at individual differences, and at state of well-being in relation to whatever defect

may be present. What particular theory may be used to understand the problem or to manipulate the condition depends on what is wrong with a particular person at a particular time and what human function is most in need of manipulation.

Consider the following clinical example. Jason, a 15-month-old boy, was admitted to a large children's hospital with a functional transection of the spinal cord at the C-5 level. On the day he became ill, Jason appeared to be coming down with a cold. By the early evening, Jason's breathing was labored and he was limp. He was admitted to the local community hospital with a number of tentative diagnoses including meningitis and cerebral injury. He was placed on a respirator, and, when all tests for the usual causes were negative, he was transferred to the medical center about 100 miles from his home.

At the medical center a number of different specialists examined Jason: virologists, immunologists, cardiologists, and neurologists completed workups to identify a cause that might lead to an effective treatment. All failed to come up with results that explained what was happening to the young boy. Jason stabilized with a normal temperature and an alert and responsive level of consciousness but continued on the respirator, paralyzed from the cervical collar down. His parents and 4-year-old sister roomed-in on the unit.

However, as Jason's disease remained a mystery to the specialists, the nurses understood Jason more and more as a 15-month-old boy and member of a family. After Jason was hospitalized for 2 months and neither cause nor treatment had been discovered, his parents had to return to their home, visiting only on weekends. Shortly after they left, Jason suddenly began having apnea spells and losing weight. The virologists, immunologists, and neurologists again evaluated Jason and again could find no cause.

As the specialists sought to understand Jason with the maps of their specialties, nursing was focused on providing care to Jason as a 17-month-old with a major disruption to his functioning. They were working with Jason both in the context of the disorder and in terms of activities and needs normal for a young child. They recognized that separation from his parents could have been a major factor in the change of his condition and attempted to reduce the impact of his loss.

When Jason began losing weight, nursing asked a question different from those of the other specialties. Instead of examining the weight loss as an indication specific to a particular disorder (such as viral illness or immunological disorder) the nurses examined the weight loss in terms of Jason's behavior and response. They asked, "How can we help him to eat more, to eat better, to enjoy eating, to show the eating behaviors appropriate for a child of 17 months?"

They discovered that Jason ate best when one particular nurse fed him. They carefully examined what she did and how that differed from what the others had done when they fed him.

Jason had a habit of closing his eyes and pursing his lips on occasion during mealtime. At these times most of the nurses would place the spoon gently at his lips and urge him to eat. The one nurse most successful in feeding Jason did something different. She would take the spoon away and talk to him in a low, lulling voice saying, for example: "I'll bet you want the fruit instead of the carrots" and so on. When Jason opened his eyes and looked at her, she would begin to feed him again. Through this exchange, Jason often finished most of his meal.

What was the significance of the questions that the nurses asked? What was learned through their analysis that would not otherwise have been discovered? First, an effective technique was discovered—a technique that worked for Jason. But more important, a different, relevant, theoretic perspective, a different map was brought into Jason's case. Through the examination of their practice and Jason's response, the nurses could understand his behavior as an attempt to control his environment. The concept of controllability and the related research and interventions were now recognized as being salient to understanding Jason and to deriving strategies for care. By introducing the notion of controllability, nurses were able to design interventions to improve his eating behavior.

Jason was using his gaze and closed lips to control the feeding situation. The nurse who "read" this behavior correctly was able to alter the environment in tune with Jason's need. Jason was engaging in reciprocal exchange at his own level of functioning. Once the nurses had employed this new map (ie, controllability, behavioral reinforcement), they realized its relevancy to other areas of Jason's functioning. Because Jason was limited to movement of his neck, eyes, and facial muscles, gaze direction and lip movements became a code for Jason to ask for toys, Sesame Street on television, and favorite foods. Jason even created his own code—a pouting look—as a sign of protest and anger. As a pièce de résistance, an electric train was rigged to run around the crib rails directed solely by Jason's gaze, which completed an electric-eye circuit. In a healthy, age-appropriate manner for an 18-month-old, Jason used the train to act out against the rules of bedtime and mealtime!

Besides illustrating creative interventions, this story exemplifies the effect of asking a functional question. When the nurses asked "What helps Jason to eat more?" they asked a fundamentally different question from "Why is Jason losing weight?" First, the question directed attention toward specific eating behaviors at specific meals—information that would be more or less irrelevant when the perspective of interest is total weight gain or gastrointestinal abnormality. Second, the question focused on the developmental, psychologic, and situational factors in combination. Finally, the functional question provided the opportunity to view Jason's situation through perspectives from such seemingly unrelated areas as conditioning, behavioral analysis, and reinforcement theory. The nurses did not invent new theory through their questions; rather they accessed knowledge that would have not been available to the problem solving in this case had a disease orientation and questions of cure, pathology, and defect guided the definition of relevant observations and perspectives.

Jason remains paralyzed. No cause has been uncovered and no cure found for the transection. However, there is ongoing analysis of Jason's care needs. Perspectives relevant for a 4-year-old, still respirator-dependent, who has vulnerabilities from his disorder and strengths from his cognitive ability, his strong family, and his remarkable personality are now the factors that define the relevant information in planning care interventions.

Along the way many theories have been tapped, many different disciplines have been consulted, and many different maps have been followed. Obviously, much of the knowledge used to direct Jason's care was borrowed; however, in the borrowing and application of the knowledge, the nurses created something different than that which was invented by other perspectives.

The case of Jason depicts nurses as being more than consumers of theory, appliers of information that comes preassembled and packaged for use. Nurses are rather the agents who assemble the package, using different perspectives, or different maps. The focus of nursing on function and on care defines the phenomena of a case in ways far broader than a focus on disease, cure, emotional response, or reaction to stress. In the process of focusing on function and identifying strategies for care, nursing uses information from many different

perspectives and maps from many different disciplines. Whether this use of information is merely application (leading to no new knowledge) or a different level of theory development is currently the question at the core of the definition of nursing as a discipline.

GLITCHES, GULLIES, AND CLIFFS

Part of the controversy surrounding the question of the theory base for nursing comes out of misunderstandings about the nature of the theoretic perspectives and their application. Theories invented in the certainty of a laboratory or an academic circle may need considerable adjustment when applied to the more ambiguous and rigorous demands of practice. The goodness-of-fit becomes the responsibility of the map user not the mapmaker, and the task can be a difficult one. Certain common traps present particular problems for theory users.

A Rose by Any Other Name

The significance of scientific maps cannot be overstated, particularly in this time of burgeoning information, which directs specialties into a narrower and narrower slice of the general territory and deeper and deeper into their own domain. Because there is too much to know, maps provide a handy way of directing attention and energy toward the mastery of a particular aspect of a phenomenon of interest. Just as maps include that which is relevant to a particular purpose, they also leave out that which is deemed irrelevant by the particular mapmaker. What appears on one map by necessity is absent from another. The effectiveness of maps depends on their ability to abstract accurately the essential aspects of the territory. However, the abstraction has a cost: The territory is reduced to that which is relevant to the purpose of the particular map; all other information about the territory is lost.

Viewing the world through different maps can produce strange twists to a territory with which we are familiar. For example, consider the effects of using a chemical map that provides a biochemical analysis to describe one's mother. When a territory is represented according to the specifics of one particular perspective, much of the information relevant to other dimensions is lost.

In applying theories, the limitations of their representation must be respected. If not, one finds a theory stretched beyond its ability to explain accurately or to predict reliably.

We have many examples in clinical practice of the application of a particular map beyond its limits. These are the situations in which one fails to shift perspectives in response to new facts and observations. Instead the new information is forced into the old map. Consider the following example. A 9-year-old boy is admitted with a fractured femur subsequent to a bike accident. Four days after admission, while the child was in traction and recovering from a number of less serious injuries, he began complaining of abdominal pain. The orthopedic and nursing staff identified the source of the pain as being "fracture related"—referred pain from the leg injury, or the 9-year-old's difficulty in managing pain and immobilization. The child later presented with a fever and vomiting, which were evaluated by the orthopedic surgeons as symptoms possibly related to emboli, wound infection, or vessel necrosis—again secondary to the fracture. Laboratory tests and X rays were ordered to rule out these diagnoses.

Antibiotics were prescribed to ward off a developing wound infection, and increased analgesics and muscle relaxants were added to the medication regimen. Additional efforts were made by the nursing staff to encourage fluids and employ methods of pain management such as distraction and play. Within 48

hours, the child developed a rigid abdomen and underwent emergency surgery for a severely inflamed appendix.

In retrospect we can focus on the errors in management—the antibiotic therapy, the failure to do a physical examination, and so on. But let us examine the assumptions that led to the faulty decisions. When the child was first admitted, he undoubtedly received a complete evaluation. There was an effort to understand his injury in terms of cause and effect, predictable outcomes, and effective interventions. The discovery of the fractured femur in the absence of internal injuries led to a series of medical and nursing interventions that were based on concepts and theoretical propositions called "orthopedic medicine" and "orthopedic nursing." These theoretic constructs directed the kinds of assessments that the child would undergo and the care that he would receive.

Then along the way abdominal pain occurred. It is not a common symptom of fractured femurs, but it is not so uncommon that the notion of referred pain cannot comfortably explain it. Then there was the fever, which often occurs with fractures; and vomiting might easily have been associated with the pain, which also accompanies fractures.

With the theoretical construct of "fractured femur" in place, the other information was fitted into plausible places in the construct. With the governing construct determining the focus and the meaning of the information that was collected, it became difficult to reorganize the new information into a different perspective. Should a 9-year-old child without a fractured femur present with abdominal pain, a fever, and vomiting, a highly probable diagnosis would be appendicitis. However, because an inflamed appendix and a fractured femur rarely occur together, have no causal relationship connecting them, and require different theoretic perspectives to diagnose and manage, the presence of the perspective used to organize the information for the one interfered with the perspective needed for the other. In other words, abdominal pain means one thing to an orthopod and something different to a pediatrician!

In this example, the effect of misdiagnosis was discovered when the new syndrome compelled a reevaluation of the information. However, many times misassessments are not discovered. A particular perspective dominates and all information from the environment is forced into its framework. Such distortion of the territory to fit the map interferes with accurate assessments and the development of effective interventions.

The Dark Side of the Straight and Narrow

Theoretic maps attain their usefulness by paring down the limitless environment to relevant aspects. All other information becomes background, filler, "noise." This paring down of information serves a gatekeeping function, directing our attention to valuable information and helping us to ignore that which is not important. But once again, the aspects of value, importance, and relevancy are not inherent in the information; they are determined by the purpose. Because maps are inventions that have more or less validity, established over time, they are neither foolproof nor error free. And most definitely they are rarely up to date. New information, new technology, and new discoveries often outdate previous perspectives. Just as maps can fall behind the state of the art in representing all that is known, map users, enamored with a particular map (sometimes the one introduced in the learning period), often fail to update themselves with new maps of the same territory. The result can be a narrow view of the phenomenon and a restricted repertoire of intervention strategies.

Even when maps are up to date, they cannot allow for individual variations of a phe-

nomenon. Therefore, information that may be valuable in a particular case may be missed. Consider a clinical example. Nurses working on a short-term surgery unit admitted a young child named Bobby for a tonsillectomy. The nurse who did the admission and preparation noticed that, although the boy was only 7, he seemed to "take charge." On the other hand, his mother seemed overwhelmed by the experience and sat quietly, often tearfully, by while her son answered questions and interacted with the staff members.

The child listened attentively to the preparation done by his primary nurse and was interested in learning all that was to happen the following morning. The next day he went off to the operating room reassuring his mother that he would be back soon.

After returning from the recovery room, Bobby was quietly cooperative during the readmission procedure and smiled reassuringly at his mother before falling asleep. However, in a short while an aide reported to the nurse that Bobby was "agitated." The nurse went back to the room expecting to see the usual postanesthesia thrashing and random discomfort. Instead, she found Bobby sitting up in bed holding his throat and croaking in a hoarse voice, "Something's wrong!"

The nurse tried to reassure Bobby, but he was so insistent that she examined his throat. There was no evidence of bleeding. She reminded Bobby that his throat would be sore for a while and offered him a sip of water. He would not be dissuaded. "Something's wrong," he insisted.

The nurse, puzzled by his response, called the resident from ENT. After hearing her description he asked about vital signs, vomiting, and other signs of bleeding. Then finding no signs and symptoms of hemorrhage, he ordered Vistaril for restlessness postanesthesia. The nurse objected. She, like Bobby, insisted that what was occurring was not restlessness. Something else was going on.

The resident came to examine Bobby and similarly found no evidence of bleeding. After his examination he again ordered the Vistaril. He agreed, "It doesn't look like your usual restlessness, but what else could it be, he's not bleeding?"

The nurse was still uncomfortable with the order. She had known Bobby's response to the hospitalization in general, his ability to understand what was happening, and his management of anxiety and fear. In light of that information, his insistence that something was amiss convinced her that there was a problem, even in the absence of concrete signs.

In a final attempt to understand the problem, the nurse took Bobby to the operating room suite to be seen by the surgeon who performed the tonsillectomy. As the surgeon came irately to the door, Bobby suddenly gagged and spit up enough blood to fill an emesis basin. He sighed and announced "I feel better now" as he was taken back into surgery for cautery. Bobby had been bleeding into the nasopharyngeal cavity, but a clot had blocked the passage of the blood to a location where it could have been seen.

This case could be incorrectly used as an example of the superiority of nursing judgment and the irascibility of physicians. However, the case illustrates a much more subtle and important difference between the professionals of medicine and nursing and their use of theory. For the ENT surgeon, the interaction between the mother and son was irrelevant to the successful removal of the tonsils. For the nurse, that information was important for the provision of care. In the theoretic perspective of nursing there was room for that information; in the ENT perspective, there was not.

To the physicians, who specialize in ears, noses, and throats, the possible domain of untoward responses after surgery includes there being something wrong with the surgery or something wrong with the anesthesia. There are definite signs of each: bleeding or infection for surgery, agitation or respiratory problems for anesthesia. Information that applies to something other than these (such as the child's coping ability or response to stress) is not useful in diagnosing the problem. For nurses who specialize in individuals who have a variety of problems, the signs of bleeding, infection, agitation, and respiratory problems (as well as the child's coping ability), studying their response to stress and seeking much more information are relevant to teasing out aspects of the problem.

The essential point in this case is not about personality differences between nurses and physicians; it is about differences in the use of theoretic maps. The way in which nurses use theories in practice allows them to use more of the information from the environment to inform their analyses and guide their interventions. For nursing, theory is not restrictive; for specialties that are based on the application of a particular theory or set of theories, it is.

Primacy and Certainty

Nursing does not always take advantage of the flexibility that the perspective of care gives it in choosing a map to guide the analysis of a problem and direct the planning of interventions. A common view held about theories and disciplines suggests that there is an order of primacy with regard to theoretic perspectives. The view can be summed up with several propositions, overstated to make the point.

The first proposition that governs the view of primacy can be stated as the more basic the science, the better is the science. Similarly, the more absolute the techniques of the science, the more important is its domain. The popularity of this proposition stems in part from the nature of the basic sciences. They offer more certainty, and certainty in turn offers more comfort. The trap here is recognizing the limitation of the certainty offered. In the laboratory, certainty is obtained by simplifying the conditions under which a phenomenon is considered; so we can be certain that a particular chemical reaction produces specific results. Outside of the laboratory, however, the simplicity disappears, and certainty is no longer as easily obtainable. The organism may produce the disease but not in everyone at all times; or the chemical reaction occurs less than 50 percent of the time.

In health care and the treatment of illness, the certainty of the laboratory cannot answer the questions important to patients and central to the delivery of their care: Why me? Why now? And what am I to do about it?

The second proposition that is used to order the importance assigned to theories deals with the way one comes to know about the different domains. The information found in those sciences that do not deal with anatomy, physiology, or pharmacology can be intuited and does not require systematic study. An example of this proposition can be found during any medical or nursing rounds where speculation about the impact of the patient's personality and home conditions is a topic of sideline information, if discussed at all.

A more serious and lamentable example can be found in the way patient care assignments are sometimes made: nurses handle the highly technical procedures dealing with machines, IVs, and monitors, while aides are assigned to persons awaiting surgery. It is as if the technical demands of the preoperative patients are minimal, and anyone who speaks the language can answer the questions of the person and family!

A particularly troubling example of this proposition comes from examining the curricular offerings of some graduate programs in nursing in which there are established courses for pharmacology, advanced physiology, and even suturing and spinal tap procedures, while at the same time the curricula have few courses in family theory, effects of culture, and theories of care and nursing. Even more disconcerting is the deficit in courses in developmental theory and nutrition.

Few in nursing or even in medicine would argue that the psychologic, social, cultural, and spiritual aspects are unimportant. But what is believed is that the knowledge in the domain of these perspectives is "common knowledge" that is available to the caregiver merely through living. The unfortunate result of this belief is the loss of valuable information and ideas for the delivery of care.

The last proposition deals with the separation of theoretic perspectives that relate to the division of mind and body. Information found in the nonbiological sciences sheds absolutely no light on either the occurrence of disease or response to illness. This final proposition serves as a gatekeeper in warding off the integration of different perspectives and information from different disciplines. The best recent example is found in the ramifications of one study on the relationship between psychosocial variables and outcome in patients with advanced stages of cancer, which was reported in the *New England Journal of Medicine* (Cassileth, Lusk, Miller, Brown, & Miller, 1985). The results of the study, which demonstrated no relationship between these variables, were quickly cited in the medical community as being definitive evidence of the dichotomy between the physical and mental realms of a person's existence. That is, on the results of one study, a major part of the scientific community was overprepared to accept categorically that person-related variables such as personality style, family support, and so on have little effect on the recovery of cancer patients. It is important to note that the original study examined the relationship in the advanced stage of the disease only and made no assumptions about either disease onset or recovery in earlier stages and their relationship to psychosocial variables. The interpretation in the medical community far exceeded the bounds of the study and touted it as being conclusive scientific evidence to undermine the folklore of the interaction between mindstates and disease (Angell, 1985).

Nursing has made remarkable headway refuting this proposition in theory. However, in practice, nursing care often subjugates its convictions about the importance of the person-related variables to the hierarchy of theory adhered to by the medical community. Even when nurses govern their own practice, they succumb to a belief that the "soft stuff" such as feelings and beliefs and support are not quite as substantive as the hard data from laboratory reports and sophisticated monitoring.

At times, the view of certain perspectives as being inherently better than others interferes with the delivery of optimal care. Recently a 5-year-old girl was scheduled for a liver transplant. With much effort a clinical specialist had worked with her and the family to prepare them for the unpredictable wait, the number of invasive procedures, and the involved recovery. On the day of surgery, in the flurry of preparation, the child was with her family in the last minutes before going to the operating room. A nurse entered and announced that the parents had to leave while she and two others inserted a urethral catheter. As they began the procedure, the child became more and more distraught. Her screams of protest upset the parents, and finally the clinical nurse specialist was called to intervene. She decided, much to the staff nurses' surprise and dismay, that the catheter could easily be inserted after the child was under anesthesia with no effect on the timing of the surgery. The nurses reluctantly went along with the plan but commented: "There's a time to be nice and a time to get serious about the care."

This example is a disturbing one that illustrates a common belief that providing an atmosphere that supports a person's coping and mastery is not instrumental in the caregiving processes. A care intervention that should have been central to the caring process was seen as a gratuitous overindulgence. In this case, the staff nurses gave the physiologic map primacy over maps that explain and predict coping, response to stress, and the relationship between psychologic distress and physiologic recovery.

In addition to interfering with optimum care, the propositions that support the idea of primacy in theories interfere with the systematic investigation of the many factors that contribute to disease and to health. Such an investigation could begin to build theoretical bridges between such disparate constructs as tumors and beliefs, heart disease and temperament, immunodeficiency and hope. What better area do we have for building this kind of integration than nursing practice? What better discipline is there for examining the phenomena surrounding persons and their health from different perspectives than nursing—the discipline which is privy, through its unique intimacy, to knowing people on many different dimensions, in many different situations?

ON TO UNCHARTED TERRITORY

Nursing has been examined in this paper from the perspective of map users. Theory has been described as invented representations of our existence. Theories bear the hallmarks of their inventing disciplines and provide accurate explanations and reliable predictions of phenomena when used within their limits.

Nursing uses theory to direct the exploration and manipulation of its domain—providing care. The particular theories used depend on the demands of the care situation. Because care needs are amorphous in terms of particular content, nursing's use of theoretic perspectives is eclectic. No one scientific theoretic base is adequate to describe its domain.

In application, theory is limited in its scope. When these limitations are respected, distortions of information from the environment are reduced. With the recognition that any theory is a temporary, working draft of an idea about the world, exploration of new possibilities and different perspectives are encouraged. With the understanding that theory is an amalgamation of particular perspectives, there is no confusion that theory is truth; theory remains a tool with which to understand and alter the world.

Because of the focus of nursing on phenomena, nursing asks questions for which there are not yet answers. Its focus on individual differences and on the interaction of the many different variables relevant to health and its interest in long-term adaptation place its domain in unmapped territory. It is at this point that nursing becomes a mapmaking endeavor, charting the domain of its practice. It is at this juncture—between the questions derived from practice and the need for new information, for rules for integrating borrowed knowledge, and for the invention of new perspectives—that nursing's disciplinary work of conducting research and building theory lies.

REFERENCES

Angell, M. (1985). Disease as a reflection of the psyche. *New England Journal of Medicine, 312* (24), 1570.

Bateson, G. (1979). *Mind and nature: A necessary unity*. New York: E. P. Dutton.

Casselith, B. R., Lusk, E. J., Miller, D. S., Brown, L. L., & Miller, C. (1985). Psychosocial correlates of survival in advanced malignant disease? *New England Journal of Medicine, 312* (24), 1551.

Leininger, M. (1984). *Care: The essence of nursing and health*. Thorofare, NJ: SLACK, Inc.

Reichenback, H. (1968). *The rise of scientific philosophy*. Berkeley, CA: University of California Press.

Watson, J. (1985). *Nursing: Human science and human care*. Norwalk, CT: Appleton-Century-Crofts.

33

Theory-based Advanced Nursing Practice

JANET W. KENNEY, RN, PhD

All professional disciplines are based on their unique knowledge, which is expressed in models, and theories that are applied in practice. The focus of nursing knowledge is on humans' health experiences within the context of their environment and the nurse-client relationship. Theory-based nursing practice is the application of various models, theories, and principles from nursing science and the biological, behavioral, medical, and socio-cultural disciplines to clinical nursing practice. Conceptual models and theories provide a broad knowledge base to assist nurses in understanding and interpreting the client's complex health situation and in planning nursing actions to achieved desired client outcomes. "Explicit use of conceptual models of nursing and nursing theories to guide nursing practice is the hallmark of professional nursing"; it distinguishes nursing as an autonomous health profession (Fawcett, 1997:212).

This chapter describes the value and relevance of theory-based nursing for advanced practice nurses and discusses some underlying concerns about applying theories in nursing practice. The structure of nursing knowledge and the transformative process for theory-based practice are explained, along with the importance of critical thinking. An overview of various models and theories of nursing, family, and other disciplines is provided. Lastly, the process for selecting and applying appropriate models and theories in nursing practice is thoroughly described.

RELEVANCE OF THEORY-BASED PRACTICE IN NURSING

The value of theory-based nursing practice is well documented in numerous books and journal articles. Although many articles illustrate the application of a nursing model or theory to clients with a specific health problem, Alligood (1997b) recently reviewed the nursing literature and found that about 68% of the articles reflect a medical approach to nursing. She also noted that most nurses described their practice in terms of a specialty area, types of care or health problems, and nursing interventions.

All nurses use knowledge they acquired during their formal education and clinical experience to guide their practice. Some nurse practitioners consistently use models and theories to guide their practice, but most nurses are unaware of existing theories and models or do not know how to apply them. Many nurses are not aware of what knowledge they use or where they learned it, thus, their implicit knowledge tends to be fragmented, diffused, incomplete, and greatly influenced by the medical model (Fawcett, 1997). Although graduate nurse practitioner students learn about nursing models and theories, their education often emphasizes application of medical knowledge as the base for their nursing practice. Thus use of medical knowledge and policies of health care delivery systems have replaced nursing knowledge and influenced some nurses to become "junior doctors," instead of "senior nurses" (Meleis, 1993).

Theories and models from nursing and behavioral disciplines are used by advanced practice nurses to provide effective, high quality nursing care. Many nurses believe that use of nursing theories would improve the quality of nursing care, but that they do not have sufficient information about them or the opportunity to use them (McKenna, 1997b). According to Meleis (1997), theories improve quality of care by clearly defining the boundaries and goals of nursing assessment, diagnosis, and interventions, and by providing continuity and congruency of care. Theory also contributes to more efficient and effective nursing practice, and enhances nurses' professional autonomy and accountability. Aggleton and Chalmers (1986) claim that providing nursing care without a theory base is like "practicing in the dark." Kenney (1996) reported that professional nurses can effectively use theories and models from nursing and behavioral disciplines to:

- collect, organize, and classify client data
- understand, analyze, and interpret client's health situations
- guide formulation of nursing diagnoses
- plan, implement, and evaluate nursing care
- explain nursing actions and interactions with clients
- describe, explain, and sometimes predict clients' responses
- demonstrate responsibility and accountability for nursing actions

- achieve desired outcomes for clients (p. 9)

As we enter the next millennium, the health care revolution requires that nurses demonstrate efficient, cost-effective, high quality care within organized delivery systems. "Nursing theory-based practice offers an alternative to the dehumanizing, fragmented, and paternalistic approaches that plague current delivery systems" (Smith, 1994:7). With changes in the current third-party reimbursement systems, nurses will be paid for effective theory-based practice that enhances clients' health and their quality of life. To accomplish this, nurse practitioners must use critical thinking skills combined with theory-based knowledge and clinical expertise to achieve desired client outcomes.

Issues related to theory-based nursing practice

In recent years, the enthusiasm for using nursing models and theories in practice has waned due to criticisms about the "theory-practice gap" and the lack of relevance to clinical practice. Also there are philosophical concerns about whether only nursing models should guide practice and whether models and theories of nursing and other disciplines may be integrated in practice. This section discusses some of these issues.

The "theory-practice gap" refers to the lack of use or inability of nurses to utilize nursing and other theories in clinical practice. McKenna (1997b) claims that theories are not being used in a systematic way to guide nursing practice, although using theories may improve the quality of care. He believes nurses do not use nursing theories because they do not know about them, understand them, believe in them, know how to apply them, or are not allowed to use them. Professional nursing practice more often reflects the medical or organizational model of care than application of relevant nursing models or theories.

According to Rogers (1989:114), "Nursing knowledge . . . is often seen as being unscientific, intuitive, and highly subjective." Some nurses believe that conceptual models and theories are too abstract to apply in nursing practice: they do not provide sufficient information to guide nursing judgments, are subject to different interpretations, are incomplete, and lack adequate testing and refinement (Field, 1987; Firlet, 1985). Others argue that some nursing theories were never meant to be directly applied in nursing practice but were intentionally abstract to stimulate thinking, provide new insights, and develop creative ways of viewing nursing (McKenna, 1997b).

As a practice discipline, nursing models and theories should be useful in practice, or their value is questionable. When models and theories are logical and consistent with other validated theories, they may provide the rationale and consequences of nursing actions, and lead to predictable client outcomes. There are numerous articles and chapters describing application of various models to clinical nursing practice. However, rigorous research studies on how nursing models and theories contribute to desirable nursing actions and client outcomes are lacking.

Another issue is whether only nursing models and theories are appropriate for the discipline, since nursing is an applied science. Most professional nurses are familiar with theories from other disciplines, such as systems theory, family theories, developmental theories, and others; in clinical practice, nurses often combine their nursing and medical knowledge with theories from other disciplines. Some nurse scholars argue that nursing practice must be based on nursing models and theories, since they are consistent with nursing's view of human science and provide the structure for explaining nursings' unique contribution to health care (Cody, 1996; Mitchell, 1992). Since nursing models or theories represent the theorist's unique beliefs about persons, health, and nursing and guide how nurses interact with clients, McKenna (1997b) believes that an eclectic approach, combining theories from nursing and other disciplines, may compromise nursing theories if the concepts are removed from their original context and interwoven with other theories.

In contrast, Meleis (1997) argues that because nurses study other disciplines, nursing theory tends to reflect a broad range of perspectives and premises. Many nursing theorists have incorporated or "borrowed" theories from other disciplines, then transmuted them to fit within the context of nursing, so that their nursing theories comprise shared knowledge used in a distinctive way (Timpson, 1996).

A related issue is whether professional nurses should consistently use only one nursing model, or use various models and theories from nursing and other disciplines in their practice. Most professions, like nursing, have multiple theories that represent divergent and unique perspectives about the phenomena of concern to their practice. Within nursing, conceptual models and theories range from broad conceptual models, or grand theories, to specific practice theories. There are advantages and disadvantages to using one or more theories in clinical practice. Depending on the nurse's knowledge and clinical practice area, some nursing models and theories may be more appropriate than others. However, some would argue that use of only one nursing theory limits the nurse's assessment to only those things addressed by the theory, and the nurse may be forced to "fit" the client situation to the theory.

Others believe that nurses should consider a variety of nursing theories and select the model or theory that best "fits" the client's health problems. The majority of early nursing theories were based on traditional scientific methods and reflect a reductionistic perspective of humans as passive beings, consisting of elementary parts that respond to external stimuli in a linear, causal, and predictive way (Benner & Wrubel, 1989). Nursing models based on this perspective ultimately dehumanize individuals into disparate parts and systems and lead to fragmented, non-holistic nursing care (Aggleton & Chalmers, 1986). More contemporary nursing models view humans as continuously changing during reciprocal interactions with their environment, thus individual's reactions to nursing care are not predictable, nor can they be controlled. However, these newer nursing models are more abstract than earlier models and are less likely to offer specific guidelines for nursing actions. Professional nurses are expected to develop unique, creative nursing actions suitable for each client's health problem and lifestyle. And, theories from other disciplines may be integrated to complement and strengthen some limitations in both early and contemporary nursing models.

Cody (1996) contends that eclecticism, or selecting the best theory from other sources, is not necessarily wrong, but constantly borrowing theories from other disciplines does not contribute to the science of nursing or differentiate nursing from other professions. He believes that nursing practice ought to reflect a coherent, nursing theoretical base to guide practice in specific ways and contribute to the quality of care.

Since professional nurses provide health care for a variety of clients, each of whom is unique yet may have similar health concerns, nurses must use a broad knowledge base from nursing and other disciplines to select and apply relevent models and/or theories that are congruent with the client's situation. Health care, based on appropriate nursing models and theories, that integrates appropriate family, behavioral, and developmental theories, is most likely to achieve desired client health outcomes.

STRUCTURE OF NURSING KNOWLEDGE AND PERSPECTIVE TRANSFORMATION

Advanced practice nurses must first understand the structure of nursing knowledge and the process of transforming nursing models and theories into useful perspectives prior to implementing theory-based practice. In her recent book, Fawcett (1995) described the structural hierarchy of nursing knowledge, or nursing science. Nursing's metaparadigm, which includes the major concepts of person, health, environment, and nursing, provides the foundation from which nursing philosophies, conceptual models, and theories are derived. Each nurse theorist developed unique definitions of her major concepts, based on her education, practice, and personal philosophy (values, beliefs, and assumptions) about humans, health, nursing, and environment. The theorist's philosophy also influenced her conceptual model, which describes how the concepts are linked: the model explains the relationships among client-health-nursing situations (Sorrentino, 1991). Conceptual nursing models are usually called "grand theories," because they are broad and abstract and may not provide specific directions for nursing actions. Some nurse theorists have developed mid-range or practice theories from their models that describe specific relationships among the concepts and suggest hypotheses to be tested.

According to Rogers (1989), an individual's personal "meaning" perspective or conceptual model provides a frame of reference or lens that influences how one perceives, thinks, and behaves in the world. Yet, most people are not aware of how their perspective influences and affects their view of themselves, others, and their world because underlying beliefs are held in the unconscious mind. In practice, nurses' perceptions, thoughts, feelings, and actions are guided by their personal framework or perspective of nursing, which provides a cognitive structure based on their assumptions, beliefs, and values about nursing (Fawcett, 1995). Many nurses unconsciously use a medical or institutional model as their perspective for organizing care. The prevalent values of such models or perspectives are efficiency, standardized care, rules, and regulations, such as "critical care pathways" (Rogers, 1989). As nurses become aware of the differences between the present and potential possibilities of nursing practice, they experience a cognitive dissonance or discomfort from an awareness of "what is" versus "what could be" (Rogers, 1989). Thus, only when nurses experience cognitive dissonance in practice will they change their frame of reference and use nursing models and theories.

For professional nurses to apply conceptual nursing models and theories, a dramatic change, or "perspective transformation," must occur (Rogers, 1989; Fawcett, 1995). Perspective transformation is the process of moving from one frame of reference or perspective to another, when unresolved dilemmas arise and creat dissonance in one's current perspective (Mezirow, 1979). It is a process of critical reflection and analysis of other explanations or perspectives that might resolve the dilemma and explain or guide one's understanding and actions. The process involves gradually acquiring a new perspective that leads to fundamental changes in the way nurses experience, interpret, and understand their world and their relationships with others (Fawcett, 1995).

Fawcett (1995) describes nine phases leading to "perspective transformation." Initially, the prevailing *stability* of the current nursing practice is disrupted when use of a nursing conceptual model or theory-based practice is introduced. *Dissonance* occurs as nurses consider their own perspective for practice and the challenge of changing to a new conceptual model or theory. Some nurses identify discrepancies between their current practice and how the new model or theory could affect their practice. *Confusion* may follow as nurses struggle to learn about the model or theory and how to apply it in practice. Nurses often feel anxious, angry, and unable to think during these phases and may grieve the loss of familiar perspectives of nursing. Their former perspective no longer seems useful, yet they have not internalized the new model or theory well enough to use it effectively. While *dwelling with uncertainty*, nurses acknowledge that their confusion is not due to personal inadequacy, and as their anxiety diminishes, they begin to critically examine former practice methods and explore the possibilities of implementing a new model or theory (Rogers, 1989; Fawcett, 1995).

With the discovery that a new model or theory is coherent and meaningful, *synthesis* occurs. As ways to apply the new model become clearer, new insights assist nurses to understand the usefulness of the conceptual model or theory in nursing practice (Fawcett, 1995). *Resolution* occurs as nurses become comfortable using the new model; they may feel a sense of empowerment and view their practice differently. Gradually nurses consciously change their practice during *reconceptualization*; they shift from their former patterns to new ways of thinking and acting within the new model or theory. The final phase, *return to stability*, occurs when nursing practice is clearly based on the new nursing model or theory. Acceptance of a new perspective or paradigm, along with the corresponding assumptions, values, and beliefs concludes the transformation process.

Models and theories from nursing and other disciplines provide the cognitive structures that guide professional nursing practice. This body of knowledge helps nurses explain 'what they know' and the rationale for their nursing actions that facilitate the client's health (Fawcett, 1997). Theory-based nursing practice depends on the depth of nurses' knowledge of models and theories and their understanding about how to apply them in practice (Alligood, 1997a). Nursing models and theories represent ideal, logical, unique perspectives or 'maps' of the person and health. They provide a structure and systematic approach to: examine clients' situations, identify relevant information, interpret data for nursing diagnoses, and plan effective nursing care through critical thinking, reasoning, and decision-making ((Mayberry, 1991; Timpson, 1996; Alligood, 1997a).

Nurses must use *critical thinking skills* to apply models and theories to their clients' health concerns. Paul and Nosich's (1991) definition of critical thinking is a commonly accepted one:

> Critical thinking is the intellectually disciplined process of actively and skillfully conceptualizing, applying, analyzing, synthesizing, or evaluating information gathered from, or generated by, observation, experience, reflection, reasoning, or communication, as a guide to belief and action (p. 4).

According to Cradock (1996), it is *not what they know* that makes nurses advanced practitioners, but *how they use what they know*. They must make expert clinical decisions based on reflection, complex reasoning, and critical thinking to apply theoretically based knowledge to diverse client situations (Sparacino, 1991). Critical thinking incorporates ideas from both models or theories with clinical experience, and provides the structure for unique, creative nursing practice with each client (Alligood, 1997a; Field, 1987; Mayberry, 1991; Sorrentino, 1991). Several nurse authors believe that nursing theories will become the stimuli for reflection and critical thinking, leading to realms for creative expressions in nursing practice (Chinn, 1997; Marks-Moran & Rose, 1997). Theory-based nursing and critical thinking are the foundations of advanced nursing practice (Mitchell, 1992). Specific critical thinking skills for each component of the nursing process are identified in Table 33.1.

MODELS AND THEORIES APPLICABLE IN ADVANCED NURSING PRACTICE

Theory-based nursing practice is the creative application of various models, theories, and principles from nursing, medical, behavioral, and humanistic sciences. Models and theories from relevant disciplines provide the knowledge base to understand various aspects of the client's health concerns and guide appropriate nursing management. In advanced nursing practice, the client may be an individual, familys or an aggregate, such as a community or special population. Knowledge of relevant models and theories from nursing and other disciplines enables the nurse to select those that 'best fit' each client. This section provides a brief overview of some nursing, family, community, and other models and theories that may be relevant and useful to nurse practitioners.

Table 33.1. Application of Critical Thinking Skills to the Nursing Process

Components & definitions	Critical thinking skills & activities
Assessment An ongoing process of data collection to determine the client's strengths and health concerns	Collect relevant client data by observation, examination, interview and history, and reviewing the records Distinguish relevant data from irrelevant Distinguish important data from unimportant Validate data with others
Diagnosis The analysis/synthesis of data to identify patterns and compare with norms and models A clear, concise statement of the client's health status and concerns appropriate for nursing intervention	Organize and categorize data into patterns Identify data gaps Recognize patterns and relationships in data Compare patterns with norms and theories Examine own asumptions regarding client's situation Make inferences and judgments of client's health concerns Define the health concern and validate with the client and health team members Describe actual and potential concerns and the etiology of each diagnosis Propose alternative explanations of concerns
Planning Determination of how to assist the client in resolving concerns related to restoration, maintenance, or promotion of health	Identify priority of client's concerns Determine client's desired health outcomes Select appropriate nursing interventions by generalizing principles and theories Transfer knowledge from other sciences Design plan of care with scientific rationale
Implementation Carrying out the plan of care by the client and nurse	Apply knowledge to perform interventions Compare baseline data with changing status Test hypotheses of nursing interventions Update and revise the care plan Collaborate with health team members
Evaluation A systematic, continuous process of comparing the client's response with the desired health outcomes	Compare client's responses with desired health outcomes Use criterion-based tools to evaluate Determine the client's level of progress Revise the plan of care

From: Christensen, P.J. Kenney, J.W., eds: *Nursing process: Application of conceptual models,* ed 4, St. Louis, 1995, Mosby, p. 8.

Nursing Models and Theories

Numerous nursing models and theories have been reported in the literature since the 1950s. Some well-known nurse theorists' works are cited: readers are encouraged to seek other sources for more information about their models and theories. The early nurse theorists's conceptual models focused on individual clients and described nursing goals and activities. Peplau's "Interpersonal Model" described a goal-directed, nurse-client interpersonal process to promote the client's personality and living. Orlando's model explained a deliberative nursing approach to understand nurse-patient relationships and the communication process. Hall's "Core-care-cure Model" expanded and clarified nursing actions to promote clients' health. Levine's model identified four principles of human conservation to guide nursing activities.

More contemporary nursing theories have been published since 1970, when Rogers introduced her "Science of unitary man." She described mutually evolving relationships between humans and their environment that are expressed as changing energy fields, patterns, and organization. Orem's "Self-care Model" identified requisites for an individual's self-care, and specific nursing systems to deliver care according to the client's self-care needs. King designed a systems model that included the individual, family, and society, then developed her "Theory of Goal Attainment," which described nurse-patient transactions to achieve the client's goals. Roy's "Adaptation Model" identified three types of stimuli that affect a patient's four modes of functioning. She described how the nurse identifies maladaptive behaviors and alters stimuli to enhance the client's adaptation. Paterson and Zderad developed a model of "Humanistic Nursing." Leininger's "Transcultural Nursing Model" explained differences between universal and cultural specific views of health and healing, and how nurses can provide culturally congruent health care. According to Watson, nursing is the art and science of human care: nurses engage in transpersonal caring transactions to assist persons achieve mind-body-soul harmony. Johnson's "Behavioral Systems Model" focused on nurturing, protecting, and stimulating the individual's seven subsystems to maintain balance and stability. Neuman designed a complex "Health Care Systems" model that identified different types of stressors and levels of defense: nursing actions were based on three levels of prevention. Parse developed a "Man-living-health Theory" in which nurses assist individuals to explore their past-present-future life experiences and illuminate possible lifestyle choices to enhance their health and lives. Newman's theory of "Health as expanding consciousness" considers disease as part of health, and explores time and rhythm pattern recognition with changes in life and health.

Family Models

Although most nursing models were originally designed to focus on individual clients, a few are applicable to families. King views the family as a social system or group of interacting individuals, and family health as dynamic life experiences. Roy views the family as part of the client's immediate social environment, whereas Neuman's concept of family is harmonious relationships among family members. These nurse theorists focused on the individual client with the family seen as context. If the family is viewed as the client, the nurse must decide what the model should focus on—family development, interactions and stress, family systems, structure and function, or a combination of these models, such as the Calgary Family Model.

Family development models are based on the premise that the life cycle of families follows a common sequence of events from marriage through childrearing, retirement, and bereavement. Most are based on the typical nuclear two-parent family and emphasize the stages and adult's responsibilities to accomplish desired goals. Duvall's (1977) model is well-known, and Stevenson (1977), a nurse theorist, also designed a family model.

Family interactional models view family members as a unit of interacting personalities within a dynamic life process. These models focus on how members' perceptions and interpretations of themselves and other family members determine their behaviors and actions. Also, these models consider how members' roles affect their interaction with others. Satir's "Family Interaction Model" is an example. Family stress and coping models, based on the work of Lazarus and Folkman, were developed by Moos and Billings (1984) to identify how the family appraised the situation, dealt with their problems, and handled the resulting emotions. McCubbin and McCubbin (1993) designed the "Double ABCX Model," which examines family life stressors and resources, along with changes that affect their adaptation to health problems, and ability to manage family crises. Curran's (1985) "Healthy Family Model" identified characteristics of healthy families and common stressors affecting families.

Family systems models view the whole family as greater than and different from the sum of its parts or members. These models focus on the family with a hierarchy of subsystems (mother-father, parent-child) and supersystems in the community (social, occupational, recreational, and religious networks) that interact with the family system. Olson, Russell, and Sprenkle's (1983) model identifies 16 types of family systems based on the premise that a balance must be maintained in family *cohesion*, so that members do not become too enmeshed or too distant, and *adaptability*, wherein too much change creates chaos and too little change leads to rigidity.

Communication between family members is the third dimension. The "Beaver's System Model" (Beavers & Voeller, 1983) examines the *structure*, *flexibility*, and *competence* of a family and its members. Centripetal families enjoy close family relationships, while centrifugal families seek satisfaction outside the family.

Family structural-functional models view the family as a social system composed of nuclear and extended family members, and their social-communicative interactions to achieve family functions. According to Friedman (1992), the structural components include family composition, values, communication patterns, members' roles, and the power structure. Functional components of this model include physical necessities and care, economic, affective, and reproductive behaviors, socialization and placement of family members, and family coping abilities. The structural and functional components are interrelated, and each part is affected by changes in other parts.

A model that combines many of the above models is the Calgary Family Model, developed by Wright and Leahey (1994). The major components include the internal and external family structure, similar to Friedman's (1992) model, along with family context, such as race, ethnicity, social class, religion, and environment. Family functions are viewed as "instrumental" or daily living activities, and "expressive" activities, including communication (emotional, verbal, and behavioral), problem-solving, roles, influences, beliefs, and alliances or coalitions. Family developmental stages and tasks, similar to Duvall's (1977), are also part of this comprehensive model.

Any family model may be combined with and complement a nursing model since nursing practice may involve individual clients or families. Nurses with knowledge of various family models are more likely to select the most appropriate and relevant one to meet the family's health concerns.

Community Models

There are many community models that are useful to nurses, but they differ according to whether "community" is considered a target population or aggregate or a geographical area. McKay and Segall (1983) described an aggregate model, in which the focus is on a group of individuals who share common characteristics, but may not interact with each other. Shamansky and Pesznecker (1981) identified three interdependent factors that constitute a geographical community: 1) *persons* who reside in an area; 2) *space and time*, which includes the community's history and environmental features; and 3) *purpose* factors that explain functional processes such as government policies, educational services, and forms of communication. The "Community-as-Client Model," designed by Anderson, McFarlane, and Helton (1986) combines both the aggregate and geographical community. It addresses the following eight subsystems of the aggregate in the community: physical environment, education, safety and transportation, politics and government, health and social services, communication, economics, and recreation. A community nursing process model was developed by Goeppinger, Lassiter, and Wilcox (1982) that examines the following eight processes in a community: commitment of members, awareness of others' views, articulation of community needs, effective communication within and among members, conflict containment and accommodation, participation in organizations, management of relations with the larger society, and mechanisms to facilitate participant interactions and decision-making. Knowledge of several community models facilitates selection of the most appropriate one.

Other Useful Models and Theories

Nurses, and theorists in other disciplines, have developed many relevant models and theories that are useful in advanced nursing practice. Some of these models include Maslow's Hierarchy of Needs, Erikson's "Stages of Development," Piaget's "Cognitive Development of Children," Pender's (1987) "Health Promotion/Disease Prevention" model, and Loveland-Cherry's (1989) "Family health promotion" model. In addition, there are numerous theories of stress, crises, coping, grief, berevement, death, and dying developed in psychology and behavioral disciplines. Nurses have transformed some of these theories to encompass a health-illness context. Nurses who are cognizant of a variety of nursing, family, community, and behavioral models and theories are more likely to select the "best fitting" model for their clients.

SELECTION OF RELEVANT MODELS AND THEORIES

This section provides an overview of several nurse scholar's criteria and guidelines for selecting models and theories. Meleis (1997) identified six criteria to guide selection of suitable models and theories for practice. McKenna (1997a) described seven selection criteria based on a review of the literature. Kim (1994) constructed a framework for practice theories with four dimensions to consider in selecting nursing models and theories. Fawcett and associates (1992) suggested that nurses consider three questions to determine the best "fit" between the client's health concerns and various models and theories. Relevant criteria from the above scholars' work were integrated with the author's prior work to delineate five guidelines for selecting appropriate models and theories (Christensen & Kenney, 1996).

Meleis (1997) wrote that selecting models and theories for nursing practice is both a subjective and objective process. She identified six criteria for nurses to consider in the selection process.

- *Personal* the nurse's comfort with the theory and congruency with the nurse's own philosophical views of life
- *Mentor* the model or theory learned from a nurse mentor or educator
- *Theorist* their reputation in the discipline and degree of recognition
- *Literature support* the amount of literature available about the theory and the theory's significance for one's specialty
- *Socio-political congruency* the model or theory's acceptability within the nurse's workplace and whether major structural or practice changes are required
- *Utility* the ease in which nurses can understand and apply the model or theory in practice settings.

McKenna (1997a) reviewed the literature and identified the following seven criteria for selecting models and theories.

- *Type of client* the client's needs should direct the choice since the theory provides guidelines to achieve the client's goals
- *Health care setting* the type of clinical setting and nursing practice are contextual factors that affect selection of theories
- *Parsimony/simplicity* simple and realistic theories are more likely to be understood and applied in practice
- *Understandability* nurses must understand a theory if they expected to use it
- *Origins of the theory* the credibility, prior use, and testing of the theory should also be considered

- *Paradigms as a basis for choice* nurses must decide between the totality or simultaneity paradigm, as each provides a different view of clients and nursing actions
- *Personal values and beliefs* the theory must be congruent with the nurse's own views about humans, health, and nursing.

In her article on practice theories, Kim (1994) defined two dimensions of theories, which include four "sets of practice theories" relevant to selecting models and theories. One dimension is the "target," which addresses both the philosophy of care for the person and the philosophy of therapy for the client's problems. The other dimension is the "nurse-agent," which includes two phases, deliberation, and enactment. The four "sets of practice theories" serve to guide nurses in choosing theories that will: 1) explain the patient's problems and ideas about therapy for the problems; 2) provide ideas about how the nurse should approach the patient, such as through communication, caring, or empowerment; 3) explain how to make decisions about appropriate nursing actions for the patient; and, 4) explain what happens during enactment of nursing actions. Kim proposed that a science of nursing practice could be developed from this framework.

Fawcett and associates (1992) identified questions to guide nurses' selection of appropriate theories and models. The nurse must understand the differences among various models and theories in nursing and other disciplines to answer these questions. The following three questions will help the nurse identify the most appropriate model:

1. Does the theory or model address the client's problems and health concerns?

2. Are the nursing interventions suggested by the model consistent with the client's expectations for nursing care?
3. Are the goals of nursing actions, based on the model or theory, congruent with the client's desired health outcomes?

These questions help nurses decide which models and theories will assist them to organize the data into patterns, identify other health concerns, and determine congruency of the client's and nurse's view of nursing and health.

The first step toward theory-based nursing practice is the *conscious decision to use theories in practice* (Fawcett, 1997). The second step is recognizing that use of conceptual nursing models and theories requires a major change in how the nurse thinks about and interacts with clients to alleviate their health concerns. This change, referred to earlier as a "perspective transformation," occurs gradually as the nurse discards one framework of practice and learns another perspective. Adopting and applying new models and theories in practice depends on nurses having knowledge of various models and theories and understanding how these models and theories relate to each other (Alligood, 1997a).

GUIDELINESF FOR SELECTING MODELS AND THEORIES FOR NURSING PRACTICE

After deciding to implement theory-based nursing practice, the author believes that each nurse must engage in the five steps described below.

1. *Consider your personal values and beliefs about nursing, clients, health, and environment.*

Each nurse has a personal frame of reference or perspective of nursing practice, based on his/her conscious or unconscious assumptions, beliefs, and values about nursing. One's perspective of nursing provides a cognitive structure that guides one's perceptions, thoughts, feelings, and nursing actions (Fawcett, 1995). Clarifying one's own values and beliefs about clients, health, and nursing practice is necessary before a "perspective transformation" can occur.

2. *Examine the underlying assumptions, values, and beliefs of various nursing models, and how the major concepts are defined.* After clarifying one's own values and beliefs, the nurse examines the definitions of major concepts in various models and theories to determine whether they are congruent with one's own beliefs (Alligood, 1997a). Nursing models and theories are based on different values and beliefs about the nature of the client's behaviors and abilities, what is health and environment, and what nursing actions facilitate clients' health.

Each nursing model and theory provides a unique view for specific nursing practice. Some nursing models reflect a "totality" paradigm, and view humans as having separate biological, social, psychological, and spiritual parts that respond to environmental stimuli or change, and the nurse's role is to facilitate adaptation or equilibrium to maintain health. Other nursing models reflect a "simultaneity" paradigm, and believe humans are intelligent beings, capable of making informed decisions about their lives, and that they continuously engage in a dynamic, mutual interaction with their environment. In this paradigm, the nurse's role is to guide clients in choosing lifestyles and/or therapies that are acceptable to them and facilitate their growth and life-health process.

3. *Identify several models that are congruent with your own values and beliefs about nursing,*

clients, and health. Each nurse must consider whether the theorist's underlying values are congruent with one's own personal values and beliefs about clients, health, and nursing because the theorist's values guide the nurse's critical thinking and reasoning processes (Alligood, 1997a). Models and theories reflect the theorist's views about people and nursing. They directly effect how nurses approach their clients, what information they gather, how that information is processed, what nursing activities are appropriate, and, what client outcomes are expected based on the model. For example, some traditional nursing models define the person as a bio-psycho-social being who responds to environmental stimuli, and health results from nursing actions that lead to predictable changes. These models would be incongruent for contemporary nurses who believe that people are free agents, dynamically interacting with their environment as a whole, and capable of making rational decisions, and that the nurse's role is to assist clients to explore various options and choose ones that are acceptable with their values and lifestyle.

4. *Identify the similarities and differences in client focus, nursing actions, and client outcomes of these models.* Nursing models and theories consist of concepts with specific definitions, and statements that describe how the concepts are interrelated. Some propose specific nursing actions and expected client outcomes. The major concepts guide what data is collected during the assessment and how the data is organized to identify and interpret bio-behavioral patterns and determine nursing diagnoses. Nursing models also guide development of the nursing care plans and designate desired outcomes to evaluate. By comparing various models, nurses recognize which ones are congruent with their values and beliefs about nursing and offer the best "fit" with the client's health concerns.

5. *Practice applying the models and theories to clients with different health concerns to determine which ones best "fit" specific situations and guide nursing actions that will achieve desired client outcomes.* The nurse explores specific models in depth, and may analyze their usefulness before implementing them. By comparing several models and examining the attributes of the client, the focus of nursing actions, and the proposed outcomes, the nurse will acquire a more in-depth understanding of different models. Each nursing model describes different areas for assessment, unique nursing diagnoses, and specific nursing interventions to assist the client toward health. The nurse must decide which models and theories are most appropriate for each client. Which one offers the best 'fit' for the client's health concerns? Selecting appropriate models and theories for each unique client health situation requires nurses to use their broad knowledge base from various disciplines, critical thinking skills, clinical expertise, and intuition to identify the best 'fit' between the client's health concerns and nursing models (Fawcett, et al., 1992).

APPLICATION OF THEORY-BASED NURSING PRACTICE

The choice of theories and models suitable to the client's health concerns occurs during the initial data assessment process. The initial data focuses on the client's primary expressed concerns and how they are related to or affect the client's lifestyle and patterns of living. These data assist the nurse to identify and understand the client's common and unique patterns. The client's view of health, along with past and present "lived experiences," and future lifestyle and health concerns, are also considered. Using this information, the nurse considers various models and theories from nursing and other disciplines that are relevant to the client's unique health concerns, and congruent with the nurse's own beliefs. Then,

TABLE 33.2. Theory-Based Nursing Practice

Component	Nursing process Use	Nursing model Use
Assessment	Describes *how* to collect data	Guides *what* data to collect
Diagnosis	Describes *how* to process data	Guides organizing, categoriz- ing, and interpreting data
	Provides format for nursing diagnosis	Provides concepts for nursing diagnosis
	Describes *how* to plan	Guides *what* to plan
	Facilitates development of care plan unique to client	Designates appropriate types of nursing interventions
Implementation	Describes phases of implementation	Directs model-specific nursing actions
Evaluation	Identifies *how* to evaluate	Guides *what* to evaluate
General	Requires accountability through use of systematic approach to nursing practice	Enhances accountability of theory- based practice
	Process enhances continuity of care	Provides a comprehensive, coherent approach to care of client

From: Christensen, P.J., Kenney, J.W., eds: *Nursing process: Application of conceptual models*, 4th ed., St. Louis, 1995, Mosby, p. 21. Adapted with permission from Wealtha Y. Helland.

the nurse selects those models and other theories that best "fit" the client's situation and health concerns and will systematically direct nursing practice.

The major concepts of the chosen models and theories guide each component of the nursing process, as shown in Table 33-2. The concepts serve as categories to guide additional data collection. They suggest, either directly or indirectly, *what* information is relevant and should be collected. The models and theories assist the nurse to organize, categorize, and interpret pertinent data that illustrate the client's bio-behavioral patterns and identify appropriate nursing diagnoses that are linked to relevant etiological factors.

Nursing and other models and theories guide development of a care plan by suggesting appropriate types of nursing interventions and specific nursing actions. Desired client outcomes are derived from the models and theories and define what changes in the client

should be evaluated. For example, if Roy's model is chosen, data about the client's physiological needs, self-concept, role mastery, and interdependence, along with related stimuli would be collected, and used to identify adaptive and maladaptive behavioral patterns. The nurse who uses Orem's Self-Care Model would assess and judge clients' ability to meet their universal and developmental self-care requisites and whether they had any health deviations. From analysis of this data, the nurse would diagnose self-care deficits and determine appropriate nursing plans for partial, compensatory, or health education nursing care. Nursing care plans are based on the model and describe the client's desired outcomes, along with nursing actions to achieve the client's outcomes. Nurses who use Johnson's Behavioral Systems Model would consider ways to nurture, protect, or stimulate the client to facilitate health, whereas the Neuman's Health Care System's model assists the nurse to explore ways to reduce stressors within the three levels of disease prevention.

Some nurses believe that family models complement nursing models and provide a more holistic and comprehensive perspective of clients and their health concerns. Selection of a family model occurs after the nurse gathers preliminary data about the family and identifies its unique and common patterns. Then the nurse decides whether the "family as context" or "family as client" would be more appropriate and best "fit" the client's situation. Also the nurse's perception and definition of family and health guide the selection of a family model. For example, a pediatric nurse who works in an outpatient clinic may choose Orem's Self-Care Model to guide care of a nine-year-old child with an ear infection and the mother's treatment of the child. Friedman's Family System model may complement Orem's model and enhance understanding the family's structure and functions. The nurse may also use Erikson's Developmental Framework to help the mother recognize and encourage her child's normal developmental behaviors. Pain management theories may also be applied to reduce the child's earache.

This example illustrates how nurses examine and judge the value of various models and theories and select those which are most congruent and useful and best 'fit' the client's health concerns and the nurse's perspective of practice. Gradually nurse practitioners develop an expertise in selecting theories and models that are appropriate and relevant to their client's health concerns and congruent with their own views of advanced practice.

SUMMARY

This chapter described the importance and value of applying models and theories from nursing and other disciplines in advanced nursing practice. Issues related to the nursing theory-practice gap were discussed, along with concerns about using only one nursing model in practice and about integrating models and theories from other disciplines with nursing models and theories. The structure of nursing knowledge was explained and the need for a "perspective transformation" to occur prior to implementing theory-based nursing practice. Critical thinking, logical reasoning, and creatively applying nursing models and theories was emphasized. Different types of nursing, family, community, and other models and theories were discussed. Lastly, the process of selecting and applying models and theories was thoroughly described.

In the last few decades, the emergence of nursing models and theories has illuminated several nursing paradigms and explicated their underlying assumptions, beliefs, and values that guide nursing practice. The science of nursing and empirical patterns of knowing are represented by these nursing models and their theories. Application of models and theories from nursing and other disciplines depends on nurses having a broad knowledge base and understanding how models and theories are interrelated. Empowerment of nurses through 'perspective transformation' and the use of nursing models and theories is essential. They provide the framework for critical thinking within the context of nursing and guide the reasoning that professional nurses need to survive in an era of cost containment and evidence-based practice. Use of models and theories from nursing and related health disciplines enables nurses to demonstrate accountability for their decisions and actions through scientific explanation and provides a coherent approach to theory-based nursing practice.

REFERENCES

Aggleton, PJ, & Chalmers, H. (1986). *Nursing models and the nursing process*. Basingstoke: Macmillan.

Alligood, MR. (1997a). Models and theories: Critical thinking structures. In MR Alligood and A Marriner-Tomey, *Nursing Theory: Utilization & Application*, St. Louis: MO: C. V. Mosby. pp. 31–45.

Alligood, MR. (1997b). Models and theories in nursing practice. In MR Alligood and A Marriner-Tomey, *Nursing Theory: Utilization & Application*, St. Louis: MO: C. V. Mosby. pp. 15–30.

Anderson, ET, McFarlane, JM, & Helton, A. (1986). Community as client: A model for practice. *Nursing Outlook*, 3(5):220

Beavers, WR, & Voeller, MN. (1983). Family models: Comparing and contrasting the Olson circumplex models with the Beaver's systems model. *Family Process*, 22:85–98.

Benner, P, & Wrubel, J. (1989). *The primacy of caring*. Menlo Park, CA: Addison-Wesley.

Chinn, PL. (1997). Why middle-range theory? *ANS*, 19(3):viii.

Christensen, PJ & Kenney, JW. (1996). *Nursing process: Application of conceptual models*, 4th ed., St. Louis, MO., C. V. Mosby.

Cradock, S. (1996). The expert nurse: Clinical specialist or advanced practitioner? In Gary Rolfe, (Ed.) *Closing the theory-practice gap: A new paradigm for nursing*. Butterworth-Heinemann Ltd., Oxford, UK.

Cody, WK. (1996). Drowning in eclecticism. *Nursing Science Quarterly*, 9(3):86–88.

Curran, D. (1985). *Stress and the healthy family*, Minneapolis, MN., Winston Press.

Duvall, EM. (1997). *Marriage and family development*, 5th ed., Philadelphia, PA., Lippincott.

Fawcett J, Archer CL, Becker D, et al., (1992). Guidelines for selecting a conceptual model of nursing: Focus on the individual client, *Dimen Critical Care Nursing*, 11(5):268–277.

Fawcett, J. (1995). Implementing conceptual models in nursing practice. In J. Fawcett, *Analysis and evaluation of conceptual models of nursing*, 3rd ed. Philadelphia, PA., F. A. Davis.

Fawcett, J. (1997). Conceptual models of nursing, nursing theories, and nursing practice: Focus on the future. In MR Alligood and A Marriner-Tomey, *Nursing Theory: Utilization & Application*, St. Louis: MO., C. V. Mosby. pp 211–221.

Field, PA. (1987). The impact of nursing theory on the clinical decision making process, *Journal of Advanced Nursing*, 12:563–571.

Firlet, SI. (1985). Nursing theory and nursing practice: Separate or linked? In J. McCloskey & HK Grace (Eds.) *Current issues in nursing*. Boston: Blackwell Scientific Publications. pp 6–19.

Friedman, MM. (1992). *Family nursing: Theory and practice*, 3rd ed. New York, Appleton & Lange.

Goeppinger, J, Lassiter, PG, & Wilcox, B. (1982). Community health is community competence. *Nursing Outlook*, 30(8):464.

Kenney, JW. (1996). Relevance of theory-based nursing practice. In P. J. Christensen & J. W. Kenney, *Nursing Process: Application of Conceptual Models*, 4th ed. St. Louis, MO: C. V. Mosby. pp 1–23.

Kim, HS. (1994). Practice theories in nursing and a science of nursing practice. *Scholarly Inquiry for Nursing Practice: An International Journal*, 8(2):145–158.

Loveland-Cherry, CJ. (1989). Family health promotion and health protection. In P. Bomar (Ed.) *Nurses and family health promotion: Concepts, assessment, and interventions*. Baltimore, MD., Williams & Wilkins.

Mayberry A. (1991). Merging nursing theories, models, and nursing practice: More than an administrative challenge, *ANS*, 15:44.

Marks-Moran, D, & Rose, P. (Eds.) (1997). *Reconstructing nursing: Beyond art and science*. Philadelphia, PA., Bailliere Tindall.

McCubbin, MA, & McCubbin, HI. (1993). Families coping with illness: The resiliency model of family stress, adjustment and adaptation. In C. B. Danielson, B. Hamel-Bissell, & P. Winstead-Fry (Eds.), *Families, health and illness: Perspectives on coping and intervention* St. Louis, MO., Mosby (pp. 21–65).

McKay, R, & Segall, M. (1983). Methods and models for the aggregate. *Nursing Outlook*, 31(6):328

McKenna, H. (1997a). Choosing a theory for practice. In Hugh McKenna, *Nursing theories and models*. New York, Rutledge, pp. 127–157.

McKenna, H. (1997b). Applying theories in practice. In Hugh McKenna, *Nursing theories and models*. New York: Rutledge, pp. 158–189.

Meleis, AI. (1993). *Nursing research and the Neuman model: Directions for the future*. Panel discussion conducted at the Fourth Biennial International Neuman Systems Model Symposium, Rochester, NY.

Meleis, AI. (1997). *Theoretical nursing: Development and progress*, 3rd ed. Philadelphia, PA. Lippincott.

Mezirow, J. (1979). Perspective transformation. *Adult education*. 28(3):100–110.

Moos, RH, & Billings, AG. (1982). Conceptualizing and measuring coping resources and processes. In L. Goldberger & S. Breznitz (Eds.) *Handbook of stress*. New York, Free Press.

Mitchell, G. (1992). Specifying the knowledge base of theory in practice. *Nursing Science Quarterly*, 5(1):6–7.

Olson, DH, Russell, CS, & Sprenkle, DH. (1983). Circumplex models of marital and family systems: VI. Theoretical update. *Family Processes*, 22:69–83.

Paul, RW, & Nosich, GM. (1991). Proposal for the national assessment of higher–order thinking (revised version). The United States Department of Education Office of Educational Research and Improvement, National Center for Education Statistics.

Pender, NJ. (1987). *Health promotion in nursing practice*. New York, Doubleday.

Rogers, ME. (1989). Creating a climate for the implementation of a nursing conceptual framework. *Journal of Continuing Education in Nursing*, 20(3):112–116.

Shamansky, SL & Pesznecker, B. (1981). A community is . . . . *Nursing Outlook*, 29(3):182–185.

Smith, MC. (1994). Beyond the threshold: Nursing practice in the next millennium. *Nursing Science Quarterly*, 7(1):6–7.

Sorrentino, EA. (1991). Making theories work for you. *Nursing Administration Quarterly*, 15(3):54–59.

Spiracino, P. (1991). The reciprocal relationship between practice and theory. *Clinical Nurse Specialist*, 5(3):138.

Stevenson, J. (1977). *Issues and crises during middlescence*, New York, Appleton-Century-Crofts.

Timpson, J. (1996). Nursing theory: Everything the artist spits is art? *Journal of Advanced Nursing*, 23:1030–1036.

Wright, LM, & Leahey, M. (1994). *Nurses and families: A guide to family assessment and intervention*, 2nd ed. Philadelphia, PA., F. A. Davis.

Frederickson, et al. (1997). Nursing theory-guided practice. *Nursing Science Quarterly*,10(1):53–58.

Gioiella, EC. (1996). The importance of theory-guided research and practice in the changing health care scene. *Nursing Science Quarterly*, 9(2):47.

Huch, MH. (1988). Theory-based practice: Structuring nursing care. *Nurs Science Quarterly* 1:6.

Huch, MH. (1995). Nursing science as a basis for advanced practice. *Nursing Science Quarterly*, 8(1):6–7.

Huckabey, LH. (1991). The role of conceptual frameworks in nursing practice, administration, education, and research. *Nurs Admin Quarterly* 15(3):17–28.

Jacobs, MK, & Huether, SE. (1978). Nursing science: The theory-practice linkage. *Advances in Nursing Science*, 1(1):63–78.

Kappeli, S. (1994). Why not practice-based theory? *Clinical Nursing Research*, 3(1): 3–6.

Koziol-McLain, J, & Maeve, MK. (1993). Nursing theory in perspective. *Nursing Outlook*, 41 (2):79–81.

Kristjanson LJ, Tamblyn R, & Kuypers JA. (1987). A model to guide development and application of multiple nursing theories. *J Adv Nurs*, 12:523.

Oberst, MT. (1995). To what end theory? *Research in Nursing & Health*, 18:83–84.

Rolfe, G. (1996). Nursing praxis: Integrating theory and practice. In Gary Rolfe, *Closing the theory-practice gap: A new paradigm for nursing*. Butterworth & Heinemann Ltd.: Oxford, UK.

Wardle, MG, & Mandle, CL. (1989). Conceptual models used in clinical practice. *Western Journal of Nursing Research*, 11(1):108–114.

Wilkinson JM. (1992). *Nursing process in action: A critical thinking approach*. Menlo Park, CA.: Addison-Wesley.

ADDITIONAL REFERENCES

Birx, EC. (1993). Critical thinking and theory-based practice. *Holistic Nursing Practice*, 7(3):21–27.

Chinn, PL, & Kramer, MK. (1995). *Theory and nursing: A systematic approach*, 4th ed., St. Louis, MO., Mosby Year Book Co.

Cody, WK. (1994). Nursing theory-guided practice: What it is and what it is not.*Nursing Science Quarterly*, 7(4):144–145.

Derdiarian, AK. (1991). Effects of using a nursing model-based assessment instrument on quality of nursing care. *Jr of Nurs Admin*, 15(3):1–16.

Index